Penny and Andrew Stanway

Breast is best

A common-sense approach to breastfeeding

PAN BOOKS

First published 1978 by Pan Books

This revised edition published 1996 by Pan Books
an imprint of Macmillan Publishers Ltd
25 Eccleston Place, London SW1W 9NF
and Basingstoke

Associated companies throughout the world

ISBN 0 330 34753 5

1 3 5 7 9 8 6 4 2

A CIP catalogue record for this book is available from
the British Library.

Typeset by CentraCet Ltd, Cambridge
Printed and bound in Great Britain by
Mackays of Chatham plc, Chatham, Kent

To Susannah, Amy and Ben

Acknowledgements

We would like to thank all the many breastfeeding women and their helpers around the world whose shared experiences have enriched this book.

Thank you too to Susanne Baumgartner and Leo who grace the cover.

Contents

Appendix 441

Index 467

Preface

Breast is best. What an extraordinary claim!

Surely, at the turn of the twenty-first century, it hardly matters whether babies in developed countries are breastfed or not. They all seem to do equally well, so why bother?

There's an element of truth in this. But when looked at more closely, it is indisputable that breastfeeding offers many advantages to babies, their mothers and families, even in the most highly developed of countries.

Breast Is Best is for all those who want to know more about breastfeeding. Its practical guidelines, based on shared experiences, handed-down wisdom, common sense and the latest research from around the world, will, we hope, be invaluable both to mothers and their helpers.

If a woman decides to bottle-feed, having weighed up the pros and cons of breastfeeding as she perceives them, she has the right to make that choice. But our personal, clinical and academic experiences have persuaded us not that breast *might be better* but that breast really *is best*! Everything being equal, we think the optimal way of nurturing babies and young children involves the kind of mothering that naturally accompanies successful breastfeeding. This sort of breastfeeding may involve a rather different way of thinking – a paradigm shift.

If you agree – or would like to explore these ideas further – *Breast Is Best* should help.

ONE

So you want to breastfeed

'Why on earth should I need a book to teach me how to breastfeed?' you may ask. 'Haven't women fed their babies for millions of years? And anyway, how do mothers in developing countries get on? Most of them breastfeed and they don't learn from books!'

FASHION, INSTINCT AND EDUCATION

These are the kinds of question people have been asking us over the twenty years or more that we have been personally and professionally involved with breastfeeding. Unfortunately, the answers are often not that simple.

Although more than nine out of every ten women in the world breastfeed, women in industrialized countries live in a society in which bottle-feeding is very common and, indeed, the norm in some areas. We're going through a time when families are small and many young pregnant women have never had the opportunity of seeing other women breastfeed. And we're seeing a large proportion of women give up breastfeeding sooner than they intended.

Because breastfeeding has lost favour with many modern women, it no longer comes naturally to many of them and has to be learnt like any other skill. In the past, other women helped and taught the new breastfeeding mother. This ensured that breastfeeding was almost universally successful ('success' in this context meaning that a baby received the nourishment and comfort he needed from the breast, and a woman could go on breastfeeding until she and/or her baby were ready to stop).

Evidence from many parts of the world shows that in the past, babies of women who didn't produce enough milk simply died. This alone was a considerable incentive for women to help each other breastfeed – as indeed they nearly all did, helping to feed other people's babies, if necessary, as well as their own.

Your baby almost certainly won't need to be taught how to feed, because it's an instinct that usually comes naturally. But most women need help and encouragement if they are to succeed.

Before we go any further, let's get one thing straight. With the right advice and encouragement nearly all women *can* breastfeed successfully for as long as they or their babies want.

In 1975 the US had the lowest breastfeeding rate in the world. Fewer than one in four babies was being breastfed at one week old and by six months the figure had fallen to one in twenty. Back in 1916, however, 60 per cent of North American babies were still being breastfed at one year. In evolutionary terms, 1916 is not very long ago. These changes are so large and have occurred so quickly that as far as medical science is aware no genetic explanation is acceptable. Clearly the fall in the number of American women breastfeeding must have stemmed from social or psychological factors rather than biological ones.

The swings in the popularity of breastfeeding this century have been truly amazing. In a campaign over fifty years ago to encourage and support breastfeeding in Minneapolis, 96 per cent of nearly 3000 women were fully breastfeeding their two-month-olds, and 84 per cent were still breastfeeding at six months. During the five years between 1978 and 1983, following massive publicity about the benefits of breastfeeding and its endorsement by the American Academy of Pediatrics and the World Health Organization, the breastfeeding rate in the US rose to 62 per cent of newborn babies. By 1995, however, it had fallen again and now only 56 per cent of women giving birth in hospital choose to breastfeed at all.

The picture is much the same in the UK. In 1974 the Department of Health and Social Security recommended encouraging women to breastfeed for a minimum of two weeks and preferably for at least four to six months. Two out of every three newborn babies were put to the breast in 1980 compared with one in two in 1975 – a big difference in anyone's terms.

But how many women actually breastfeed now in the UK? The Office of Population Censuses and Surveys (OPCS) organized large surveys in 1975, 1980, 1985 and 1990. These are the breastfeeding statistics at different ages in England and Wales:

	1975 %	1980 %	1985 %	1990 %
Birth	51	67	65	64
1 week	42	58	56	54
2 weeks	35	54	53	51
6 weeks	24	42	40	39
4 months	13	27	26	25
6 months	9	23	21	21
9 months	0	12	11	12

These figures show that women are nowhere near achieving the Department of Health's goal. In 1990, only half of the newly delivered mothers in the survey breastfed for even two weeks and only a quarter breastfed for four months or more. Scottish babies fared even worse: at two weeks old only two in five were breastfed in 1990, and by four months the proportion had fallen to one in five.

Clearly, breastfeeding statistics change surprisingly quickly. The changes have sometimes been even more dramatic. For example:

— A study in France showed that the number of babies getting no breast milk at all rose from 31 to 51 per cent in five years.

Now let's look at the very different proportions of women breastfeeding in two other European countries.

— Recent research in twenty-one European countries revealed that in Greece almost nine out of ten one-month-old babies were fully breastfed, whereas the Irish figure was fewer than one in five!

What lies behind this and other similarly huge differences in breastfeeding rates from one country to another? There are probably many answers, including differences in cultural and religious history, in the man–woman relationship, and in women's expectations and experiences. But there's something more. The final clue comes when women who believe they are unable to breastfeed – usually because they think they can't make enough milk – receive help and encouragement and go on to feed their babies successfully. Clearly, most women who fail to breastfeed do so because of a lack of information and support.

Why, though, should modern women need so much help and encouragement? The answer is that women have always benefited from skilled support but many need it all the more now that they have to choose between breastfeeding and bottle-feeding.

Milk-producing animals have only been reared for the last 10,000 or so of man's five million years on earth. Only in the last sixty years has the use of cows' milk as a source of infant food become widespread. This unnatural change in diet from breast milk to cows' milk at so crucial a period in a baby's life is a modern intervention without parallel in the history of mankind. So massive and uncontrolled a change is it that one researcher calls it the greatest uncontrolled trial ever to have been done on human beings. We have become strangely obsessed with cows' milk and ought seriously to question our obsession. The trouble is that in the West the advertising industry, nutritionists and dietitians have made cows' milk out to be a food with almost magical properties. This overemphasis on the goodness of cows' milk is closely tied (albeit unconsciously) to the fact that we willingly deprive our babies of the very milk they were meant to get.

But why should all this worry a woman who decides to breastfeed? Today, if a mother has any problems at all with breastfeeding she may be handicapped further by a sense of guilt and personal failure. Then, because formula feeds are so readily available and carry no possibility of personal failure, she soon starts her baby on the bottle. At a stroke she transforms herself from a 'failure' into a 'success'. It's easy to see how compelling this is in a world in which women are brought up to be winners.

The sad thing is that most people consider breastfeeding simply as a way of getting food into a baby whereas in reality it's so much more.

The first doubts about bottle-feeding arose as new facts about the disadvantages of even the newest modified cows' milk formulae came to light. Cows' milk preparations were found to lack vitamin B_6, vitamin E and linoleic acid and to be too high in protein, sodium and phosphorus; to cap it all, it was discovered that there were many more protective antibodies against disease in breast milk than had ever been thought. It was also clear that whole protein molecules from cows' milk could leak through a baby's gut wall into the bloodstream and that these foreign proteins could lay the foundation for allergic problems in both infancy and later life.

Infant formula manufacturers speedily changed their formulae to keep pace with these new discoveries and there was talk about vaccinating herds of specially bred cows to give them immunity against human diseases. But by this time the damage had been done. When mothers demanded to feed their babies with the best baby food of all – breast milk – they found that the womanly art of breastfeeding had been all but lost. Mothers had lost confidence in their natural ability and common sense. Health professionals too had seen few mothers breastfeed successfully and were brainwashed by rigid advice on breastfeeding schedules. Hospitals had forgotten that they existed to do their best for the patients, not to idolize the new god, 'routine'. And even the mothers' own mothers were often little help, as they were among the first to use cows' milk formula when they fed their babies.

RECENT CHANGES

Thankfully, things have changed a lot over the twenty years or so since we wrote the first edition of this book in 1978. Breastfeeding education has improved for mothers- and fathers-to-be, as well as for doctors, midwives, health visitors (in the UK) and other professional breastfeeding helpers. Breastfeeding information and advice in the community are now more accurate and helpful, and public attitudes are marginally more encouraging.

In other words, there's an increased general awareness of the benefits of breastfeeding, how to do it successfully, and how to manage when problems occur.

However, some women still receive poor advice. And when they do get good advice, it tends to stop as soon as they appear to be managing on their own. While the new mother might like the *idea* of breastfeeding (and millions really do believe that breast is best) as soon as any problem, however small, crops up, she'll be lucky to continue because she'll be showered with conflicting advice from all sides. A lack of good, consistent advice and information frequently leads to a woman's milk drying up. Once she's put her baby on the bottle, she's likely to feel very disappointed. Indeed, many women experience a deep and lasting sense of failure after doing so. After all, there are few things that a mother can do for her baby that so uniquely build their relationship. Countless women who successfully fed later babies but failed with their first have told us over the years how sad they felt at what both they and their first babies missed out on. For some it is a wound that never heals and for others a source of rage that they were never helped in the way they needed. Most say they feel cheated out of something that could so easily have been theirs.

WHY YOU MAY NEED HELP

Today's society isn't geared to encouraging and enabling women to breastfeed. For a start, it's considered normal for babies to be bottle-fed, which means that if you breastfeed you are to some extent 'abnormal'. Though many mothers in the UK start off breastfeeding, the vast majority of babies are soon completely or almost completely bottle-fed. One reason is that women – and men – are simply more familiar with bottle-feeding. Another is that breastfeeding is much more likely to produce challenging situations than is bottle-feeding. Given the poor help and support some women receive, it's hardly surprising that they choose the easier route, even if deep down they know it's not the best one for their babies.

Lack of education

Nowadays, unless a forward-thinking school-teacher asks a breastfeeding woman to come in and talk to her class, a girl can still reach motherhood and a boy fatherhood without ever having seen a baby at the breast. Up-to-date teachers make sure children have an opportunity to discuss breastfeeding in biology and parentcraft classes. The subject can be introduced to young children of any age, and teachers can be creative in the way they and their class learn. If the topic of breastfeeding is left until the teenage years, many girls and boys in mixed classes are too embarrassed to learn anything much.

— A survey of teenagers' attitudes to infant feeding in Liverpool (1989) found that those who had been breastfed themselves, or who had seen a baby breastfed, were much more likely to choose to breastfeed.

A series of breastfeeding education packs for teachers to use with children of different ages has been put together by the Norwich Joint Breastfeeding Initiative (see Appendix).

Family attitudes

Many of a woman's older relatives will be far more familiar with bottle-feeding, and while not actively discouraging her from breastfeeding, may make a very good job of persuading her that bottle-fed babies are as contented and healthy as breastfed ones – after all, they did it and their children came to no harm.

Women's role as workers

Perhaps more insidious, in this context, is the fact that today's young woman is most often brought up and educated to think of herself mainly as a wage-earner and career woman. When she leaves her parents' home, she'll almost certainly need her earned income to start a place of her own and it may be difficult for her and her husband (or partner) to give this up when a baby comes along. In any event, women when they're pregnant tend to think of themselves not so much in relation to their baby as to their husband (or partner) and career or job.

As all of us who are involved with ante-natal education know, it is very hard to get pregnant women to focus on the realities of baby feeding. For many such women the birth is as far as they wish to see. When the baby does arrive, however, things change and they confront the reality of the choice between caring for it, going out to work or somehow combining the two.

It's often claimed that many of today's mothers don't breastfeed because they go back to work so soon. In fact, however, the results of a large British survey in 1990 showed that only a few women actually return to work while their children are very young (see page 292). It also found that the working mothers breastfed for as long as those who didn't work.

The status of mothers in society

Western society doesn't seem to value its mothers as it once did, possibly because of the world population explosion. The world simply doesn't need as many babies and as a result mothering is everywhere being downgraded as a meaningful and rewarding career in itself. With society's devaluation of motherhood and the increase in the number of working women, it's widely accepted that substitute mothers, be they child-minders, nursery nurses, au pairs, mother's helps or nannies, are just as good as the mothers themselves at looking after their babies. So not only have many of us accepted the concept that breast milk is no longer essential for a baby, but we also seem to have bought into the notion that mothers aren't important either.

The women's movement may be the saving grace for motherhood and breastfeeding, strange though this may seem! Perhaps, instead of being looked down on, women who choose to have children and breastfeed will be encouraged not only to think well of themselves for doing a job which is unique for each child and an invaluable contribution to society, but also to enjoy what they are doing and so raise its profile.

More women are showing an interest in breastfeeding today. Unfortunately, their success rates are poor and most put this down to 'not having enough milk'. This gives breastfeeding a bad press, which is entirely unjustified, as has been shown in studies all over the world. Very, very few women have too little milk if they go about breastfeeding in the right way. All they need are some simple, proven guidelines.

At this point some readers may say that there's already a lot of help available to pregnant and nursing mothers. However, a large amount of this advice is frankly lukewarm, unhelpful and contradictory. Why? Mainly because health professionals are influenced by society, fashion and their own upbringing, like the rest of us. Some pay lip-service to breastfeeding but don't tell mothers that it's the very best thing, often because they are afraid of making women feel guilty if they don't do it (see page 457).

—A national survey (1995) of doctors specializing in paediatrics, obstetrics and family medicine in the US found that they rated their

training in the benefits and management of breastfeeding as inadequate. Astonishingly, the curriculum of the American Accredita-
tion Council for obstetric and family medicine fails to mention
breastfeeding even once!
— A survey of American paediatricians showed that they advised
mothers according to the breastfeeding experience of their own
wives. If their wives had had a difficult time or were unsuccessful,
they anticipated difficulties with their patients and so put them off
breastfeeding.

However, when health professionals take an interest in how
women are going to feed their babies, it makes a big difference.
Midwives (and, in the UK, health visitors) can have an enormously
influential role in encouraging women to breastfeed and supporting those who do so. Studies show that a paediatrician who is
enthusiastic about breastfeeding can make all the difference to the
numbers of women who breastfeed. He or she can also have a big
influence by encouraging all the members of the hospital or
community team of health professionals, not to mention others in
contact with mothers (such as cleaners, clerks, orderlies and so on),
to work together to make sure that theirs is a Baby-Friendly
Hospital (see page 144). Women need to know about the benefits
of breastfeeding and those who wish to breastfeed need good
information and support if they are to do so successfully – that is,
for as long as they wish.

WHAT HELP IS THERE?

At some stage most women need help with breastfeeding. It may
be the odd practical tip or a total overhaul of technique. Some
mothers have a problem deciding where to go for this help and
knowing who to trust when they receive conflicting advice. To a
great extent a woman's choice is governed by her personality and
previous life experiences.

Medical, nursing and midwifery help

If you are the sort of person who looks to professionals for answers to such things then you'll probably start with your doctor, midwife (or, in the UK, health visitor). The level of advice will depend almost entirely on the particular individual you happen to encounter. For example, a female GP who has breastfed successfully herself, or a male or female doctor with a professional and personal interest in the area, may indeed be very useful. However, many doctors are not well informed about the practicalities of day-to-day breastfeeding and disappoint and confuse some of the women they deal with.

Much the same applies to midwives and (in the UK) health visitors. Although many of these are far better informed about infant feeding than is the average GP, their advice can still be very patchy, depending on the personality and individual experience of the professional involved, as well as on the quality of their original professional education and continuing in-service training.

Friends, relatives and neighbours

If you don't see breastfeeding as a 'medical' matter at all, then you'll probably talk to a friend, relative or neighbour. Seeking help from your mother might seem a good idea but clinical experience shows that this can be tricky. If you are lucky she'll be up-to-date and modern in her outlook but some mothers are rooted in the past and believe that what they did thirty years ago is the right way for their daughters to behave today. This can provoke conflict, especially if at some unconscious level either woman is still embroiled in her own infantile past with her mother.

Self-help groups (see page 152)

Some of the best helpers are breastfeeding counsellors or leaders in organizations such as the National Childbirth Trust (NCT) and La Leche League. These women have not only themselves breastfed for prolonged periods but have also learnt a great deal from practical experience with many women as well as from books and courses. They are also deeply committed to positive breast-feeding attitudes and practices in a way that professionals can find hard to equal. They have the time and the desire to focus on breastfeeding and are able to provide a level of one-to-one support that few professionals can match because of their other commitments.

The NCT Breastfeeding Promotion Group has a network of mothers throughout Great Britain who have breastfed their children and are trained as breastfeeding counsellors. They will help on the phone if you have problems and will visit you at home if necessary.

La Leche League (LLL) is an international organization started by a small group of mothers who realized that the only people who seemed to know what they were doing when breastfeeding were other mothers who had breastfed their babies and overcome any problems on the way. LLL's slogan is 'Good mothering through breastfeeding'. Its groups hold meetings and discussions and its trained group leaders give help on the phone or in person when necessary.

The Association of Breastfeeding Mothers is a UK self-help organization with local groups and counsellors who offer information and support to all those who are interested in breastfeeding.

Breastfeeding isn't always easy, especially in the early days. However, a lot of help is available now, so there's no need to stop unless you really want to.

You can also teach yourself how to breastfeed successfully for as long as you want. We'll show you how – but first let's look at how breastfeeding works.

TWO

How breastfeeding works

This chapter and the next will give you an idea of how breast-feeding works and why your milk is best for your baby. The practical details of breastfeeding are outlined in Chapter 6 but the next few chapters fill in the essential background knowledge you'll need to understand how to breastfeed and be aware of what can go wrong. They'll bring you right up to date with the major research carried out into breastfeeding over the last thirty years.

Let's start by looking at the breasts themselves.

THE BREASTS

A year or so before a girl's periods start, changes begin in the shape and size of her breasts, nipples and areolae. These changes continue until her late teens. After this a young woman's breasts remain the same (if her weight stays steady) until she gets pregnant. Humans are the only mammals in which the breasts enlarge before pregnancy. Breasts also have a sexual role in courtship that isn't seen in other mammals and it's this that helps colour our attitudes to breastfeeding in the Western world.

The increase in size of the breasts during adolescence results from the laying down of fat and the lengthening and branching of the milk ducts. At this stage there's very little glandular tissue but buds which will later develop into milk glands now begin to form.

The breast is made up of fifteen to twenty segments, each containing a gland leading to a main duct which, in turn, opens at the nipple. This means that between fifteen and twenty ducts open at each nipple. You can see their openings as little crevices and if you stop for a moment when you're feeding your baby, you'll notice drops of milk coming from them. Sometimes you'll see fine sprays or drops of milk coming from several ducts at the same time. Some ducts may merge within the nipple, so there are often fewer openings at the nipple than there are ducts.

In a pregnant or breastfeeding woman the glandular part of each segment of the breast is rather like a bunch of grapes on a stalk. Each 'grape' is called an alveolus or milk gland and has a tiny duct leading to the 'stalk' or main milk duct. The milk gland is lined with milk-producing cells, each bordering on the tiny duct. Milk produced by these cells goes from the tiny duct to one of the fifteen to twenty larger ducts and thence to the nipple. Around each milk gland is a network of branching, star-like muscle cells. These can contract, squeezing the gland and forcing milk from the cells into the ducts.

The main duct from each segment of the breast widens as it reaches the areola and enters one of the fifteen to twenty milk reservoirs (lactiferous sinuses) under the areola. These distend as they fill with milk, the diameter of a full reservoir being between a half and one centimetre. It's easy to see that they can store a lot of milk ready for the baby at the beginning of each feed. These reservoirs are capable of storing even more milk after several weeks of breastfeeding, which is why some mothers notice that any leaking they have stops after six to eight weeks as their storage capacity increases.

BREAST CHANGES IN PREGNANCY

During pregnancy many women notice tingling and fullness of their breasts as early as their first missed period. Indeed, breast sensations are often the first symptom of pregnancy. Little prominences around the areola called Montgomery's tubercles become more noticeable at about six weeks. These contain glands that produce a substance that lubricates and protects the skin of the nipples during breastfeeding. Some women also produce milk from one or more tubercles. This is quite normal because the tubercles are anatomically like tiny breasts.

By five months most women find they need a larger bra. In a first pregnancy the nipples and areolae now begin to darken. If you lose your baby after five months, you'll lactate just as if you had given birth at full term.

These changes are all caused by hormones (some of which are present only in pregnancy) circulating in the blood. (See 'Milk production', page 16).

Breast size in pregnancy

On average, each breast weighs 1½ pounds more at the end of pregnancy, mainly because of the development of milk glands and proliferation of milk ducts.

The size of your breasts before pregnancy has no bearing on your ability to breastfeed; some small breasts contain more milk-producing glands than do larger ones. However, the increase in the size of your breasts during pregnancy is quite a good indicator of your ability to feed easily. As a general rule, if you need a bra one or two sizes larger by the end of pregnancy, you should have little trouble getting off to a good start with breastfeeding. The younger a woman is when she has her first pregnancy, the greater is the increase in size of her breasts. This may explain why women having their first babies young tend to produce more milk than do older ones at first. Women with very small breasts may be at a slight disadvantage early on because their breasts can become overfilled more quickly than larger breasts and may leak unless offered to the baby more frequently. However, as their storage capacity increases during the first few weeks this becomes less of a problem.

BABIES' BREASTS

While on the subject of breast size, it's interesting to note that mothers often comment on the size of their babies' breasts. Newborn babies often have enlarged breasts because of the effects of maternal hormones travelling across the placenta before birth. Sometimes milk comes out of them. This is called witches' milk and is seen in both boys and girls. The swelling and the milk eventually disappear, though sometimes this takes several months or even longer.

NIPPLES

Not only do a woman's nipples become larger during pregnancy but they also become more protractile (able to be lengthened), which makes it easier for the baby to take hold of them with his mouth. There are a few women whose nipples don't change like this and their babies may at first have problems 'latching on' (see page 167).

MILK PRODUCTION

Production of milk by the milk glands is under the influence of the hormones prolactin, growth hormone, the corticosteroids, thyroxine and insulin; there may be other hormonal influences too. Each milk gland is surrounded by a fine network of blood vessels which carry hormones to the milk-producing cells. Blood provides the materials from which the cells make milk.

Prolactin

This hormone is present in the blood in extremely small amounts in women who are neither pregnant nor breastfeeding. Its level increases from the eighth week of pregnancy onwards, reaching a peak at birth, and then gradually decreases during the time a woman breastfeeds. During pregnancy it stimulates breast growth but other hormones (oestrogen, progesterone and human placental lactogen) prevent it from producing milk in any volume.

After a baby is born these 'brakes' disappear and high levels of prolactin, the hormone that 'turns on the taps', trigger milk production and, in particular, the production of casein and lactose. Milk usually starts to be produced ('comes in') between the second and fourth days after delivery but can start earlier in women feeding their babies frequently and in an unrestricted way from birth, and in those having second or subsequent babies. Milk usually comes in slowly but there may be a deluge.

The hormone prolactin is produced by the brain's pituitary gland. Nipple stimulation during a feed sends messages along nerves to this gland to tell it to make more prolactin. It's the holding and squeezing of the nipple and areola by a baby's mouth that stimulate the nipple rather than the suction. However, pumping the breast with an electric pump doesn't raise prolactin levels. It's possible, though as yet unproved, that a baby who sucks and milks the breast strongly raises his mother's prolactin level more than does one with a weaker sucking and milking action.

Nipple stimulation immediately boosts prolactin, which reaches a peak within thirty to forty-five minutes of starting a feed. Over the next two hours it gradually decreases to its resting level. A raised prolactin level increases the milk supply, so the more her baby is at the breast, the more milk a woman makes. In other words, each time a baby feeds, he places an order for more milk to be made, ready for the next feed. Waiting longer between feeds doesn't produce more milk because it doesn't increase prolactin levels – only more frequent (or longer) feeds do this. Prolactin levels fluctuate throughout the day and are highest at night.

Research suggests that nipple stimulation encourages the development of the breasts' prolactin receptors – tiny structures in the milk glands that 'capture' and remove prolactin from the blood and allow it to increase their milk production. This removal of prolactin may explain why the hormone's level in the blood is not directly related to the amount of milk produced. *Put in another way, nipple stimulation is necessary for the breast to respond to prolactin and make milk, and the more frequently a woman feeds from either breast, the more sensitive and responsive does that breast become to prolactin.* This may account for why, when a woman feeds her baby only or mainly from one breast, as a few do (see page 339), the milk in her little-used or unused breast gradually decreases or even dries up, despite high prolactin levels produced by plenty of stimulation of the other nipple. A woman can produce milk during a second or subsequent pregnancy if nipple stimulation continues because her older baby or toddler goes on breastfeeding.

So far we've considered only the milk-producing effects of prolactin but it may have other actions too. For example, many breastfeeding mothers experience feelings of happiness and tranquillity. These emotions are boosted by an increase in the blood concentration of endorphins – natural hormone-like chemicals which are also stimulated by breastfeeding. Research shows that the hormones in lactating rats buffer them against stressful situations. This may also be true in humans. Some people go so far as to call prolactin the 'mothering hormone' or 'happiness hormone'.

Fore-milk and hind-milk

As the milk glands make milk, it trickles into the milk ducts and gradually fills the reservoirs under the nipple. This milk, known as fore-milk, is low in fat and hence in calories. Fore-milk is available immediately whenever a baby wants to feed. However, at any one time the bulk of the milk – the hind-milk – remains in the milk glands and is available only if the let-down reflex operates to squeeze it from the glands into the ducts and hence to the nipple (see below).

Getting milk into a baby in large enough amounts is a skill that needs to be learnt and, like most skills, is acquired all the more quickly if you understand what's involved. There are two vital mechanisms: one is the let-down reflex and the other is the law of demand and supply. Let's look at each in turn.

THE LET-DOWN REFLEX

After a feed, milk-producing cells in the milk glands gradually enlarge, becoming round and full as they produce more milk. The fullness and slight lumpiness you may feel some time after a feed are caused by these swollen milk glands with their laden cells and ducts.

When the muscle cells around each gland contract, the milk in the cells is released into the ducts very quickly and the milk is said to have been 'let down'. Without the let-down, the milk in the gland cells – the hind-milk – stays put and the baby has access only to the fore-milk which is readily available in the reservoirs and ducts. Hind-milk is rich in calories, containing 30 calories per 30 ml (1 fl oz) compared with only 10 in fore-milk. Most babies who don't get hind-milk don't thrive.

Oxytocin

This hormone is responsible for the let-down reflex. When an experienced breastfeeder knows her baby is ready for a feed, she automatically releases oxytocin. This sometimes happens even before the baby gets to the breast. This is because the let-down is a physiological reflex conditioned by her past experience. The baby's presence is a powerful stimulus but many women find that their let-down is triggered simply by the sight, sound or even the thought of their baby (or possibly someone else's), particularly if they haven't breastfed for some time.

Stimulation of the nipple skin and the tissues under the areola during suckling is another important oxytocin-trigger. Messages travel along nervous pathways from the nipple to the pituitary gland where they trigger the release of oxytocin into the blood. Oxytocin then travels to the breast where it makes the muscle cells around the milk glands contract and squeeze milk into the ducts. This cycle (of suckling or another trigger listed above – messages to the pituitary – oxytocin release – contraction of muscle cells – release of milk into the ducts) is why the let-down is called the let-down *reflex*. It is outside conscious control.

The let-down reflex usually takes some weeks to become reliable. When people talk about 'establishing' breastfeeding, they are referring to the establishment of a reliable let-down reflex.

The time the let-down takes to work varies from woman to woman and also depends on many other factors, including a woman's surroundings and how she feels. From when a baby is put to the breast the let-down can take a minimum of thirty to fifty seconds to work but often takes longer. Some women need two to three minutes of nipple-stimulation before their maximum milk flow occurs. This means that a hungry or thirsty baby may finish the fore-milk before any hind-milk is let down, which can be frustrating. The let-down is a fairly sensitive mechanism and is easily disturbed, especially in the early weeks. If her baby cries and becomes restless, perhaps turning away and fighting at the breast, an inexperienced mother may become so anxious that she won't let her milk down at all.

Being anxious, over-stressed or embarrassed can inhibit the let-down in two ways. First, it can prevent oxytocin from making the muscle cells around each milk gland contract. And, second, it can prevent oxytocin being released from the pituitary gland.

The let-down is usually a pleasant feeling and has been described as 'something between a sneeze and an orgasm'. When milk is let down, it spurts through the ducts so quickly that it may spray or drip from the nipples. In any one let-down there's a series of spurts with a gap between each and there may be several let-downs within each feed. This is why researchers find that oxytocin levels during a feed change rapidly from one minute to the next. One study found that the first let-down is associated with a higher level of oxytocin in the blood than subsequent let-downs in any one feed. The level of oxytocin in a woman's blood falls extremely rapidly and is all gone within about four minutes of the start of the let-down.

In the early days it's often easy to know when your let-down is working because of tingling, tension and warmth in your breasts; leaking, dripping or spraying of milk; and womb contractions which are rhythmical and one cause of 'afterpains'. Many women say the removal of the milk by the baby sucking after the let-down reflex produces a welcome feeling of relief as the tension in their full breast diminishes.

Some women have none of these sensations yet have a very good let-down reflex, and any individual mother can experience different let-down sensations from baby to baby. Other women report that the feelings they experience as their milk is let down change or even disappear completely throughout the months of breastfeeding one baby. One mother described a sensation of cold water trickling down her breastbone when she let her milk down in the first few weeks of breastfeeding. In later weeks this was replaced by tingling throughout her breasts and, later still, by itching beneath her areolae. (See also page 275.)

Leaking

Warmth from a hot bath or your baby's mouth can cause initial leaking without a true let-down. Elastic muscle fibres in the nipple and areola are usually contracted, keeping the duct openings closed. Warmth lengthens these fibres, releases their tight hold on the ducts and allows milk to escape. If your breasts are full of milk, simply leaning forward or to one side can cause leaking too, as can sexual arousal (see page 203).

HOW YOUR BABY GETS MILK

So much for the production and let-down of milk, but how does it get to the baby? There are many old wives' tales about this but the most common is that a baby gets the milk by sucking. Actually, a baby obtains milk from the breast by a combination of methods: sucking, milking and allowing let-down milk (or leaking milk from a full breast) to drip or spray into his mouth.

Holding the breast in his mouth

A baby holds the breast in his mouth between his upper gums and his tongue with the tongue covering his lower gums.To do this he sticks the front of his tongue out beneath the nipple as far as his lower lip, curls it up slightly, then pushes the back of his tongue up against the nipple and areola. He then sucks and this helps him hold the breast in place.

Sucking

When the nipple touches a baby's palate in the roof of his mouth, he automatically starts sucking. This sucking reflex is instinctive and at its strongest twenty to thirty minutes after birth. If a baby isn't put to the breast during this time, the sucking reflex temporarily becomes much weaker, but after forty hours it becomes stronger again.

A baby sucks to draw the nipple and areola into his mouth and to keep them there. The sucked nipple is about twice as long as usual. The nipple and areola together in the baby's mouth form a sort of 'teat' – and it's on the shape of this that manufacturers based the design of a feeding bottle's teat. The vacuum created by the baby sucking draws milk into his mouth and encourages the milk reservoirs to refill with milk. However, the actual sucking involved is relatively unimportant, although the cheeks do exert measurable suction. The 'milking' a baby does is more important.

Milking

A baby gets milk mostly by milking (or 'stripping') the nipple and areola with his tongue. With the breast in his mouth, his whole tongue moves backwards, pressing against the nipple and areola as it does so. Then it contracts rhythmically in horizontal waves or undulations of muscular movement known as peristalsis. This milking action squeezes milk from the reservoirs under the areola. During this milking the baby's jaws open and close to help his tongue compress the nipple and areola. The further he draws the teat he makes from nipple, areola and reservoirs under the areola into his mouth, the better he empties the reservoirs.

If you could see inside your baby's mouth (and this has been done with X-ray studies), you'd see that your nipple goes way back, as far back as where his hard and soft palate join. You'd also see a furrow down the length of the upper surface of his tongue. The teat made from the nipple and areola fill this furrow. The baby's milking action stimulates your let-down reflex which ejects milk from the nipple in fine jets towards the back of his mouth. All he needs to do now is swallow.

Nutritive and non-nutritive sucking

Many babies start a feed by sucking and milking continuously for around thirty seconds. They then fall into a pattern of inter-mittent, long bursts of this sucking and milking action. This is because milk lets down in spurts. If oxytocin levels in the blood are continuously monitored during a feed they can be seen to rise and fall in waves corresponding with the spurts of milk.

When the milk is flowing well, the baby carries out 'nutritive sucking' in which he sucks slowly and purposefully at a rate of about one suck per second. However, when the milk isn't flowing, he does 'non-nutritive sucking', which is characterized by short sharp bursts of sucking at a rate of two sucks per second.

As a baby rests, his lower jaw drops, releasing the pressure of the tongue on the nipple and areola and allowing the reservoirs to refill with let-down milk.

The swallowing reflex

This is essential for a baby to get the milk from his mouth into his stomach. All three reflexes seen in breastfeeding babies – the rooting reflex (see page 165), sucking reflex and swallowing reflex – may be temporarily absent in pre-term babies or impaired in those infants who have brain damage, jaundice or an infection. Mechanical problems such as a cleft palate may also interfere.

DEMAND AND SUPPLY

All the time a baby is feeding, he stimulates the nipple and areola, causing his mother's pituitary gland to release prolactin and oxytocin. Since prolactin helps controls milk production it's easy to see that the more you have your baby at your breast, the more prolactin you'll make and, in turn, the more milk there'll be. Also, the more often you feed him, the more reliable your let-down reflex becomes. This is the basis of the second mechanism of successful breastfeeding – that of demand and supply. There would be far fewer breastfeeding failures if those caring for new mothers understood the mechanisms of both the let-down reflex and of demand and supply.

The converse, 'supply and demand', isn't such a good term because with breastfeeding, the demand produces the supply, not the other way round. Nor, incidentally, is 'demand' a particularly good word to use at all, first, because many babies let their mothers know they're ready for a feed simply by becoming slightly restless or nuzzling at the breast. They 'ask' gently, rather than cry in a 'demanding' way. And, second, a few babies don't 'demand' or ask in any way at all, especially if they've often been left to cry in their mother's mistaken belief that they should be made to wait for a set time before the next feed. These babies seem 'happy to starve' (see page 269) and become quieter and quieter though their bodies are in desperate need of milk. Without attention to their needs they rapidly become ill and gain the impression that the world is an unfriendly place that produces feelings of unhappiness.

In general, the more feeds your baby asks for and gets in a day, the more milk you'll have (though see also page 211). This has been proven in many surveys. For example, in one survey in Sheffield as long ago as 1952, demand-fed babies gained weight faster than those fed according to a schedule, proving that mothers produced more milk by feeding more often. There are no limits to the number of feeds you can give your baby. Every time he asks, you can offer the breast. This doesn't mean, though, that you should feed *only* when he asks. You may want to do so because your breasts feel full, you want the pleasure of a close cuddle, or it's a convenient time.

Successful or natural breastfeeding puts no rules or limits on suckling time (see page 271). 'Suckling', by the way, is something a mother does to her baby. A mother suckles and a baby sucks – and a baby is called a suckling.

Babies allowed to feed as often as they want take very variable numbers of feeds during the twenty-four hours. In the early days some want something every hour or so. The greatest number of feeds often occurs on the fifth day after birth. In the Sheffield survey mentioned above, 29 per cent of babies fed on demand wanted eight feeds on the fifth day and 10 per cent wanted more than nine.

In a textbook for doctors published in 1906, when successful breastfeeding was the norm, the following schedule of feeds was recommended per day:

First day	4 feeds
Second day	6 feeds
Rest of the first month	10 feeds
Second and third months	8 feeds
Fourth and fifth months	7 feeds
Sixth to eleventh months	6 feeds

Some years later, many hospitals recommended a breastfeeding schedule of every four hours for a large baby and every three hours for a small one. Unfortunately, with the increasing medicalization of childbirth and mother and baby care, and with the tight control exerted over women and their babies in hospitals, this bad advice remained widespread for many decades and is still given in some out-of-date, non-'baby-friendly' (see page 144) hospitals today.

However, women's experiences and scientific evidence agree that any sort of schedule which restricts the number of feeds by day or night produces notoriously poor results.

Completely unrestricted, natural breastfeeding involving very frequent feeds in the early days is best. The woman who wants to breastfeed successfully should discard any schedule which restricts the frequency of feeds.

Having said this, two 'schedules' are worth considering:

1 Not leaving more than a certain number of hours between feeds if you need to make more milk for your baby (see page 273).
2 Restricting the length of a feed by discouraging 'non-nutritive' sucking if you have sore or cracked nipples (see page 311).

— A survey in Africa throws light on this subject. Researchers watched mothers sleeping with their babies over many nights to see how often the babies fed while their mothers slept. No baby went longer than twenty minutes without feeding.

Contrast these lucky babies with the many in developed countries who are rationed to one feed a night at most until their mother's milk dries up completely.

One sure way of reducing the number of feeds your baby asks for (and thus decreasing your breast stimulation and therefore your chances of breastfeeding successfully) is to keep him apart from you. In countries where mothers carry or hold their babies by day and lie next to them at night, and where few clothes are worn by baby or mother, infants spend very much more time at their mother's breast than do Western ones. It's not surprising that babies who are allowed virtually unrestricted access to their mother's breasts are almost always breastfed fully and successfully for a long time. The supply of milk in these circumstances continues for an average of three years until the baby no longer wants to be at the breast.

A word of warning. Never compare your baby with that of your neighbour. Every baby is unique and should be allowed to be so. Some settle into a self-created routine of a certain number of feeds a day within a few weeks but this is certainly not a goal to aim at, it's just one of many patterns your baby may adopt in time.

And another word of warning. One leading authority in the UK has said that in her experience if a baby has five or fewer feeds a day, the likelihood is that his mother's milk will dry up within a month through lack of stimulation of the breasts.

LENGTH OF FEEDS

The length of a feed is also a matter for the individual baby–mother pair and shouldn't be dictated by doctors, midwives or other health professionals. The average time at one breast is about ten minutes but averages are worked out from observing many babies. Some get all they need in five minutes and some need twenty or much longer at each breast before they are satisfied. Others like a break before coming back for another go!

Feeding times vary for several reasons. First, the let-down may be slow to work so a baby doesn't start getting hind-milk for some minutes. Second, some babies are much hungrier or much greedier than others, so they suck more strongly and get all they need in a shorter time. Third, some babies – especially in the early days – may not be very alert and so need to take their time over a feed. All these situations are discussed in more detail later.

'FEEDS'?

Although we have been conditioned into talking about the periods of time a baby spends at the breast as 'feeds', it would be far more helpful to change this concept because it inevitably makes us think of a baby's 'feed' purely as a mealtime – a time to get milk down in as businesslike a way as possible. Many babies, however – especially in the early days – like to drink their milk in a very leisurely, long-drawn-out way, snoozing between bouts of sucking. While snoozing, they may let go of the breast only to wake again in a short while, or they may hold the nipple in their mouth and give an occasional gentle, 'fluttering' sort of suck for minutes at a time. It's not uncommon for a young baby sometimes to spend hours at the breast in this fashion, if allowed. Such behaviour, which can be perfectly normal, makes the counting of feeds meaningless. It isn't difficult to understand that a baby allowed to behave like this stimulates the breast much more than a baby allowed only a certain number of 'proper' feeds of a certain length.

It's important not to curtail the length of feeds in the first few days particularly, because it's all too easy to take the baby from the breast before the let-down starts to work. Many hospitals insist on very short suckling times in the first few days to prevent sore nipples but, as we'll see later, this is a fallacious argument. Short suckling times often prevent or delay the establishment of successful lactation and benefit mother or baby only in very occasional circumstances.

Now that we've taken a look at the breasts and how breastfeeding works, we'll look in the next chapter at breast milk itself.

THREE

Breast milk – the perfect food

Thirty years ago doctors recognized only a few advantages of breast milk and summed them up to medical and nursing students as follows: 'It's at the right temperature; it contains exactly what the baby needs; it's bacteria-free; it comes in such cute containers; and the cat can't get at it!'

For years this was the sort of level at which doctors and nurses were taught about breast milk. Small wonder then that when infant formula manufacturers kept coming up with yet more modified and 'improved' products, both mothers and the health professionals thought they were getting something every bit as good as breast milk – possibly even better. Only later did researchers show that they were wrong. However much manufacturers modify infant formula – and whether they make it from cows' milk (like most), from soya beans or whatever – it is different from breast milk. We'll look later in the chapter at just how different it is, but first, let's see why.

OTHER MAMMALS' MILK

The outstanding characteristic of mammals is that they suckle their offspring with milk at least until the young can feed themselves. As mammals are so different one from one another, it isn't surprising that their milks differ too. If an elephant, rat, sheep, whale and human ate similar diets, and if their young grew at the same rates and had similar digestive tracts and body composition, it would be reasonable to expect their milks to be similar. But they don't, so their milks are different. Over scores of thousands of years each mammal has developed a unique type of milk to suit its own young.

All milks

The basic similarity between all milks is that they contain the same groups of substances: water, proteins, fats, carbohydrates, minerals, vitamins, anti-infective substances, hormones, enzymes, live cells and other factors. The differences occur because these substances are present in different amounts and in varying proportions. In addition, apart from water, these substances are not single entities but are often made up of whole families of different substances – and the proportions of each of these can differ too.

For example, there are many different types of fat and their proportions vary from one animal's milk to another, including women's and cows'! Whales' milk has a very high fat content which gives it a huge calorific value, making it richer than double cream. This is essential for an infant whale which needs to form a thick layer of blubber very quickly to protect it from the cold water.

The protein content of rabbits' milk is very high at 14 per cent, compared with 1.2 per cent in human milk (see 'Proteins', page 34). This is necessary because the growth rate of the young rabbit is so fast. A rabbit doubles its birth weight in six days, whereas a human baby takes about 140 days to do so. High milk-protein levels are a must for every newborn mammal that grows quickly, because protein provides the basic building blocks for the growth of tissues. Compared with most other young mammals, human babies grow very slowly. As a result, breast milk has correspondingly little protein.

Animals whose milk contains large amounts of fat and protein (such as seals, rabbits and deer) tend to feed their young much less frequently than those (such as dogs) with less. And those with very low protein and fat concentrations (such as monkeys and other primates) carry their young around and feed them almost continuously.

Interestingly, human milk contains more carbohydrate (mainly in the form of milk sugar – lactose) than any other mammalian milk.

Cows' milk

The first time one group of mammals used another's milk to any great extent was when more than the occasional few humans started giving their babies cows' milk this century. Of course, over the centuries the occasional baby has been fed on the milk of another animal (Romulus and Remus were supposedly reared by a wolf) but the widespread use of cows' milk is a new phenomenon. Nearly all types of infant formula today are made from cows' milk.

But why did we in the West choose cows' milk as the main substitute for breast milk? It's a good question because this milk is by no means the nearest in composition to human milk – donkeys' milk is much closer! People in various countries have used milk from goats, donkeys, buffalo, sheep, llamas, reindeer, mares and camels for their babies over the years but the great move towards artificial feeding came from the West. Cows were already being reared for meat and dairy produce, so it was convenient and economically sensible to use their milk. Cows are also docile, easily herded animals which produce large volumes of milk. Add to this the fact that their four teats make for easy milking and the original and continuing attraction of their milk as the basis of milk formula for babies is clear.

Just a note in passing here as to why we call it cows' milk rather than cow's milk. The product that the milk industry markets is pooled milk from many cows – not the milk of one cow. We shall see later that human milk changes greatly from day to day and within a feed, and of course it is exactly the same with cows feeding their calves. Pooled milk from many cows is thus a very much more homogenous product than are sample's of milk taken from a breastfeeding mother at different times.

Before this century, if a mother didn't want to feed her baby, another woman had to take over as wet nurse if the baby was to have a good chance of surviving. Now millions of babies grow up on cows' milk formula. However, even today in some countries a baby has a high risk of dying if the mother doesn't feed him herself.

Difference between cows' milk and breast milk

Ordinary cows' milk – whether it's pasteurized or raw, full-cream, semi-skimmed or skimmed, liquid or dry – is not suitable for babies under six months old. This is because cows' milk is very different from breast milk.

One of the most obvious differences is that cows' milk contains more protein and less sugar. This led doctors and food scientists to modify it earlier this century so that it resembled breast milk more closely. They did this by diluting it with water and adding sugar. This basic modification was used for years and mothers either adapted ordinary liquid cows' milk by diluting it with water, adding sugar and then boiling it, or they bought dried, evaporated or condensed milk and made their own formula by adding water and sugar. Modern dried milk formulas need only to have water added.

However, over the years more and more differences between the two milks have come to light and scientists have had to make one modification after the other in their quest for the ideal formula. We now know that some of these differences have led – and a few still can lead – to medical problems in bottle-fed babies. We'll consider these in Chapter 5.

WHAT MILK CONTAINS

Milk – or 'white blood', as it's called in parts of India – is a fascinating fluid which is as much a food as a drink.

Water

Our bodies are composed of 80 per cent water and this fluid is vital for every body cell. A lack of water causes dehydration and cell damage. Certain cells are particularly susceptible to dehydration, with brain cells being especially at risk.

The liquid part of milk which makes up its main bulk is water. All the other constituents are either dissolved or suspended in this water, making milk appear white, creamy, translucent or yellow, depending on their proportions.

Breast milk is the perfect food for human babies because the proportions of water and other constituents are just right. Many women worry that their own milk might be too 'watery'. This is very unlikely (unless they aren't letting down their hind-milk – see page 275) and anyway you can tell very little about the nutritional value of your milk simply by looking.

A thirsty baby given enough breast milk gets the right amount of water to satisfy his thirst. A breastfed baby who drinks enough breast milk never needs to drink water. However, in very hot weather a breastfeeding mother needs to drink more so that neither she nor her baby becomes dehydrated.

A thirsty bottle-fed baby who drinks a lot more formula than usual may risk getting too much of certain substances because their concentration is higher in formula than in breast milk. This can occur if bottle-feeds are made up too strong – particularly dangerous if a baby is dehydrated from diarrhoea, vomiting or sweating from a fever. Such a baby needs more drinks of water, not formula – and certainly not extra-strong formula. Recent modifications of cows' milk formulas have made them safer but the proportions of the substances in them are still very different from those in breast milk.

The bowel motions of bottle-fed babies contain less water than those of breastfed ones, which is one reason why they are more likely to suffer from constipation.

Proteins

About 1.2 per cent of breast milk is protein. This is made up of whey proteins – including lactalbumin, lactoglobulin (immuno-globulins, or antibodies), lactoferrin, folate- and vitamin B_{12}-binding proteins, enzymes, hormones and growth factors, and curd protein (casein). All proteins are, in turn, composed of amino acids. Cows' milk has 3.3 per cent protein (necessary because a calf grows fast, doubling its birth weight in fifty days) and this extra is composed of six times as much casein as there is in human milk.

When milk enters a baby's stomach it becomes curds and whey, with casein forming the curds. Cows' milk curds are much bulkier than those of breast milk. They are so tough, rubbery and bulky that many babies get indigestion if they drink ordinary unmodified cows' milk. This is the main reason behind the basic modification of cows' milk when making formula: its dilution with water. Adding water dilutes tough indigestible casein. Boiling, homogenization and the addition of various chemicals also alter casein, making it less tough and more digestible.

In contrast, breast milk protein forms finely separated curds in the stomach. These pass quickly and easily into the small intestine where they are broken down. This means a breastfed baby's stomach empties more quickly than that of a bottle-fed one, which is why a breastfed baby gets hungry more quickly and needs more frequent feeds. Cows' milk curds stay in the stomach for about four hours but breast milk only for about one and a half hours. *So four-hourly feeds for a bottle-fed baby are reasonable but breastfed babies need feeding more often.*

A bottle-fed baby uses only about half the 'nutritional' protein available in cows' milk formula, whilst a breastfed baby uses nearly all (95 per cent) of the nutritional protein in breast milk, with virtually no waste. Not all milk protein is primarily there for nourishment – lactoferrin, for example, helps bind surplus iron, and the antibodies are there for defence purposes. The protein a bottle-fed baby doesn't use is partly passed out in the stools (which makes them bulkier than those of a breastfed baby) and partly broken down before being excreted by the kidneys in the urine.

Because there is so little waste from breast milk, breastfed babies need less milk than bottle-fed ones. If this is forgotten, test-weighing a breastfed baby (to see how much milk he's taken during a feed) can easily be misleading; *the amount a breastfed baby drinks should never be compared with the amount drunk by a bottle-fed one.*

Amino acids – Besides proteins, which are made of amino acids, there are free amino acids in both human milk and cows' milk, but their proportions differ. Breast milk contains, for instance, more of an amino acid called cystine compared with cows' milk, which, in turn, contains more of another called methionine. This is important for pre-term babies who are incapable of using methionine until they become more mature. Cows' milk contains less taurine (an amino acid found in many body fluids, particularly in the eye and nervous system) than breast milk, which is why it's now added to cows' milk formula.

Nucleotides – These building blocks for proteins are present in human milk but only in minimal amounts in cows' milk. They may also encourage the growth of helpful bowel bacteria. Most babies can make nucleotides, but pre-term and some full-term babies can't make enough. Although scientists don't yet know whether this is important and aren't aware that any babies have had problems from a deficiency, there's enough concern for manufacturers to have added nucleotides to some formulas.

The main nucleotide in cows' milk, orotic acid, isn't found in human milk at all.

Fats

The fats in mature breast milk provide more than 50 per cent of a baby's energy. They mostly occur in milk as globules of tri-glycerides but there are also phospholipids (including lecithin), cholesterol and free fatty acids. Fatty acids are the building blocks of fats and are classed as saturated, monounsaturated and poly-unsaturated, depending on their molecular structure.

Certain fatty acids are little changed as they pass from a woman's blood into her milk; others are made from scratch by breast cells from glucose. By and large, the proportions of fatty acids in a well-nourished woman's milk reflect the types of fat in her diet.

The amount of milk fat varies from one woman to another. While the average fat content is between 2.6 and 4.5 per cent, levels of 1.2 and 12 per cent have been reported.

The fat content of a woman's milk varies during a feed, with two to three times as much at the end than at the beginning. It also varies from when her baby is born to the later stages of breastfeeding.

— A group of German researchers reported that the fat level changes throughout the day, with English mothers' milk having the highest levels in the evening and that of German mothers in the afternoon. This possibly reflects the fact that English people tend to have their main meal in the evening and Germans at lunchtime.

However, other researchers report that breast milk fat levels stay fairly constant throughout the day. Perhaps this is because some breastfeeding women use fatty acids from their fat stores to make milk; the fatty acid pattern in their milk then reflects that of their stored fat.

Essential fatty acids – While our bodies can make some of the particular types of fatty acid they need, there are others (some of the polyunsaturated fatty acids, or PUFAs) which we must have in our food. This is why they're called *essential* fatty acids.

Fats in general, and PUFAs in particular, are necessary for many aspects of growth, especially the development of PUFA-rich nerve-coverings in the brain and the spinal and peripheral nerves.

Breast milk contains a higher percentage of PUFAs, including the essential fatty acid linoleic acid, than cows' milk. But whilst cows' milk contains less linoleic acid, cows' milk formula contains enough to prevent deficiency symptoms (poor growth and thick, scaly skin). However, some formula manufacturers were so concerned about their products' low PUFA levels that they replaced some of the saturated fat with vegetable oil PUFAs. At first they added linoleic acid in far greater quantities than are found in human milk and some babies developed severe anaemia. The manufacturers speedily had to rectify their mistake.

There are two groups of PUFAs, the *omega-6* and *omega-3* fatty acids; the amounts and ratio of these groups and the amounts and pattern of their individual fatty acids differ in breast milk and cows' milk formula. Researchers recently found that these differences have important implications for a baby's brain and eye development (see page 97).

Certain PUFAs are found only in breast milk. These are the PUFAs whose molecular structure scientists describe as 'long-chain', such as DHA (docosahexaenoic acid, an omega-3 fatty acid) and AA (arachidonic acid, an omega-6). These fatty acids are sometimes also referred to as LCPs – long-chain polyunsaturated fatty acids. Milk formula also contains highly variable amounts, if any, of alpha-linolenic acid.

Even if a formula does contain enough alpha-linolenic and linoleic acids – the 'parent' PUFAs of the omega-6 and omega-3 groups from which healthy full-term babies make DHA, AA and other long-chain PUFAs – some bottle-fed babies, both full-term and pre-term, can't make them fast enough. This means that, for them, DHA and AA join the ranks of fatty acids which are essential for a baby to have in his milk.

Neither full-term nor pre-term bottle-fed babies necessarily get enough DHA from the usual types of formula for the optimal development of their eyesight. And pre-term bottle-fed babies may not get enough AA for optimal growth or mental development. Breastfed babies, in contrast, get all the DHA and AA they need from breast milk.

World Health Organization experts recommended as long ago as 1978 that AA and DHA are desirable components of milk formula but nothing was done. Recently, however, and after more research, other scientists recommended that manufacturers should add DHA and AA to pre-term formula – and preferably add these and other PUFAs in exactly the same proportions as in breast milk. They are also questioning whether full-term bottle-fed babies might benefit from a similar change in formula. However, making the PUFA-profile of formula similar to that of breast milk is expensive and considerably increases the cost of bottle-feeding. None the less, some formulas – including most of those especially made for pre-term babies and, in the UK, one made for full-term babies – are now enriched with these fatty acids.

As yet it is not known whether the amounts and ratio of saturated and monounsaturated fats and PUFAs in breast milk protect a baby against heart disease and other arterial disease later in life. But we do know there's more of another fat, cholesterol, in breast milk than in cows' milk and that breastfed babies have higher cholesterol levels in the early months.

You may ask whether cholesterol-rich milk is best for babies. Ironically, though, it looks as if breastfed babies' higher levels of cholesterol accustom them to handling it. This could stand them in good stead in the future and it's possible that it might even prevent or reduce the risk of later heart disease (see page 101).

Enzymes in the gut called lipases split fats into simpler fatty substances. The digestion of cows' milk fat by lipase releases a fatty acid called palmitic acid which combines with calcium in the gut and leaves the body in the bowel motions, so removing calcium. In human milk, palmitic acid is built into fat particles in such a way that when fat is digested by lipase, the acid isn't released as a free fatty acid but is absorbed into the blood together with part of the broken-down fat particle. This means there is no calcium loss, which is important because when babies are growing fast they need a plentiful supply of calcium to build strong bones and teeth.

Human milk contains some lipase of its own, unlike cows' milk which relies solely on lipase in the baby's intestine for its digestion. The fat in breast milk starts being digested by milk lipase even before it reaches the gut. This means that valuable fatty acids are available sooner from breast milk than from cows' milk.

Digestion of both breast and cows' milk fats in a baby's stomach produces fatty acids as well as other, simpler fats which help protect babies from infection.

— Researchers in New York pointed out in 1990 that some fatty acids have more anti-viral activity than others. They suggested that changes in a woman's diet that alter the fatty acids in her milk might make it even more protective against infection.

Lastly, less important but more practical is the fact that if a breastfed baby brings up any milk, the smell isn't particularly unpleasant, whereas a bottle-fed baby's vomit has a much sourer smell which quickly permeates clothing. The difference is due to the presence in formula of a fatty acid called butyric acid which smells unpleasant when partially digested.

Carbohydrates

Both breast and cows' milks contain lactose (milk sugar) but breast milk has more (7g (¼oz) per 100g (4oz) of milk compared with 4.8g in cow's milk). Between 84 and 95 per cent of breast milk's carbohydrate is in the form of lactose, which is why it tastes so sweet. Babies like sweet tastes even more than adults do and the taste-buds at the tip of a baby's tongue – the ones which detect sweetness – are more concentrated than on an adult's tongue. Given the choice between breast milk and formula, babies prefer breast milk, probably simply because it's sweeter.

Some lactose is split into two simple sugars, galactose and

glucose, in the gut. The rest travels through undigested. This undigested lactose improves calcium absorption and encourages a healthy balance of micro-organisms in the gut. Galactose is an important part of the myelin coating of nerves, and besides getting it from breast milk a baby can make it from glucose in his liver.

Both breast milk and formula contain glucose, although some other sugars in breast milk are completely absent or present in much lower quantities in formula.

Breast milk contains twenty-five or more sugars called oligo-saccharides. Formula contains only a very small amount of some of these and none of others. Oligosaccharides encourage a healthy population of micro-organisms in the gut and protect against infection by preventing bacteria from sticking to the gut lining. Also, when there's breast milk in the baby's mouth and throat during and after a feed, the oligosaccharides in the milk prevent bacteria such as pneumococci and *Haemophilus influenzae* (both of which can cause respiratory infections) from sticking to the back of the throat. Oligosaccharides also help prevent urine infections. Interestingly, some of these sugars vary according to the mother's blood group.

The bifidus factor is a mixture of about ten oligosaccharides and offers valuable protection against gut infection (see page 45).

Minerals

Whole, unmodified cows' milk contains almost four times as many minerals as breast milk, which is one reason why it might easily overload a baby's kidneys.

Cows' milk formula has been processed to have a much lower mineral content but even so there's no formula which has as low a content of minerals as breast milk. As minerals are so important to a baby's health, we'll discuss some in more detail.

Sodium – The amount in breast milk is ideal for human babies. The level in cows' milk formula is lower than that in fresh cows' milk but still higher than in breast milk. Sodium is closely linked with water in the body and an imbalance of either can be serious and even fatal. This is why bottle-fed babies need particular care if they become dehydrated as the result of diarrhoea, vomiting or a fever, and why bottle-feeds must not be made up too strong.

Calcium and magnesium – There are higher levels of both these in cows' milk than in breast milk, although modification has reduced them in modern formulas. Several problems arose from older high-calcium formulas, including a higher risk of the muscular spasm known as neonatal tetany in bottle-fed babies, as well as convulsions, and poor development of tooth enamel followed by severe dental decay. Although there's a little less calcium in breast milk than in modern formulas, babies absorb breast milk calcium more efficiently than that from formula, possibly because high levels of lactose in breast milk promote its transfer from gut to blood.

Phosphorus – There's less phosphorus in breast milk than in cows' milk formula. Also the amount in breast milk changes as time passes, whereas that in formula obviously remains the same.

Iron – This is one mineral present in larger amounts (twice as much) in breast milk than in cows' milk, although the levels in milk formula are higher than in breast milk because formula is fortifed with iron. However, a fully breastfed full-term baby of a healthy mother almost never becomes anaemic in the first six months and the amount of iron in breast milk remains the same even in mothers who have an iron deficiency, whether or not they receive iron supplements. Research indicates that breast milk iron is better absorbed by a baby than that in formula. Breastfed babies absorb about half the iron present in breast-milk, whereas bottle-fed babies probably absorb only one-tenth of that in formula. Vitamins C and E, lactose and copper, present in higher amounts in breast milk, encourage more efficient absorption, and breast milk's relatively low concentration of proteins, calcium and phosphorus helps too.

Test-tube experiments show that adding iron to breast milk

reduces the anti-infective activity of an important iron-absorbing substance called lactoferrin (see page 45), found in very much greater amounts in breast milk than in formula, so the lower breast-milk iron levels shouldn't be seen as inferior to the higher levels in formula.

Fluoride – See page 90.

Trace elements – These minerals include copper, zinc, manganese, chromium, cobalt, molybdenum, selenium, iodine, silicon and boron. Many form parts of enzymes (see page 51) and are known to be essential for babies. As far as we know, there's generally enough of most of them in breast milk and in cows' milk formula. Selenium, an anti-oxidant (see below), can be an exception: if women don't eat enough selenium-containing foods, they may have low levels in their milk; it's also possible that some cow's milk formulas could be improved by having more selenium.

Vitamins

Breast milk contains more of the vitamins A, C and E than does cows' milk, but less vitamin K. In mothers who are well nourished in pregnancy and eat a well-balanced diet while breastfeeding, there's scant evidence that their fully breastfed babies normally need any vitamin supplements in the first six months.

In general, the principle should be to give any additional foods and vitamins necessary for a baby's well-being to the mother, not to the baby direct.

Vitamin A – Both breast milk and cows' milk provide vitamin A and carotenoids (used by the body to make vitamin A). Carotenoids are yellowish substances which the body can turn into vitamin A and also use as anti-oxidants to protect cells from being damaged by free radicals during illness and physical and mental stress.

Breast milk provides substantial amounts of vitamin A. Beta-carotene forms 24 per cent of the carotenoids in breast milk and 85 per cent in cows' milk; other carotenoids in breast milk include lycopene and beta-cryptoxanthine, but many remain unidentified. The amount of carotenoids varies considerably from one woman to another; it also varies in any one woman according to how many babies she's had, what she's eaten, and when the milk sample was taken.

Vitamin C – This vitamin is concentrated in breast milk and the baby of a healthy mother who eats a healthy diet needs no extra. Even women suffering from scurvy don't produce babies deficient in vitamin C. If a mother's diet is deficient in this vitamin, it is she who needs supplements of vitamin C rather than her baby.

Vitamin C passes readily from a mother's blood into her milk. If she has a food or drink containing vitamin C, the level in her milk rises within half an hour.

Vitamin D – This vitamin helps minerals such as calcium enter and strengthen bones and helps prevent rickets (soft, bendy bones). Colostrum contains more vitamin D than does mature milk, but vitamin D-fortified formula has very much more than either.

Fattty fish, eggs, butter and soft margarines all contain vitamin D but, interestingly, the amount of this vitamin in a breastfeeding woman's diet has little, if any, influence on her baby's vitamin D level. Sunshine on the skin is a far better source for a breastfeeding mother than any food. Skin produces vitamin D after exposure to daylight and the body stores the vitamin for use in the darker months.

There isn't always enough vitamin D in breast milk to strengthen a baby's bones, which is why pre-term and some full-term breastfed babies may benefit from a supplement. This is important for breastfed babies if their mothers are malnourished or eat a vegetarian diet containing a lot of chapattis (chapatti flour contains substances which prevent calcium from being absorbed). A supplement may also be important for breastfed babies whose mothers go outside very little, or who always cover their skin out of doors and so get little ultraviolet light from bright daylight. However, some such mothers can solve the problem simply by getting more daylight on their skin. Babies whose bare skin is exposed to direct daylight for only a short time every day make their own vitamin D. Even exposing just their faces to daylight has been shown to be enough.

Vitamin K – Breast milk contains less of this vitamin than cows' milk does. Some babies suffer from a condition called haemorrhagic disease of the newborn, which is due to a shortage of vitamin K. This makes the gut lining bleed and is more common in breastfed babies. Many doctors recommend that all newborns should receive vitamin K after birth, by injection and/or by mouth, whether or not the mother is going to breastfeed. If it's given by mouth, some babies, including those who are breastfed, need more doses than others. It's worth pointing out that a woman who feeds her baby frequently is likely to produce more milk – and therefore more vitamin K – more quickly than a woman who schedule-feeds.

Anti-infective factors

We've already mentioned breast milk antibodies but many other substances also help fight infection and some are more plentiful and active in breast milk than in formula.

Proportions of nutrients – The very proportion of nutrients in breast milk compared with those in formula prevents the growth of certain organisms, including *E. coli* and dysentery and typhoid bacteria, in the baby's gut. The high lactose, low phosphorus and low protein levels are particularly helpful.

Micro-organisms – A baby's gut contains a large number and bulk of micro-organisms. These vary from one baby to another and account for the unpleasant smell of a bottle-fed baby's bowel motions compared with the sweeter smell of those of a breastfed baby. Many researchers (though not all) report that the organisms in the breastfed baby's bowel are predominantly lactobacilli (also known as bifidobacteria). Lactobacilli produce acetic and lactic acids which together prevent the growth of many disease-producing organisms such as *E. coli* (a common cause of gastroenteritis in bottle-fed babies), the dysentery bacillus and the yeasts which cause thrush. However, the balance of different micro-organisms may vary in pre-term babies and also according to the type of delivery and whether the baby has had antibiotics.

The bifidus factor – The bifidus factor (also known as gynolactose) is a mixture of about ten oligosaccharides, present in breast milk but virtually absent from cows' milk. In fact there's about forty times as much bifidus factor in human milk as in cows' milk. The bifidus factor promotes the growth of lactobacilli, encouraging a healthy balance of micro-organisms in the gut. There's a possibility that it interferes with the flu virus too.

Lactoferrin – Colostrum – the very first milk made in the few days after delivery, see page 53 – and mature milk are unusually rich in this important anti-infective, iron-binding whey protein. Lactoferrin makes up between 10 and 25 per cent of the protein in breast milk and there's very much more (ten to twenty times more) in human milk than in cows' milk (see page 42). There's also some in tears, saliva, pancreatic juice and other secretions.

Lactoferrin has several important actions. It mops up a potentially harmful excess of iron, so probably helps regulate the amount of iron a baby absorbs; it may also absorb excess iron in a breastfed baby eating iron-rich solids.

Test-tube experiments show that together with one of the immunoglobulins (IgA), lactoferrin inhibits the growth of many potentially harmful organisms, including *E. coli*, yeasts, *Staphylococcus aureus* and possibly even viruses, by robbing them of the iron they need for growth. It also kills various micro-organisms directly and makes some bacteria more susceptible to damage from lysozyme (see page 48). Up until recently it hasn't been clear whether lactoferrin is actually active in this way in a baby, partly because we don't know whether stomach acid interferes with its action. However, we do know that lactoferrin is largely broken down in the gut into fragments called peptides.

— Japanese researchers reported in 1994 that one of these peptides, lactoferricin, has an even more powerful anti-infective action than lactoferrin itself.

Scientists think that giving a breastfed baby iron supplements – or even formula with its added iron – may encourage gut infection because lactoferrin can't mop up enough of the extra iron to prevent infecting micro-organisms from growing and dividing. To any mother whose baby has had gastroenteritis this is far from simply academic!

Lactoferrin, like antibodies and enzymes, loses its anti-infective activity when milk is boiled, so the small amount naturally present in fresh cows' milk becomes useless as cows' milk is processed into formula.

Dutch scientists are currently breeding dairy cows descended from a 'transgenic' bull called Herman. Transgenic means that the genetic material contains an implanted human gene. And in Herman and his daughters the gene makes them produce lacto-ferrin. The scientists hope that the milk from transgenic cows will contain high levels of lactoferrin so that it can be used to make milk formula with a high lactoferrin content more like that of breast milk. The cattle will effectively become bovine lactoferrin factories.

Immunoglobulins (antibodies) – For years scientists thought that babies obtained antibodies from their mothers only before birth, across the placenta. We now know that breastfed babies continue to receive them from breast milk.

Antibodies are specialized proteins. The main one is immuno-globulin A (IgA); the others are IgD, IgE, IgG and IgM.

Colostrum contains especially large amounts of antibodies, which is one reason why it is so important. Breast-milk IgA differs from the IgA in a woman's blood partly because its structure makes it resistant to a baby's stomach acid and digestive enzymes, and partly because its antibodies are specifically geared to combat gut infection.

Breast-milk IgA antibodies are programmed with information which helps protect a baby against those bacterial, fungal and viral illnesses from which his mother has suffered. They may also protect him against infections to which she has been immunized. And they can protect him against certain food antigens (food proteins that can lead to ill-health in sensitive babies). If the relevant antibodies are present – that is, if a mother has some degree of immunity to any one infection – they can help protect her baby from tetanus, whooping cough, pneumonia, diphtheria, *E. coli* gastroenteritis, typhoid, dysentery, flu and various other viral illnesses, including rubella and polio. However, it's important to point out that whatever infections or immunizations you've had, you can't rely on your breastfed baby being protected; any protection, good as it may be, is unpredictable.

Breast-milk antibodies can be absorbed into a baby's blood and also act in his gut. IgA in colostrum and milk coats the gut lining in the first few days after birth and prevents many infective organisms and other large protein molecules from entering the blood.

A growing baby only gradually begins to manufacture antibodies in response to infection or immunization. Cells in his gut lining may begin to make IgA from around twelve days if he is full-term. However, seven out of every ten bottle-fed babies still have no IgA in their bowel by four weeks old. When the cells eventually make enough, the mother's IgA becomes unnecessary, but for the first few months the coating of breast milk IgA prevents some infections and food allergies. The concentration of IgA-producing cells in a baby's gut doesn't reach the adult level until he is two years old. The early period of absent and then gradually increasing antibody formation by the baby has been called the 'immunity gap', a gap that can be filled only by breast milk. We'll say more about this in Chapter 4.

Cows' milk contains antibodies too but these, of course, are effective against cows' infections, some of which differ from human ones. Antibodies in cows' milk are also altered so much by heating during the treatment of fresh milk to make formula that they lose their activity. So formula doesn't contain active antibodies. The ultimate irony is that calves reared on heat-treated milk or dried milk powder get more enteritis than those drinking fresh, untreated milk. This enteritis is effectively treated by fresh cows' milk!

An interesting parallel was seen in a nursery in Belgrade where an epidemic of *E. coli* gastroenteritis could not be stopped even when the previously bottle-fed babies were fed with donated breast milk. However, at first this milk was boiled before use. Not until the breast milk was given fresh and unboiled was the epidemic controlled.

Lysozyme and complement – These two proteins interact with IgA to kill bacteria. Lysozyme is present in breast milk in amounts 300 times greater than in cows' milk. Lysozyme is also present in other body secretions such as saliva and tears, where it helps prevent infections of the eyes and eyelids. Breast milk's lysozyme level falls in the first few months, then starts rising until at six months there is more than there was in colostrum. At one year there is an even higher level.

Anti-staphylococcal factor and *hydrogen peroxide* – Together these, plus vitamin C, kill bacteria such as *E. coli*.

Lactoperoxidase – This is an enzyme (see page 51) which inhibits the growth of bacteria.

Fibronectin – This is present in large amounts in colostrum. It encourages some of the white cells to mop up harmful bacteria and also reduces inflammation.

Live cells – These are white cells similar to some of those in the mother's blood. This means that breast milk is a living fluid. Fresh cows' milk contains living cells too but these are killed as the milk is processed into formula. Research suggests that some white cells from breast milk pass from a baby's gut into his bloodstream. It has also been found that white cells from a single feed of mother's milk stick to the gut lining or nestle into this lining and remain there for sixty hours.

Lymphocytes make antibodies as well as the anti-viral substance interferon and can be absorbed from a baby's gut into the blood to continue making IgA. Researchers believe that hormonal and other factors in breastfeeding women send IgA-producing T-lymphocytes ('T-cells') from the lymph tissue in the gut to the breasts. This means that the breast milk lymphocytes know about the potentially harmful organisms in the bowel and can protect the baby from them. What's more, they 'remember' past infections and protect against new attacks for many years.

Neutrophils, granulocytes and epithelial cells are the names of other live cells in breast milk. They are present in even larger amounts in colostrum.

Macrophages are large cells which actively engulf foreign particles such as bacteria. They also produce lactoferrin, lysozyme and complement, may help transport antibodies, and are thought to protect against necrotizing enterocolitis (see page 71).

Anti-viral substances – Various other substances act against viruses including polio, mumps, herpes simplex and encephalitis viruses.

Mucins: One group of substances newly recognized in breast milk (and probably responsible for half its anti-viral activity) are proteins called mucins, present elsewhere in the body in slime. Mucins are large molecules containing protein and carbohydrate that can stick to unwanted bacteria and viruses, bind viruses to certain sugars, and carry these organisms out of the body in the bowel motions. They are especially active against the rotaviruses which are so often responsible for diarrhoea. Older babies make mucins in their gut. The mucins in cows' milk are removed during formula manufacture. One reseacher has suggested that if mucins could be synthesized they would make a useful addition to formula.

An interesting new field of research lies with certain viral infections in breastfeeding women. Viruses such as cytomegalovirus and rubella may enter breast milk and give a baby an infection which, because of antibodies in his mother's milk, is generally very mild. The baby is immunized by breast milk against his mother's infection.

Hormones

Breast milk contains many hormones, hormone-releasing factors and hormone-like factors, including insulin, prolactin, corticosteroids, relaxin, oestrogens, progesterone, gonadotropins, gonadotropin-releasing hormone, thyroid hormones (T_3 and T_4), thyroid-releasing and thyroid-stimulating hormones, parathyroid hormone and erythropoietin. Some come from the mother's blood and, of these, some are concentrated in her milk. Others are made in the breast.

The primary action of some milk hormones may be in the mother's breast, for example, to help make milk proteins and enzymes. However, others, including insulin, prolactin, thyroxine and thyroid-stimulating hormone, are thought to be important to the baby.

At one time breast milk's thyroid hormones were thought to protect hypothyroid babies but they are no longer considered sufficient. Hypothyroidism needs to be detected and treated as soon as possible, however a baby is fed.

Erythropoietin helps regulate red cell production. Pre-term babies are particularly susceptible to anaemia and there's some evidence that giving pre-term babies drug treatment with erythropoietin may be beneficial. It's possible, though unproven, that breast milk's erythropoietin helps protect pre-term babies from anaemia.

Prostaglandins

These hormone-like substances are found in breast milk but not in formula. A baby can use essential fatty acids (omega-3 and omega-6 PUFAs (see page 36) to make prostaglandins, but needs a good balance of omega-3s and omega-6s to make a healthy balance of different prostaglandins. However, the amounts and proportions of individual PUFAs and of the two main groups of PUFAs, the omega-6s and omega-3s, in cows' milk formula currently differ widely from those in breast milk.

The concentration of certain prostaglandins (E and F) in breast milk is 100 times that in a woman's plasma (the liquid part of blood). Their importance isn't clear but they are known to affect the gut. One function may be to help a baby absorb zinc from breast milk. This would explain the protective effect of breast milk against the rare and inherited ulcerating skin disease called acrodermatitis enteropathica (see page 83).

Growth factors

Breast milk contains many growth factors, including two which affect the growth and development of the gut lining and the nerves.

Epidermal growth factor is a hormone-like polypeptide that stimulates normal multiplication and development of several cells, including those in the gut lining. There's a lot of this in colostrum and a group of researchers in the US has suggested that it may be particularly valuable for very immature pre-term babies. There are substantial amounts of epidermal growth factor in breast milk but very much less in cows' milk formula.

Nerve growth factor helps the maturation of developing nerves.

Enzymes

Over seventy enzymes have been identified in breast milk and there may well be many more. Some originate from tissue fluid (which comes from tiny blood vessels in the breast), and others come directly from milk gland cells, where their production is under hormonal control. Some milk enzymes are there as a by-product of milk production; others are important for the baby's digestion or development.

Some enzymes help with digestion; the role of many of the others is unclear. However, most are present in highest concentration soon after birth in colostrum. Two, lipase (see page 38) and lactoperoxidase (see page 48), have already been mentioned. Others include lysozyme (see page 48), xanthine oxidase, aldolase, alkaline and acid phosphatases, anti-trypsin (see page 54), amylase, glutathione peroxidase (which may help a baby absorb an important anti-oxidant mineral, selenium) and catalase.

Enzymes are destroyed by heating, which is one reason why expressed or pumped breast milk should ideally not be heated before being fed to a baby, particularly if the baby is pre-term. Most enzymes in cows' milk are destroyed by pasteurization during its conversion to formula.

Foods, drugs and environmental contaminants

Breast milk may contain such things as alcohol, caffeine, theophylline and theobromine from coffee and tea (see Chapters 9 and 13). The concentration of alcohol in a woman's milk tends to reflect the amount in her blood, whereas tea and coffee derivatives aren't transferred from blood to breast milk to such an extent. Her milk may also contain traces of whole food protein molecules.

Certain drugs, certain dietary and environmental contaminants and radioactivity can also enter both breast milk (see Chapter 13) and formula.

Formula may also contain traces of cows' foodstuffs, drugs and environmental contaminants. One problem has arisen with the addition of vegetable oil. In 1991 four French researchers reported that eleven out of forty-five different types of formula contained peanut oil. Allergy to peanuts is now one of the four most common childhood allergies, frequently causing eczema and occasionally leading to sudden allergic shock (anaphylaxis), which can cause death if not treated promptly. Peanut oil contains peanut proteins and it's these which do the damage in susceptible babies.

So much for the substances we *know* are present in milk. Most people are astonished to learn how complex it is. There are almost certainly other things we haven't yet isolated, which is partly why it's impossible for formula manufacturers to make an accurate substitute for breast milk.

HOW BREAST MILK CHANGES

Neither breast milk nor milk direct from a cow is of constant composition. Milk's make-up varies according to the length of lactation, the time of day, and when within a feed the sample is taken. A calf which feeds directly from its mother benefits from these changes. However, a bottle-fed baby drinks milk of a highly consistent composition because many cows' milk, taken from different stages of lacatation and at different times of day, is pooled to be made into milk formula for human consumption. Breast milk, on the other hand, is supplied on a 'one-off' basis direct from producer to consumer and varies in composition considerably in any one woman at any given time and from one woman to another. These variations, far from being harmful, are of considerable importance, as we shall now see.

Colostrum

This is the first milk made by the breast before birth and for several days after. Colostrum is rich in protein (nine times as much as in mature milk), cells, certain amino acids, minerals (including calcium, magnesium and zinc), vitamins A, E, B_6 and B_{12} and epidermal growth factor, and has less sugar than later milk. It also has less fat but is particularly rich in DHA. A breast-fed baby one week old has five times the vitamin E that a bottle-fed baby has in its body. Most important, the protein in colostrum contains large amounts of antibodies – the same types as in mature milk but many more of them. These give the newborn baby resistance to infection at a time when he would otherwise be particularly susceptible.

Bottle-fed babies don't get cows' colostrum, let alone human colostrum, yet cows' colostrum ('beestings') is considered so vital for calves that farmers save it for them or even go to the expense of buying it in if necessary.

Colostrum often leaks from the nipples in the second half of pregnancy and looks thick and yellow. The colour is due to high levels of beta-carotene, a powerful anti-oxidant that helps protect cells from damage. The mother gets beta-carotene by eating cabbage, spinach and other dark green leafy vegetables, carrots and certain other vegetables, and some fruits. Her baby can use it to make vitamin A.

The low fat content of colostrum is advantageous to the newborn baby who secretes little lipase of his own. Without colostrum he would have difficulty digesting larger amounts of fat in the first day or so.

Colostrum also speeds the passage of meconium – a baby's sticky, tar-like earliest bowel motions – through the gut, so reducing the absorption of bile pigments, naturally occurring substances that might cause or worsen newborn, 'physiological', jaundice (see page 359).

An anti-trypsin enzyme in colostrum (also present in mature milk) helps prevent the digestion of antibodies by trypsin in the gut. Antibodies are proteins and without this enzyme one of the gut's own enzymes, trypsin, would break them down.

A few days after birth colostrum becomes more milky and is sometimes called 'transitional milk'. This, in turn, changes to mature milk but there is no sudden change from one to the other.

There is not a fixed amount of colostrum, as many people think, so expressing it ante-natally doesn't reduce the supply available to the baby. Letting a baby suck frequently and for as long as he wants in the first few days not only gives him more of the valuable colostrum but also hastens the production of mature milk and encourages the let-down reflex (see page 19) to become quick and efficient.

Mature milk

This contains a fifth of the protein of colostrum but more fat and sugar. It is thinner-looking and whiter or even bluish-white. During the first year of breastfeeding the protein content of breast milk gradually falls, regardless of what the mother eats. However, most babies eat increasing amounts of foods other than milk from the age of about six months and these provide the extra protein necessary for growth. Also, a baby grows at its fastest in the first six months of life when the level of protein in breast milk is at its highest. The gradual decrease in protein is paralleled by a normal and therefore expected slowing in a baby's growth rate.

As we saw in the previous chapter, the early part of a feed is made of fore-milk, which is low in fat, while the later part is hind-milk, which has twice or three times the fat and one and a half times as much protein. Some mixing occurs if the let-down operates before the baby finishes the fore-milk. This happens more in the second breast. Fore-milk tends to look relatively thin and white or bluish-white, while hind-milk is thicker and creamy-white. Hind-milk has a different 'mouth-feel' from fore-milk – it's more viscous and coats the mouth more.

The changing composition of milk during any single feed means that a baby allowed to go on feeding at the first breast as long as he or she wants, finishes with high-fat hind-milk on that side. He then carries on at the second breast with lots of thin, watery fore-milk. Babies have been seen to stop feeding at the first breast even though there is still milk there. Then, to everyone's surprise, they feed with vigour at the second breast. One researcher suggested this might be because a baby has had enough fat-rich hind-milk and wants some of the more thirst-quenching fore-milk. However, another researcher found no difference in the lengths of feed when babies were bottle-fed with breast milk of varying fat content.

The concentration of fat in breast milk is lowest in the early hours of the morning.

Regression milk

As a baby takes less and less milk as the months go by, it comes to look thicker, yellower and more like colostrum. Some women can express this milk for many months after they have stopped breastfeeding.

Monthly mid-cycle changes when your periods return

When you eventually start to ovulate again after having your baby, your milk will alter slightly in composition before and after ovulation. Five to six days before ovulation (which occurs on the twelfth day of the average cycle, beginning from the first day of a period) breast milk changes in composition for between thirty and forty hours; a similar change happens six to seven days after ovulation. In both cases there's temporarily less lactose, glucose and potassium, and more sodium and chloride (see page 255). Some experienced breastfeeders say that they detect that their baby notices these changes.

Pre-term milk

Mothers of pre-term babies produce 'pre-term milk' which has a different composition from mature milk. It changes only gradually (see page 342).

The basic thing we've tried to get across in this chapter is that breast milk is very different from formula – however much the latter is modified. No longer is it reasonable for anyone to claim that formula is very close to breast milk. Today we know better. In the next chapter we'll look at why these differences are important.

FOUR

Best for baby?

When weighing up the pros and cons of breastfeeding, the scale-pan falls decisively on the side of the pros. Indeed, when writing this and the next chapter we found it difficult to find anything much to say against breastfeeding. Even many of the 'disadvantages' that would-be breastfeeders may see are usually readily overcome if they know how.

Experts around the world, including those from the World Health Organization and the American Academy of Pediatrics, strongly recommend exclusive breastfeeding as the best way of feeding babies. One UK lactation physiologist says that 'in global health terms breastfeeding is perhaps the most significant form of preventive medicine'.

SCIENTIFIC EVIDENCE

An increasing body of scientific evidence underlines the medical advantages enjoyed by breastfed babies and by older children and adults who were breastfed as babies. However, not all reseach is of equal merit. Some studies reporting health benefits from breast-feeding did not sufficiently take into account the many factors that can cloud the issue, such as the mother smoking, her education and the socio-economic status and size of the family. And some studies have not looked carefully enough at different sorts of breastfeeding. For example, exclusive breastfeeding is different from partial breastfeeding, and some babies are breastfed for much longer than others.

More recent studies tend to be statistically sounder, which is one reason we've upgraded this chapter so comprehensively. Research into breastfeeding and breast milk continues apace around the world, with hundreds of new papers being published in the learned medical journals every year.

The first reports that breastfed babies might be healthier came early this century, soon after the mass introduction of bottle-feeding. The trickle of information that followed has developed into an avalanche in the last twenty-five years. The medical and nursing professions are not always quick to take up new information, especially if it favours sweeping changes in the management of people in hospital and in the community. This reluctance to change isn't necessarily bad and tends to protect the public from medical fads and fancies. Having said this, the staff in many hospitals have made sweeping improvements in the way they facilitate breastfeeding. Sadly, others haven't. But we think that if mothers understand the advantages to their babies of being breastfed, their pressure will do more than anything to change, improve and update the standard of help, information and advice available.

THE PERFECT FOOD

In Chapter 3 we detailed the unique composition of breast milk and how the amount and type of each of its nutrients suits babies so well. But breast milk doesn't simply provide food, as we shall now see.

GOOD FOR GROWTH

Bottle-fed babies tend to put on weight faster than breastfed ones. However, optimum growth isn't a matter of putting on weight as quickly as possible. The growth of the human infant is a complex affair. If you compare growth rates in different parts of the world you find that children in developing countries tend to grow more slowly than Western children. As prosperity increases, so do growth rates. But is it sensible to assume that babies are best off if they are growing fast?

Apparently not, if the work of a distinguished doctor in southern Africa is anything to go by. He questions whether the usual growth rate for American and British babies should be taken as normal. By these Western standards many millions of children are said to be malnourished yet they are perfectly fit and well and grow up healthier than many Western children. A hundred years ago English children reached their maximum height at the age of twenty-five; today they get there at sixteen. Among the rural Bantu in Africa, the age is twenty.

Animal experiments show that slower growth rates in the young make for slower ageing. This seems to be borne out in humans if we accept evidence from a South African study which found at least twenty times as many Bantu living over the age of 100 as whites. This is worth thinking about because by overfeeding our children we could be accelerating not only their growth but also the onset of degenerative diseases, thus decreasing their life span.

Weight

There's every reason to suppose that the proportions, types and amounts of nutrients in breast milk are perfectly geared to produce an optimum growth rate. This said, the weight of exclusively breastfed babies who are healthy and thriving increases more slowly than that of bottle-fed babies after the first few months.

Growth charts

World Health Organization experts are currently working on revising growth charts used around the world to plot babies' weights, because when breastfed babies' weights are plotted, many charts make it look as if many of them are growing more slowly than 'normal' after the first few months, whereas in fact all that's happening is that they're growing more slowly than bottle-fed ones. And bottle-fed babies may in fact be growing unnaturally fast.

This situation has come about because many growth charts are based on measurements of the growth patterns of a large number of babies in Ohio, recorded between 1929 and 1975. Some of these babies were exclusively breastfed, but generally only for a very short time before other foods such as formula or solids were introduced. The rest were bottle-fed from birth, many of them on old-fashioned cows' milk formulas.

Starting solids

Even when solid foods are introduced, breastfed babies continue to weigh less, on average, than bottle-fed ones. Studies show that this is not because they aren't offered or don't get enough nourishment. It may simply be that they know when they've had enough.

— Researchers in Washington and Maryland (1980) looked at ninety-six babies of La Leche League mothers who had breastfed exclusively for at least six months in the last two years. The average duration of exclusive breastfeeding was seven months. The babies' growth in terms of weight and length was fine and there was no difference between those breastfed exclusively for more than six months or less.

However, when considering babies in developing countries, it's important not to jump to any conclusions. In Botswana, for example, some babies over eighteen months – who are having both breast milk and solids – have a greater risk of becoming malnourished than those who are not breastfed at all, and many grow faster when they come off breast milk completely. The same has been reported in babies over twelve months old in Ghana.

In these countries the dilemma may be not for researchers and health workers to decide whether it's safer for these mothers to continue breastfeeding, or to stop so that their babies grow faster, but to see whether they can help the mothers increase their milk supply by encouraging them to breastfeed more frequently (even if their babies don't ask for feeds) and by giving them extra food, so that their babies continue to have the anti-infective and other benefits of breast milk. The answers almost certainly vary according to circumstances and more research is needed.

Less obesity

Breastfed babies tend to be slimmer than bottle-fed babies at one year old.

We've all become very weight-conscious, especially over the last two decades, partly because we know that very overweight adults are more prone to heart disease, high blood pressure, diabetes, varicose veins and gallstones, and have a reduced life expectancy. However, there's little evidence that being *slightly* overweight as an adult is detrimental to health, and only a little evidence that being *moderately* overweight can be harmful.

— Among 16,000 people born in Hertfordshire, England, between 1911 and 1930, those who weighed 28 lb or more on their first birthday were *less* likely to have heart disease fifty years later than those who weighed 17 lb or less.

The suggestion that fat babies become fat adults is an oversimplification and in many cases simply not true. However, there is an overall tendency for this to happen, especially if the rate of weight gain in early infancy is high. Studies show that 10–20 per cent of fat babies are fat when five to seven years old. And of babies whose weight is over the ninetieth percentile, about 14 per cent are obese twenty to thirty years later. This means that over 80 per cent of fat babies are likely to lose their excess fat after infancy. However, half of all obese children were fat as babies.

Whether or not mothers should try to prevent obesity in their breastfed babies by giving fewer and/or shorter feeds is dubious. A baby's fat stores act as depots in times of serious illness, so perhaps they should leave nature alone. The time to curtail feeds, though, is if you are breastfeeding to 'shut your baby up' when he might prefer, or need, some other form of attention (see page 108).

While we've all seen fat breastfed babies, there's a statistically greater chance of babies becoming fat if bottle-fed.

— In a Sheffield study (1971), 60 per cent of bottle-fed babies put on 'too much' weight in their first year compared with only 19 per cent of breastfed ones.

One reason why bottle-fed babies are more likely to be plump than breastfed ones is that the high mineral content of formula (see page 140) makes them thirsty. If their thirst is quenched by more milk, the extra calories can make them fat. The recent modification of formulas has reduced this danger by reducing their mineral content. However, some mothers put an extra scoop of powder into their baby's bottle, especially before bedtime, in the hope of making him sleep better. Not only does this not work, but it could theoretically lead to too high a weight-gain. It can also be particularly dangerous if the baby is unwell.

Another reason for weight-gain in bottle-fed babies is that some mothers add cereal powder to the bottle in a fruitless attempt to make their baby sleep longer. Breastfeeding mothers are much less likely to give their babies early solids.

Height

Finnish researchers found that healthy, well-nourished, exclusively breastfed babies grew in length more slowly than bottle-fed ones. Two doctors in the US speculated that this may be because bottle-fed babies receive more vitamin D from formula than breastfed ones get from breast milk. Whether or not this is important – and one growth rate is better than the other – isn't clear. Breastfed babies who have vitamin D supplements grow in length more quickly. However, a mother can increase her milk's vitamin D content by spending more time outside with bright daylight on her skin and by eating a healthy diet.

LESS ILLNESS

Babies who are breastfed – and especially those who are exclusively breastfed – are less likely to be ill in their first year. As a
result, they are less likely to be admitted to hospital. British
researchers reported in 1983 that *not* breastfeeding increased a
baby's risk of being admitted to hospital by 40 per cent. This risk
was independent of social factors. This means that breastfeeding
women experience less of the anxiety, disruption and to-ing and
fro-ing associated with treating a sick baby in their GP's surgery or
hospital.

Much more important, breastfeeding can save lives. In 1992 a
New York paediatrician calculated that breastfeeding could prevent 5000 infant deaths every year in the US by reducing the risk
of gastroenteritis, the sudden infant death syndrome (SIDS, or
unexlained cot deaths), pneumonia, meningitis, necrotizing enterocolitis and septicaemia. In developing countries the potential
saving of lives is measured in millions. The stark reality, according
to a World Health Organization estimate, is that bottle-feeding
kills a million and a half babies worldwide each year.

FEWER INFECTIONS

We saw in the last chapter that breast milk contains many factors
which help protect a baby from infection with bacteria, viruses,
yeasts and other organisms. Indeed, US researchers have found
that breast milk kills certain harmful organisms as efficiently as
any antiseptic, whereas cows' milk has no such effect. This all
sounds good but in practical terms how important is it today with
hygienic precautions for bottle-feeding so effective and the treatment of infections so advanced?

Developing countries

For two-thirds of the world's population, feeding babies with formula is 'tantamount to signing a death warrant', according to the United Nations Protein Advisory Group. The risk of these babies developing infective diarrhoea (gastroenteritis) is extremely high because of the lack of adequate hygiene, sanitation and facilities for sterilizing bottle-feeding equipment. There are very few anti-infective factors in formula and, frequently, poverty means that the family cannot afford sufficient milk powder to nourish their babies properly. Poorly treated dehydration from diarrhoea caused by infection is a frequent killer.

— In parts of rural China (1973) bottle-fed babies had twice the chance of dying as had breastfed babies.
— In Bangladesh (1988) severely malnourished children up to the age of three were less likely to die if they were breastfed than if they were bottle-fed.

Developed countries

But even in developed countries breastfed babies are less likely to suffer from infections than bottle-fed ones. This isn't to say that modern medicine does not treat most infections successfully, or that breastfed babies cannot get these infections, just that, statistically, babies have a reduced risk of several types of infection if they're breastfed.

Some critics believe that illness protection from breastfeeding is minimal in developed countries. However, part of the smallish DARLING study reported in 1995 – of babies born to relatively affluent families in the US and either fully breastfed or fully bottle-fed for the first year – concluded that the reduction in illness in breastfed babies compared with that in bottle-fed babies 'is of sufficient magnitude to be of public health significance'.

The vast majority of mothers in developed countries prepare feeds hygienically nowadays. So the many anti-infective factors in breast milk must be responsible in a positive way for a breastfed baby's resistance to infection. Perhaps the very act of breastfeeding is important in boosting a baby's immunity too.

Diarrhoea (infective diarrhoea/gastroenteritis)

— In California, in the DARLING study (1995, above), exclusively breastfed babies had half the attacks of diarrhoea experienced by bottle-fed babies in their first year.

— Doctors in Calcutta reported (1995) that babies and young children with diarrhoea were nearly seven times more likely to become dehydrated if they were bottle-fed.

— A study in Mexico (1992) found that breastfed babies were five times less likely to develop diarrhoea from giardia (protozoal) infection than were bottle-fed ones.

— A study from Dundee in 1990 reported that bottle-fed babies had four times as much gastroenteritis in the first three months as exclusively breastfed ones.

— Researchers in Brazil reported (1987) that babies who weren't breastfed were more than fourteen times as likely to die from infective diarrhoea as exclusively breastfed ones. And babies fed on breast milk and formula had over four times the risk of dying from infective diarrhoea as those that were exclusively breastfed.

In the rare instances when breastfed babies do get diarrhoea, breast milk helps protect them from potentially dangerous dehydration. (Poorly treated or untreated dehydration is the most important cause of death from diarrhoea in babies around the world.)

Respiratory infections

Many studies have found that breastfeeding helps protect babies from bronchiolitis and pneumonia in developing countries. The evidence from developed countries is mixed. Recent studies have generally taken into account the exclusivity or otherwise of breastfeeding, as well as other influences on respiratory illness (such as the mother smoking, the mother having a low standard of education, and a large family size). This means they are more trustworthy.

— A large Canadian study reported (1995) that breastfed babies had fewer respiratory illnesses.
— In Italy in 1994, babies with pneumonia or bronchiolitis were much more likely to be bottle-fed. (However, they had no protection against whooping cough.)
— A large study in the US reported (1993) that breastfeeding helped protect under-twos from pneumonia. However, introducing solids early made pneumonia more likely.
— A large study in Dundee, Scotland (1990), found that breastfeeding for thirteen weeks or more significantly reduced the risk of respiratory infection.
— However, the 1995 DARLING study of relatively affluent families found no significant difference in the rates of respiratory infections in fully breastfed and bottle-fed babies.
— Most studies consider only lower respiratory tract infections but Swedish researchers reported in 1994 that breastfed babies had fewer upper respiratory infections (colds, etc.) too.
— In 1966 researchers from the University of Naples in Italy reported that children who had had their tonsils out were less likely to have been breastfed. They suggested that breast milk decreased the severity of infection and inflammation when a child gets tonsillitis and may be associated with 'more tolerant tonsillar lymphoid tissue'.

Middle-ear infection (otitis media)

Many studies report less middle-ear infection in breastfed babies; the length of any protective effect depending on how long breast-feeding continues. Middle-ear infection can lead to deafness. It's also possible for bacteria from infected middle ears to slither along the Eustachian tubes and be swallowed – leading to diarrhoea – and to slide down the back of the throat into the lungs – leading to lung infection, including pneumonia.

Breastfed babies have a lower risk of middle-ear infection for three reasons.

1 Breastfeeding mothers tend to hold their babies in a more upright position than that in which bottle-feeding mothers hold their babies. This means milk is less likely to run from the back of the mouth and along the Eustachian tubes into the middle-ear cavities. Research also suggests that milk in the middle ears may make infection more likely. However, this may not be the whole story, as the next point makes clear.

2 When breast milk or formula enter the middle ear, they behave in different ways. Anti-infective and anti-inflammatory factors in breast milk seem to reduce the risk of infection developing in stagnant milk which has entered the middle ear. A study of babies with a cleft palate showed that those who were bottle-fed, but had breast milk in the bottle, had fewer days of middle-ear infection than those who were bottle-fed with formula.

3 Ultrasound monitoring of the palate during feeding by Southampton University researchers suggests that a breastfed baby's sucking and milking action tends to open the Eustachian tubes, encouraging fluid to drain from the middle ears and making infection less likely. This doesn't happen with bottle-feeding.

— In California, in the 1995 DARLING study, middle-ear infection in exclusively breastfed babies was 19 per cent lower than in bottle-fed ones, and the percentage of prolonged attacks (lasting longer than ten days) was 80 per cent lower. In their second year, babies who had been breastfed for a year – or were still being breastfed – had no fewer middle-ear infections than bottle-fed babies. However, the attacks they did get were nearly three days shorter.

— Dutch researchers reported (1994) that breastfeeding significantly reduced the risk of middle-ear infection in the first four months. When a mother stopped breastfeeding, her baby's risk of ear infection gradually increased until twelve months after stopping, when the risk was the same as if that baby had never been breastfed.

— A Swedish study reported (1994) that breastfeeding decreased the risk of middle-ear infection at two, six and ten months.

— Another Swedish study (1991) found that breastfed babies had half the number of attacks of middle ear infection in the first year compared with bottle-fed babies. Also, their risk of recurrent attacks were reduced by 61 per cent.

— A Scandinavian study noted (1982) that breastfeeding could protect a baby for up to three years – long after breastfeeding had stopped.

Urine infections

Several studies have shown that urine infections are less likely in children who are breastfed. One probable reason is that oligosaccharides (simple sugars) in breast milk make *E. coli* bacteria – a common cause of urine infection – less able to stick to the lining of the urinary tract and cause trouble.

Another is that a breastfed baby's urine contains more IgA, lactoferrin and lysozyme than that of a bottle-fed baby. These substances can't have entered the urine from the bloodstream, because they aren't absorbed by a baby's gut – so they can't have come directly from breast milk but must have actually been made in the urinary system. This means that breastfeeding must encourage a better immune response in the urinary system

— Welsh researchers noted in 1994 that breastfed babies had higher levels of the antibodies known as immunoglobulin A (IgA) in their urine when they were ten days old. High levels of IgA in the urine seem to cut the risk of urine infection.

— Another study (1992) found that bottle-fed babies had five times as many urine infections as did breastfed ones.

— A Mexican study (1992) reported that pre-term babies were five times more likely to have a urine infection if bottle-fed.

— A Swedish study (1990) reported that children with a kidney infection tended to have been exclusively breastfed for a shorter time than healthy 'controls'.

— An Italian study (1990) reported that babies of up to six months with urine infections were nearly twice as likely to be bottle-fed as breastfed.

— A UK study (1987) reported that a breastfed baby's urinary tract produces three times as much protective IgA as that of a bottle-fed baby.

Sticky eye

Bacterial infection of the front surface of the eye – conjunctivitis or 'sticky eye' – is common in newborn babies. Women in developing countries, including India, Jamaica, the Middle East, northern Africa and Brazil, often put a few drops of colostrum into their baby's eye to counter this infection. This may reduce the need for antibiotic eye drops or ointment. Such medication occasionally fosters the development of antibiotic-resistant strains of bacteria. Interestingly, the eighteenth-century *London Pharmacopoeia* says 'Breast milk . . . cureth Red Eye immediately.'

— More recently, researchers from New Delhi reported (1982) that breast milk can indeed reduce eye infections.

During an epidemic of acute haemorrhagic conjunctivitis in American Samoa in 1981, some adults treated their eyes with breast milk!

Meningitis

— A study in 1986 found that breastfed babies of three months or younger are less likely to suffer from meningitis.

Septicaemia

Breastfed babies are less likely to suffer from septicaemia (blood poisoning).

— A study in Pakistan (with the collaboration of Swedish researchers) reported in 1991 that even partial breastfeeding was a great help in protecting babies from septicaemia. Few women in this study breastfed exclusively, though the researchers suggested that this might have been even more protective.

Necrotizing enterocolitis

This bowel infection occurs in about 500 babies each year in the UK and is very serious, killing one or two in every five affected babies. It's more common in babies who are pre-term, tube-fed or bottle-fed.

— Research by the MRC Unit in Cambridge in 1990 found that necrotizing enterocolitis was six to ten times more common in babies who were exclusively formula-fed, compared with babies fed only breast milk. Babies fed both formula and breast milk had three times the risk of that of exclusively breastfed babies. And breast milk donated by other mothers and subsequently pasteurized was as effective a protection as a baby's own mother's milk. The researchers calculated that exclusive breast-feeding (or feeding with pasteurized donated breast milk) could save 500 babies from being seriously ill with necrotizing enterocolitis and 100 babies dying from it each year in the UK.

Other researchers have commented that freshly expressed or pumped milk may be more protective than frozen breast milk.

Better response to immunization

Breastfed babies make more antibodies when they are immunized, possibly because – as several studies suggest – breastfeeding makes their immune systems mature more quickly.

— A study reported in the *Lancet* in 1990 looked at antibody levels in babies who were immunized at the ages of two, four and six months with *Haemophilus influenzae* type b (Hib) vaccine. They found that breastfed babies (who, incidentally, were breastfed for an average of four to five months) had significantly higher levels of antibodies to Hib than bottle-fed babies both at seven and twelve months.

FEWER ALLERGIC DISEASES

The number of children known to be allergic is increasing yet the cause is often unclear. The role of breastfeeding is confusing here, partly because many early studies didn't consider factors later found to be important, such as a family history of allergy, parental smoking, family size, how long breastfeeding is exclusive, how long breastfeeding continues, and what breastfeeding mothers eat.

However, recent studies support the view that breastfeeding for at least six months can help prevent allergic symptoms.

Allergic symptoms

These include allergic rhinitis (an itchy, runny nose and sneezing, otherwise known as hay fever), eczema, urticaria (nettle-rash), lip-swelling, pain in the lips and/or throat, respiratory allergy (certain coughs, asthma/wheezing, and bronchiolitis), colic, diarrhoea, vomiting, anaemia (due to bleeding from the gut), restlessness, sleep problems and failure to thrive. Some parents and doctors report that allergic babies and children are particularly prone to wrinkles and dark circles under their eyes, puffy skin around their eyes, glassy eyes, red ear-lobes, perspiration, dribbling, middle ear infections, tiredness, thirst and occasional clumsiness.

Three factors make allergic symptoms more likely:

1 **An inherited risk** – If there's allergy in the family – especially on both sides of the family – a baby has an increased risk of eczema, asthma, hay fever and food allergy in general.

2 **Diarrhoea** – A large study found that babies who developed food allergy had had many more attacks of diarrhoea than non-food-allergic babies. Breastfeeding makes diarrhoea less likely.

3 **Allergy-triggers** – A young baby's immune system is immature. Exposure to allergy-triggers can sensitize a susceptible baby and make him prone to allergy either then or later. Triggers include

foreign food proteins, house-dust mite droppings, viral infections, smoky or otherwise polluted air and certain pollens and moulds. The trigger which sensitizes a baby is known as the primary allergy-trigger.

Cows' milk – the commonest primary allergy-trigger?

Cows' milk protein is the commonest primary trigger in susceptible babies. This isn't surprising as it is the first foreign food protein most babies receive. And it's given to bottle-fed babies in very large amounts. Boys are twice as likely as girls to suffer from cows' milk allergy.

The gender difference is interesting as in many Western societies breastfed baby boys are more likely than girls to be given formula early and they are also breastfed for a shorter time. One likely explanation for these observations is that if a breastfed boy shows signs of dissatisfaction, his mother may be particularly likely to interpret them as hunger, perhaps because at some level she thinks boys eat more, need more and are more delicate or precious. Unless she knows or learns how to increase her milk supply, she then readily believes she can't make enough milk and begins to give formula as well as her own milk. Without sufficient stimulation from frequent breastfeds, her milk supply then tends to decrease. Another possible explanation for a gender difference is that some women feel uncomfortable when they get physical pleasure and emotional intimacy from breastfeeding a boy, whereas they might feel easier if the baby were a girl. Cows' milk allergy is more common in families with a history of allergy.

— French researchers noted (1994) that cows' milk protein may act directly on the gut lining by stimulating an abnormal immune response, inflammation and diarrhoea.
— A Danish study (1990) suggested that 2–4 per cent of children are allergic to cows' milk
— In the US today cows' milk allergy is said to affect at least 30,000 babies a year.

Pinpointing the primary allergy-trigger can be difficult because:

1 Formula may not provoke allergic symptoms immediately – it may occasionally sensitize a baby without itself causing any symptoms.

2 A baby's cows' milk antibody level gradually falls after the initial sensitization. This means that this test isn't a reliable gauge of allergic sensitization unless measured both before *and* immediately after the very first drink of formula.

3 Breastfeeding women who drink a lot of milk may have traces of cows' milk in their milk, so cows' milk can be the primary allergy-trigger even in an exclusively breastfed baby.

4 Allergists believe that once a baby is sensitized, he then reacts more readily to other allergy-triggers. Certain allergic illnesses are more common at different ages (see below). They may also occur only when resistance is low, for example, during an illness or at times of other physical – or emotional – stress.

A previously breastfed baby can have urticaria after his first known feed of cows' milk.

— In 1987 researchers studied twenty-nine previously breastfed babies who had urticaria after their first known cows' milk feed. But their records revealed that sixteen of them had had cows' milk formula in hospital unbeknown to their parents. The researchers recommended strict avoidance of formula for breastfed babies.

Reducing allergy-triggers

All babies have to meet potential allergy-triggers at some time but it may be better to reduce or avoid them for a while. Three studies bear this out.

— A Finnish study (1995) followed 150 children from birth to seventeen years. There were three groups: those breastfed for at least six months, those breastfed for one to six months, and those breastfed for less than one month or not at all. All those breastfed for six months or more, and some of those breastfed for up to six months, had three and a half months of exclusive breastfeeding. None had solids until three and a half months, or any fish or citrus fruits in the first year. *The amount of allergic illness was related to the length of breastfeeding. Also, early bottle-feeding gave a higher risk of later allergy than an allergic family history.* Different allergic symptoms peaked at different ages:

There was most eczema at one year and most food allergy (a rash, urticaria, lip-swelling, aching in lips and throat, or severe vomiting after certain foods) at three years.

Respiratory allergy (some types of asthma, wheezing and hay fever) increased through school age and adolescence to a peak at seventeen years.

At one year and three years there was least eczema, food allergy and respiratory allergy in children who'd been breastfed for over six months. At least six months of breastfeeding (including three and a half months of exclusive breastfeeding) were required to reduce the risk of eczema in the first three years. However, exclusive breastfeeding for a month or more helped prevent food allergy and respiratory allergy.

At seventeen years there was least respiratory allergy in those breastfed for six months or more.

Also at seventeen years there was dramatically less 'substantial atopy' (allergic symptoms of more than one type) in those breastfed for six months or more (8 per cent), compared with those breastfed for one to six months (23 per cent), and those breastfed for less than a month or not at all (54 per cent).

.— In 1993 an Italian team studied 174 babies with an allergic family history. They were exclusively breastfed for six months (though bottles of soy milk were allowed). Their mothers drank no more than 150–200ml (5–7 fl oz) of cows' milk a day and ate no more than two eggs a week. In addition, house-dust mites were eliminated as far as possible from the home; pets and smoking were avoided; and no babies went into day care until three years old. Cows' milk and other dairy products were gradually introduced after six months; eggs and fish after a year. The babies had a very much reduced likelihood of allergic illness compared with that predicted from their family history. This protection continued for at least five years.

— A UK team conducted another study of high-risk babies reported in 1992. Allergy-triggers were reduced or avoided in one group and nothing was done in the control group.

Reduced or avoided triggers included:

For breastfeeding mothers:

Dairy products, eggs, fish and nuts

For babies:

Cows' milk formula (all were breastfed for at least six months; only if necessary did they have hydrolysed soy formula supplements)

All foods and drinks other than breast milk (or hydrolysed soy formula) for six months

Cows' milk and unhydrolysed soy formula for nine months

Wheat for ten months

Eggs for eleven months

Other dairy products, eggs, oranges, fish and nuts for twelve months

House-dust mites

By twelve months, only 14 per cent of babies in the reduced allergy-trigger group had one or more allergic disorders, compared with 40 per cent of those in the control group.

How might breastfeeding protect against allergy?

Breastfeeding seems to protect against allergy in several ways:

• Breast milk encourages a baby's gut lining and immune system to mature. The 'leaky gut' hypothesis suggests that foreign proteins can pass through a young baby's gut lining into the bloodstream and trigger food allergy. However, breast milk (and particularly colostrum) contains several substances (including cortisone, and epidermal and nerve growth factors) which probably encourage a breastfed baby's gut lining to mature and become impervious to foreign proteins faster than that of a bottle-fed baby. In addition, cows' milk protein may damage the gut lining and prevent it from maturing as fast as it should.

- Also, breast milk IgA may help prevent foreign food protein molecules from passing from the baby's gut directly into the blood (see below).
- A breastfed baby is in any case exposed to vastly lower levels of foreign food protein. Beta-lactoglobulin is the commonest culprit in cows' milk. However, there is no beta-lactoglobulin in breast milk.
- Breast milk influences the population of micro-organisms in a baby's gut which, in turn, may influence the development of allergy.
- Breastfeeding helps protect babies from diarrhoea – and repeated attacks of diarrhoea are associated with food allergy.
- Breastfeeding helps prevent the respiratory infections which can encourage respiratory allergy.

IgA It takes some months for a baby to make useful amounts of immunoglobulin A (IgA) antibodies. Researchers suggest that in the meantime, the IgA in breast milk may coat the gut lining, prevent large protein molecules from leaking from the gut into the blood and thereby reduce a baby's risk of developing an allergy to that foreign protein.

However, this IgA-coating probably disappears fairly rapidly after a breastfeed, as there's a rapid turnover of the cells lining the gut. This might mean that if feeds were widely spaced and interspersed with bottles of formula, or with solids, cows' milk protein molecules might enter the bloodstream. This is an argument in favour of exclusive breastfeeding for the first four to six months, especially for babies with a family history of allergy.

Bottle-fed babies have an enormous amount of cows' milk protein in their gut. However, they lack protective IgA because even if the IgA in formula were useful to them, it is spoilt by heat treatment during manufacture. This means that if the above theory is correct, cows' milk protein may leak from their gut to their bloodstream and travel to other parts of the body where, in a susceptible baby, it could trigger an immediate allergic response, or sensitize him to react to allergy-triggers in the future.

— A large UK survey (1990) reported that 45 per cent of 'breastfed' babies have formula or water in the first week. It is not sensible to give a breastfed baby formula without very good reason.

Eczema

Research into whether breastfeeding reduces the risk of eczema has produced conflicting results. However, Finnish evidence (1995, see above) suggested that exclusive breastfeeding can delay its onset and make it less severe, especially if there's a family history of allergy. Also:

— A study reported in the *Lancet* (1992) looked at breastfed babies with a family history of allergy. The researchers found that when mothers avoided eating milk, eggs, fish and nuts during the months they were breastfeeding, and also avoided giving their babies both these foods and soya, wheat and oranges up to the age of twelve months, the babies were significantly less likely to suffer from eczema at twelve months.

Wheezing

— Finnish evidence (1995 – see page 74) shows that exclusive breastfeeding can reduce the risk of wheezing and asthma.
— A study (1995) found that children who had been breastfed were much less likely to have recurrent attacks of wheezing when they were six years old.
— A large US study (1993) reported that breastfeeding had a small protective effect against asthma.
— Researchers in Arizona reported (1989) that breastfed babies were less likely to suffer from wheezing (with or without infections such as bronchiolitis) in their first four months.

Food exclusion and challenge for a bottle-fed baby

The only way to prove whether allergic symptoms are caused by cows' milk is to exclude formula from a baby's diet, see if his symptoms disappear, then, if so, reintroduce formula to see if they recur. Ideally you should repeat this challenge to make doubly sure you're right.

However, it's essential to have expert supervision from a doctor or state-registered dietitian to make sure your baby has adequate nourishment when you substitute another type of milk.

Your doctor will advise what's best. Hydrolysed soy formula is a possibility, though one in five babies with cows' milk allergy can't tolerate soy milk either. Neither whole nor diluted goat's milk has the right proportions of nutrients; also about 30 per cent of babies who are sensitive to cows' milk are also sensitive to goat's milk.

Breast milk is the best food for a baby who is allergic to cows' milk. With time and patience – even if you've never breastfed – you can build up your milk supply (see page 270) to provide your baby with some or all of his needs.

Allergy in breastfed babies

Exclusively breastfed babies are much less likely to develop allergies, especially if exclusive breastfeeding continues for four to six months. Breastfeeding women should ideally avoid large amounts of cows' milk, egg, nuts, fish, citrus fruits and wheat, as traces of these foods in breast milk can trigger allergy in susceptible babies. Breastfeeding mothers of babies with a high allergy risk should avoid cows' milk, eggs, nuts and fish completely.

'Nature's immunization'

Some immunologists say that traces of undigested foods in breast milk prepare a baby's digestive and immune systems for direct contact with these foods later.

However, 'traces' come in many sizes. Some breastfeeding women, for example, drink vast quantities of milk – as much as three, four or five pints a day. Some of them do this to encourage their own milk production. Not only does this not work but it may also encourage cows' milk protein to enter their breast milk.

Food exclusion and challenge for a breastfeeding mother

If you want to know whether your baby's symptoms could result from something you've eaten, do a trial of food exclusion and challenge.

However, do this under the guidance of your doctor or a dietitian to ensure that your diet remains sound and that neither your baby's health nor yours is put at risk.

When choosing what to avoid first, it's worth keeping a record of whether your baby's symptoms relate to the foods you eat. Cows' milk comes high on the list for many women simply because they drink it so frequently and in such large amounts.

Avoid only one food at a time, otherwise you'll be none the wiser, and avoid it for about a week. If your baby's symptoms improve, try adding it back into your diet to see if his symptoms return. If they do, repeat the 'challenge' to be doubly sure.

LESS COELIAC DISEASE

Some children develop coeliac disease (impaired digestion, a swollen abdomen, unpleasant-smelling motions and failure to thrive) when they begin to eat cereals. This condition is caused by their gut's inability to handle the gliadin fraction of the cereal protein gluten, found in wheat, barley, rye and possibly oats. Gluten damages the gut lining. Treatment consists of withdrawing gluten-containing foods from the diet.

The UK government advises that babies should not have cereals (or indeed any solids) before four months (at the earliest) so as to avoid contact with gluten when they are very young.

Although it's likely that the coating of breast-milk IgA antibodies on the gut lining of young breastfed babies may help prevent gluten damage during this time, it's still wise to avoid giving them cereals.

— A survey in western Ireland, at a time when only 3 per cent of babies were breastfed there, found that coeliac disease was about four times as common as in England at that time, where many more babies were breastfed.
— Scandinavian researchers reported as long ago as 1965 that cows' milk protein sensitivity could be a forerunner of coeliac disease.

PYLORIC STENOSIS

This is a narrowing of the opening of the stomach into the first part of the gut (the duodenum). Occasionally an operation is needed to allow food out of the stomach. The condition has been reported to be less common in breastfed babies.

— Italian researchers reported in 1996 that babies with pyloric stenosis were less likely to have been exclusively breastfed in the first week of life. They speculated that high levels of breast milk hormones (such as vasoactive intestinal peptide) may encourage relaxation of the muscles controlling the stomach outflow.

MECONIUM PLUGS AND MECONIUM ILEUS

Either of these conditions can cause a blockage of the gut which may need an operation. Both are less common and less severe in breastfed babies because colostrum encourages the easy passage of the sticky, tar-like meconium which forms a baby's very first bowel motions.

LESS APPENDICITIS

Breastfeeding may make appendicitis less likely in later life.

— Italian research (1995) found that breastfeeding for at least seven months halved the risk of appendicitis in children. This may be because breastfed babies are less likely to suffer from overactivity of lymphatic tissue in the appendix, or because of some unknown factor.

LESS ULCERATIVE COLITIS AND CROHN'S DISEASE

These two diseases of childhood or later life may be connected with the type of feeding in infancy.

— A Canadian study (1989) found that both bottle-feeding and early diarrhoea made Crohn's disease in childhood more likely.
— The same researchers studied 118 families with at least one child with ulcerative colitis but found no protective effect from breast-feeding. This contrasts with two studies of ulcerative colitis in adults (one of which found that people with ulcerative colitis were twice as likely as healthy people never to have been breastfed) but agrees with another.
— Another study showed that people with long-standing ulcerative colitis had high levels of antibodies to cows' milk protein in their blood.

One difficulty with such research is that few adults know with any accuracy how they were fed as babies, so researchers have to ask the subjects' mothers for details. This is time-consuming and unreliable, because the mothers may not accurately recall – or even know – what took place (especially if their babies were cared for in a nursery at night).

LESS ACRODERMATITIS ENTEROPATHICA

This is a rare disease, possibly caused by an inherited defect of zinc metabolism, for which breast milk provides the only treatment, perhaps because milk (and particularly colostrum) is rich in zinc, and zinc is absorbed very efficiently from breast milk.

Acrodermatitis enteropathica is almost never seen in breastfed children. In the extremely unlikely event that it does occur, it's thought to be because the breast fails to secrete enough zinc even though there are adequate levels in the blood.

FEWER UNEXPLAINED COT DEATHS

When a baby dies suddenly and unexpectedly, for no apparent reason, he is said to have succumbed to an unexplained cot death – so called because it frequently happens when babies are in their cots. An unexplained cot death is otherwise known as the sudden infant death syndrome (SIDS). The most recent and reliable studies suggest that breastfeeding is one of many factors which can help protect babies.

Unexplained cot deaths are most common in sleeping babies aged between four weeks and four months; 85 per cent of sudden, unexplained deaths occur under six months and 60 per cent under three months. In the US and the UK more babies die suddenly, unexpectedly and for no apparent reason between one month and one year than from any known cause. In the UK one in 1400 babies dies this way – that's ten every week. The suffering of their families is immense.

Risk factors

Researchers continue to put a lot of work into seeking the causes of SIDS. They now think that some risk factors can have a cumulative effect. This list includes both known and suspected risk factors:

1 **Sleeping on the tummy**

2 **Living with people who smoke** – US researchers found that breastfeeding reduces the risk of SIDS for babies of non-smoking mothers but not for those of smoking mothers.

3 **Overheating** – The danger comes from being wrapped up too warmly; and/or being in too hot a place – there's no need for a baby to be in a room warmer than 20–21° C (68–70° F); and/or wriggling down under the cot covers towards the foot of the cot.

4 **Mild infection** – Some seemingly healthy babies seem to have an unusually powerful response to infections easily overcome by other babies.

5 **Being pre-term**

6 **Bottle-feeding?** – This issue is subject to continued research. Eleven out of eighteen studies record a higher risk of SIDS in bottle-fed babies; in none is it higher in breastfed. For example:

— New Zealand researchers suggested (1991) that three factors were particularly important: sleeping on the tummy instead of the back, smoking, and not being breastfed. Breastfed babies in their study were one-third less likely to succumb to SIDS than those who were bottle-fed.
— A large US study reported (1988) that SIDS was twice as likely in babies bottle-fed from birth.

Some early researchers made no allowance for then unknown SIDS risk factors. Also, the researchers responsible for the seven studies which found no association between SIDS and bottle-feeding looked mainly at whether babies had ever or never been breastfed. They didn't consider whether breastfeeding was exclusive, how long exclusive breastfeeding continued, how long breastfeeding continued once a baby started on bottle-feeds or solids, what each baby had for his last meal, or what the mothers had eaten or drunk before giving the last breastfeed. However, even when these factors are considered, the evidence remains unclear:

— A New Zealand study (1993) considered these issues more closely. The researchers divided 'breastfed' babies into several groups according to how long they had been breastfed and how long they had been exclusively breastfed. SIDS babies were less likely to have been breastfed at all; those that were breastfed were breastfed for fewer weeks on average, and were less likely to have been exclusively breastfed – either on discharge from hospital, or during the first four weeks, or in their last two days. Babies not breastfed on discharge were nearly twice as likely to succumb to SIDS. The conclusion was that 'breastfeeding does have a significant association with a lowered risk of SIDS and that this seems to persist for several months'.

— However, one recent UK study (1995) failed to find that bottle-feeding was a significant risk factor. Breastfed babies had a lower risk of unexplained cot death but they were also more likely than bottle-fed babies to have non-smoking mothers, fathers in employment, to have been born at term, and to have slept on their backs. Bottle-feeding of itself was not a significant risk factor. However, the researchers acknowledged that they considered only a small number of babies and that larger studies might be able to distinguish a 'small independent risk' from being bottle-fed.

— In 1995 the New Zealand team criticized this UK work. They claimed the researchers had misinterpreted the statistics and that these were actually similar to those of other large, well-controlled studies (including a very large national survey reported in 1993) which show that breastfeeding halves the SIDS risk!

— The UK researchers replied that their results still did not suggest that breastfeeding had a strong, independent protective effect. They also claimed that, after extensive adjustment for maternal smoking, prematurity and sleeping position, only one published study has shown a significant protective effect of breastfeeding. Another study awaits publication.

7 Post-natal depression – At least two studies have found that having a depressed mother triples a baby's risk of SIDS, even accounting for other risk factors. However, post-natal depression is very common and SIDS is not, so there's no need to panic if you feel depressed. (See page 252 for steps to take if you're feeling low.)

8 Being a boy – Three boys to every two girls succumb to SIDS. Fewer boys are breastfed than girls and breastfed boys are generally breastfed for fewer months than are girls (see page 73). If there is a link between SIDS and bottle-feeding, this might help explain the gender factor.

9 Lower socio-economic group – This is probably significant only because of its association with other risk factors.

10 An inherited factor – An identical twin of a baby which succumbs to SIDS has a higher risk himself, which suggests that a genetic factor may be involved.

Other factors under investigation – These include the possibility of a defect in the way some babies use fatty acids. If proven, this could mean that a supplement of certain fatty acids – given directly to the baby or indirectly via his breastfeeding mother – might reduce the risk.

Current recommendations

Campaigns to diminish known risk factors have reduced the number of SIDS in the UK, New Zealand and Australia. UK advisers have not made such a strong recommendation to breast-feed as have those in New Zealand; they claim that the evidence from published studies does not consistently show that breastfeeding reduces the risk of cot death. However, they strongly recommend that breastfeeding be encouraged and are continuing to monitor the statistics of infant feeding and unexplained cot death.

Suggested mechanisms for breastfeeding's possible protective effect against SIDS

It's important to be quite clear that breastfeeding doesn't guarantee protection against SIDS. Even babies who are thriving, born at term, have non-smoking mothers (and fathers and other carers), always sleep on their backs, have no other known risk factors, and are exclusively breastfed, can still die of SIDS, but they are a tiny minority.

Food sensitivity – It's been suggested that SIDS may, in some babies, result from a sudden and overwhelming response to a foreign protein. Cows' milk protein is by far the commonest foreign food protein babies meet and bottle-fed babies consume a huge amount of it.

Viral infections – Another idea is that a baby succumbs to SIDS because he is completely unable to cope with a viral infection. Breast milk can protect babies against some viral infections.

Inability to cope with long gaps between feeds – Babies who succumb to SIDS tend to have had a relatively long gap (more than six hours) between their last feed and the estimated time of death.

If this is important, it may be significant that successfully breastfed babies have more frequent feeds than bottle-fed babies, especially early on. Frequent feeds are even more likely for babies who share their mother's bed or sleep by her at night.

Until we know more, it might be sensible to feed very young babies at least every three or four hours, if not more often. And while some older babies may happily go six hours between feeds at night, it might be wise not to let them go any longer, particularly if they're under six months.

Frequent sucking

— A New Zealand study reported (1993) that using a dummy may protect against unexplained cot deaths, whether a baby is bottle-fed or breastfed. Among the reasons suggested is that frequent dummy-sucking may help keep a baby's mouth and throat muscles active and toned, so keeping his airway well open. The researchers say that if this is confirmed, then using a dummy could halve the number of SIDS deaths. This effect was shown to be independent of breastfeeding.

However, perhaps breastfeeding in an unrestricted way, with frequent feeds and periods of non-nutritive sucking (see page 23) at night, might have the same protective effect as a dummy.

Bed-sharing

SIDS is only more common in babies who sleep in their mother's bed if the mother or mother's partner smokes. This is good news for non-smoking mothers who find breastfeeding easier if they sleep with their baby.

However, if you sleep with your baby, it's important never to go to bed drunk or drugged in any way. Alcohol, sleeping tablets, tranquillizers and recreational drugs enter breast milk and can affect breastfed babies. Also, if you were accidentally to obstruct your baby's breathing, you might not wake enough to move out of the way as he struggled to breathe. The same applies to a man who sleeps next to a baby.

One important thing about bed-sharing is that a baby can wake his mother when he wants a feed or is distressed much more easily than if he's in another room.

Room-sharing

— In 1996 New Zealand researchers recommended that babies should sleep in the same room as their parents at least until six months old to reduce their risk of unexplained cot death. This is because their studies suggested that room-sharing with a parent reduced the risk of cot death. A reason for this possible protection may be that if a baby becomes distressed because he can't breathe, his mother – who is likely to sleep more lightly than the baby – will be alerted by his sounds or movements if she sleeps in the same room. She can then pick him up immediately. The researchers did not find that sharing a room with another child was protective.

LESS DENTAL DECAY

Most studies agree that children who were breastfed have less dental decay than those who were bottle-fed. While breastfed babies can suffer from tooth decay, when it does occur it's less likely to be severe. There's a suggestion that this is because breastfeeding is more popular with women from higher socio-economic groups who are less likely to give their babies sugary snacks. But this can't be the only answer because exclusively breastfed babies not yet on solids have less decay than bottle-fed ones, and partial breastfeeding gives some protection too.

Dental decay costs a lot of money. More important, it causes children a lot of pain and increases the risk of needing false teeth. Although dental health has improved a lot in recent years because of better maternal and child health, better diets, fluoridation of water and better dental hygiene, twenty-two million people in the UK alone have false teeth!

So how can breastfeeding protect teeth?

Fluoride

The amount of fluoride in breast milk is relatively high in areas where there is plenty of fluoride in the drinking water. Milk from cows that graze and drink in fluoridated-water areas doesn't show as great an increase, though its fluoride content is slightly higher than that from non-fluoridated areas. An ample fluoride supply reduces dental decay by 50 per cent.

However, in non-fluoridated-water areas, although the amount of fluoride in breast milk and formula is nearly the same, breastfed babies still have reduced decay rates in early childhood. This brings us to another mechanism, illustrated by a survey which found a 46 per cent reduction in the incidence of dental decay in children breastfed more than three months in an area with little fluoride in the water, compared with children who'd been bottle-fed. This meant that the breastfed group had about half as many missing or filled teeth as the bottle-fed one.

Before jumping to the conclusion that this was because sugar had been added to the babies' bottles, the researchers considered the possibility but showed that sugar wasn't responsible.

In areas with low levels of fluoride in the drinking water (below 0.7 ppm), experts recomend that both breastfed and bottle-fed babies should have a fluoride supplement. The suggested starting age varies from one country to another and it's important not to give too high a dose as this can cause mottling of the tooth enamel.

Defective enamel

—Several groups of researchers, including a group in Tanzania in 1994, have found that decay is more common in front teeth showing signs of enamel hypoplasia – horizontal lines of defective development which are relatively weak and prone to decay. These lines may be chalky-white, grey-yellow, brown or black, and are even more likely to decay if there are associated pits or grooves. Enamel hypoplasia is more likely in babies who have been ill, or whose mothers ate a poor diet or were ill in pregnancy – especially if they took antibiotics.

Family history

A genetic susceptibility to decay can pass from parent to child.

Diet

Teeth are more likely to decay in babies and young children who eat a poor diet including frequent snacks of foods containing sugar or refined starch (white cereal flour). This is because they have more plaque (a sticky layer of food residues and mouth bacteria, including *Streptococcus mutans* and lactobacilli) on their teeth. Mouth bacteria produce acid as they feed on the sugar and refined starch in plaque; acid weakens enamel by removing minerals, and repeated acid attacks can lead to tooth decay.

A baby's teeth are most vulnerable to acid attack as they first appear and shortly afterwards. This is exactly the time when many babies are starting on other foods and drinks in addition to milk, so it's important to choose first foods thoughtfully. There's no need for them to contain any added sugar or white flour. This rules out white and brown bread, biscuits, cakes, many desserts, rusks and many breakfast cereals, but you'll have a huge choice from hundreds of delicious, healthier, tooth-friendly alternatives, including rice, potatoes, naturally sweet carrots and parsnips, swede, turnip and other vegetables, various fruits, and egg yolk. (Egg white, unheated cows' milk, citrus fruits, meat, fish and foods made with wholegrains are generally best left till a little later, especially if there's a family history of allergy.)

As babies grow older and eat more solids, it becomes increasingly important that these contain enough tooth-protecting nutrients. These include vitamins A, C and D, calcium and phosphorus.

Pooling of milk round the teeth at night

Many babies sleep with their mothers and breastfeed when they wish. Some doze with the breast in the mouth on and off for long periods between feeds, having a few occasional gentle sucks when they remember. Several researchers have found that a tiny number of these babies suffer from early and sometimes severe dental decay. However, this is rare and only an extremely small minority of babies who sleep with their mothers and feed on and off at night have 'nursing caries'. A few bottle-fed babies who doze with a bottle in their mouths suffer from the same condition.

Babies who doze at the breast don't suck and milk the breast very much; they also produce less saliva to wash milk from the teeth. This means that a pool of breast milk may linger around the front teeth. Babies with defective enamel are at the highest risk. Pooling of milk provides mouth bacteria with plenty of nourishment and encourages the thick film of plaque which makes decay more likely.

However, many mothers and babies like to be together and to breastfeed at night. Indeed, there are many advantages to both mother and baby from being close and having night feeds. So let's see how breastfeeding mothers can protect their babies' teeth even further.

Cleaning your baby's teeth

Dentists suggest wiping away the film of plaque from a baby's teeth after (though one expert prefers before) breastfeeds at night. This can also be done after solids containing sugars or white flour. Wiping takes only seconds and means there aren't enough bacteria or plaque left to encourage decay.

Use a cottonwool ball, a gauze square, a clean face flannel or a J-cloth moistened in warm water (or, when your baby is twelve months old, a very soft brush). Even a paper tissue would do at a pinch. Some experts recommend wiping away traces of milk from the easily accessible parts of the inside of the whole mouth as well.

It's a good idea to get into the habit of wiping clean your baby's mouth and teeth as soon as the first tooth peeps through. Even better, start wiping the gums before the first tooth appears. Daytime tooth-cleaning is important too if, like many babies, yours sometimes snoozes for long periods at the breast.

Some people suggest that frequent breastfeeding which continues for many months is likely to lead to decay.

— However, Irish dentist Harry Torney (1995) found no evidence in his research to support this view.

BETTER JAW AND MOUTH DEVELOPMENT

Many specialists report fewer problems of jaw and mouth development in children who were breastfed. Indeed, in one survey only two among nearly 500 children with such problems had been breastfed.

Breastfeeding exercises the muscles of the mouth, jaw and face more strenuously than bottle-feeding, because breastfeeding is harder work. In fact, breastfeeding uses sixty times more energy than bottle-feeding. Breastfeeding also exercises these muscles differently, because different movements are involved in sucking from and milking the breast compared with simply sucking from a bottle. Over the months, as a baby's face and jaw grow, their shape is partly determined by the strength and balance of the repeated pull of the various muscles.

Some – but not all – researchers report that the longer babies are breastfed, the more likely are their jaw and palate to grow into an optimal shape. In contrast, bottle-fed babies and those breastfed for four months or less seem more likely to develop a narrow dental arch (with less room for teeth to be properly spaced), and thus malocclusion, in which top and bottom teeth don't meet as they should. Orthodontic problems take much time and patience on the parts of orthodontist, child and parents to get right and treatment usually involves repeated trips to the dentist for years.

LESS CANCER

Research shows that children with lymphoma (lymph system cancer) are more likely to have been bottle-fed.

— Chinese researchers reported (1995) that babies breastfed for more than six months had a lower risk of lymphoma (especially Hodgkin's disease occurring before six years).
— A study (1991) found that breastfeeding for longer than eight months protected against Hodgkin's disease.
— An American group reported (1988) that breastfeeding longer than six months lowered the risk of lymphoma and of some other cancers. Children who had been exclusively breastfed for at least six

months were only half as likely to develop cancer before the age of fifteen as children who had been bottle-fed.

MORE SUCCESSFUL KIDNEY TRANSPLANTS

Children with kidney failure who receive a kidney transplant from their mother, brother or sister (but not their father) have a dramatically better chance of the transplant taking if they were breastfed as babies.

In one study, 79 per cent of children who'd been breastfed still had their transplanted kidney working well nine years later, compared with a very much lower rate in children who'd been bottle-fed, in spite of large doses of immuno-suppressive drugs.

LESS VITAMIN A DEFICIENCY

In some developing countries, such as Bangladesh, long-term breastfeeding protects children from vitamin A deficiency (including xerophthalmia, dangerously dry eyes which lead to a million children going blind worldwide each year). The traditional diet of young children in Bangladesh is short of vitamin A but breast milk has plenty.

— One study (1995) found that in Nepal bottle-fed children were twice as likely as breastfed children to get xerophthalmia in the first year, five times as likely by two years, and three times as likely by three years. And frequent breastfeeding was especially protective, with babies breastfed fewer than ten times a day having a 61 per cent lower risk than bottle-fed babies, and those breastfed more than ten times a day having an 87 per cent lower risk.
— Another study (1986) found that children with xerophthalmia in Malawi, Africa, were more than three times as likely as other children to have stopped breastfeeding before they were two years old.

DIFFERENT EMOTIONAL AND BEHAVIOURAL DEVELOPMENT

The causes of emotional and behavioural differences in later childhood and adulthood are impossible to pinpoint with certainty. However:

— One study of seven-year-olds showed that those who'd been breastfed were less fearful, nervous, jealous and spiteful than their peers who'd been bottle-fed. They were also more successful at school.
— Studies have also shown that breastfed babies spend less time in their cots and more with their mothers than do bottle-fed babies.

In communities which not only allow but actively encourage unrestricted breastfeeding, mothers don't let their babies cry even for a short time, whereas in many developed countries babies are often left to cry because 'it isn't time for a feed' or 'they might be spoilt if they're picked up'. The baby whose mother gives the breast for whenever he cries or otherwise appears to need it food or comfort would seem likely to grow up feeling secure that he'll get his needs met.

One researcher (Jean Liedloff, see page 442) wrote of two neighbouring tropical islands whose inhabitants had very different child-rearing practices. In one, babies were carried or held by the mother or someone else almost all the time. They slept with their mothers and were virtually never left alone. When they were with their mothers they could breastfeed very frequently, pretty much as often as they wanted. As these babies grew up they scarcely ever cried and appeared much happier and less aggressive than the babies on the other island. These others were reared in a way much more akin to the way in which many people in developed countries bring up their babies, not carried or held a great deal, and not breastfed on an unrestricted basis.

Research into a breastfeeding woman's behaviour before, during and after feeding shows that it differs from that of a bottle-feeder. A breastfeeder is more likely to kiss, rock and touch her baby, while a bottle-feeder is more likely to rub, pat and jiggle her baby and show much more concern over 'wind'. Breastfeeders also talk to their babies more than do bottle-feeders.

Most well-breastfed babies rarely cry because their hunger, thirst and need for comfort can immediately be satisfied by warm milk. In contrast, a bottle-fed baby is more likely to have to wait until his mother reckons it's time for his feed and then has to wait again while the formula is prepared and warmed. He may feel very real hunger and frustration by the time all this has happened.

Attachment to mother

Scientific proof of any increased attachment between a mother and her breastfed baby is hard to come by but a closer relationship seems likely if only because the baby depends on his mother for food. She's also likely sometimes to feed him to comfort him instead of just holding him or giving a dummy.

BETTER SPACING BETWEEN CHILDREN

The natural contraceptive effect of long-term unrestricted breast-feeding (see page 123) means that women using no other family planning methods have longer gaps between their children than if they were bottle-feeding. Having a longer gap between himself and the next child means that a baby in a developing country has a better chance not only of being healthy but also of surviving.

Chinese research (1989) in the largely rural Shaanxi province found that the child-spacing effect of breastfeeding had a marked effect on survival in infancy and early childhood.

BETTER BRAIN AND NERVE DEVELOPMENT?

Earlier walking

Two studies have shown that breastfed babies walk earlier than bottle-fed ones, even after allowing for differences in weight and excluding babies whose mothers went out to work (because they might have had less encouragement to walk).

Better intelligence and development tests

For many years some (but not all) research has suggested that breastfeeding is associated with higher intelligence. Before dismissing the idea as nonsense, because so many factors impinge on intelligence and how it's measured, it is worth considering that the profiles of fatty acids, amino acids, hormones, growth factors and other nutrients and substances in human milk are very different from those in formula. It is possible that only human milk provides optimal levels for the development of the human brain, which grows extraordinarily fast in the first year of life and fastest of all in pre-term babies.

— US researchers (1993) reported that out of 855 children followed until they were five, those breastfed for longest had the highest Bayley (up to two years) and McCarthy (from three to five years) scores. Also, both their English and maths grades were slightly higher!

— A report in 1984 of a very large, ongoing UK study of more than 12,000 children found that the longer a child had been breastfed, the better was the vocabulary and eye-hand co-ordination of that child at age five.

Pre-term babies

— Medical Research Council (MRC) researchers in Cambridge reported in 1988 and 1992 that pre-term babies given breast milk had better development scores (measured by the Bayley mental development index) at eighteen months and a higher IQ (intelligence quotient) at eight years, even allowing for the mothers' education, smoking (in pregnancy and after) and socio-economic status. Pre-term babies given their own mother's milk had the highest scores. To put the increase in scores into context, the researchers said it was of about the same magnitude as the advantage in terms of development score of being first-born, a girl, or belonging to a higher socio-economic class. They pointed out that although any one baby's score has a limited capacity to predict his future mental ability, the average score of a group is likely to be more predictive. And they made it clear that although their results might indicate that something in breast milk promotes brain growth and maturation in pre-term babies, there may (also or instead) be something about the mothers who choose to give their babies breast milk that benefits their babies.

— These MRC researchers said (1994) that new data 'add significant support to the view that breast milk promotes neuro-development'. They studied 502 pre-term babies given either donated mature 'drip' breast milk or pre-term formula (either alone or plus the mother's expressed breast milk), and found no difference at eighteen months in Bayley psychomotor and mental development indices. This is especially interesting because drip milk (milk that drips from the breast while a woman is feeding from the other side) is low in nutrients and calories compared with a pre-term baby's requirements for growth. The finding is particularly important because researchers previously found that pre-term babies fed standard milk formula had lower Bayley psychomotor and mental development indices than pre-term babies fed pre-term formula. But pre-term babies fed solely donated breast milk had 'significantly and substantially higher psychomotor development scores' at eighteen months than babies fed standard formula. The conclusion was that there is something about breast milk itself which has more advantages to pre-term babies than standard formula. This 'something' may be breast milk's arachidonic (AA) and docosahexaenoic (DHA) acids, and its many hormones and growth factors. Further work will try to ascertain whether pre-term babies who receive breast milk might do even better were it supplemented with certain nutrients.

— In 1992 Australian researchers reported a study of tests on children born with very low birth weights. They did several tests (Bayley mental development indices, then Wechsler IQ tests) up to eight years old. The scores of the children who received expressed breast milk were not significantly different from those of children who had no breast milk at all. However, children breastfed directly from their mother's breast had significantly higher scores. The researchers suggest it may not be breast milk itself which benefits the intellectual development of pre-term children, but something about the act of breastfeeding.

Better visual development and eyesight

— Recent research in Cambridge discovered that children who were both pre-term and breastfed had better visual development than children who were pre-term and bottle-fed. A few children who were both full-term and breastfed had better visual development than those who were full-term and bottle-fed too.

— In 1993 US researchers reported that very pre-term babies had significantly higher visual acuity if given docosahexaenoic acid-(DHA)-enriched milk formula than if given standard formula. Also, three-year-old children who'd been full-term and breastfed were better able to match letters and to use both eyes together than those who'd been bottle-fed.

— In 1994 other US researchers reported that the visual acuity of bottle-fed full-term babies was similar to that of breastfed babies, suggesting that DHA is not essential for full-term babies.

— However, Australian research (1995) found that bottle-fed babies had similar visual development to breastfed babies only if they receive milk formula enriched with DHA. Visual development in babies breastfed for less than sixteen weeks was between those breastfed longer than four months and those fed standard formula.

Further work suggests these outcomes are caused by different fatty acid profiles in breast milk and formula. Many pre-term and some full-term babies may be unable to manufacture certain omega–3 polyunsaturated fatty acids (including DHA, and arachidonic acid or AA). Experts previously didn't think these were essential fatty acids, but clearly for these babies they are. Following European recommendations, formula manufacturers are now adding certain fatty acids to some of their products.

LESS DIABETES?

Studies suggest that bottle-feeding may play a part in causing type 1, insulin-dependent diabetes – the sudden, young-onset type of the disease. However, more research is needed.

— Australian researchers reported (1995) that bottle-fed babies have half as much chance again as exclusively breastfed ones of developing diabetes. Other research found that babies with a family history of diabetes have a smaller risk of diabetes later in life if breastfed.

— Canadian research reported (1992) that a cows' milk protein known as bovine serum albumin (BSA) can trigger the production of BSA antibodies. In the first two years of their illness diabetic children have seven times more BSA antibodies than do healthy children. The production of BSA antibodies can lead, in susceptible children, to an auto-immune reaction in the insulin-producing cells of the pancreas. This reaction makes the cells self-destruct. It is possible that a viral infection sparks off this destruction.

— US researchers reported (1988) that children who'd been breastfed for more than twelve months had only half the risk of developing diabetes compared with other children. There was a significant, though marked, effect in those breastfed for shorter periods. They estimated that bottle-feeding could cause 2–26 per cent of type 1 diabetes.

— Research in the mid-1980s found a close correlation between the amount of cows' milk consumed in various countries and the incidence of diabetes. There's a theory that exclusively breastfed babies are less likely to get diabetes because they avoid exposure to cows' milk protein.

LESS HEART DISEASE?

Continuing research into whether early infant feeding influences heart disease in later life has so far thrown up many questions and provided few answers. It's an important subject because heart attacks are a common cause of early death.

— Interest was sparked by a French study (1967) of the bodies of 109 young people who died before the age of twenty and whose deaths were unrelated to heart disease. Coronary artery abnormalities were more common in those who'd been bottle-fed. The abnormalities were fatty streaks – localized areas of damage to the artery lining (which in healthy people who eat a good diet are generally continually repaired). Unrepaired fatty streaks encourage atheroma. Severe atheroma in coronary arteries leads to angina and eventually a heart attack.

— However, a British study concluded (1973) that men who'd had a heart attack were just as likely as those in a control group to have been bottle-fed.

— In 1984 the original French research (see above) was repeated when a Medical Research Council team in Wales examined 160 people under the age of thirty who had died suddenly. They found no evidence that breastfeeding protects against coronary artery disease and suggested that while some factors which encourage coronary atheroma may operate in infancy and childhood, bottle-feeding isn't one.

— And animal research in Texas (1991) found that young adult baboons who'd been breastfed had more extensive fatty streaks in their arteries than those who'd been fed with milk formula.

Cholesterol

— The whole story took on a new twist when a team of researchers in Southampton and Cambridge, England, reported (1992) how 5718 men born in Hertfordshire between 1920 and 1930 were fed as babies. Out of these men 1314 had died, 474 from a heart attack. Those breastfed for over a year were most likely to have died from a heart attack, followed closely by those who had been bottle-fed. Breastfeeding for less than a year, however, made a heart attack less likely, while a combination of breastfeeding (for less than a year) and bottle-feeding was the most protective. Among the living men, both those who were bottle-fed and those breastfed for over a year had higher blood levels of total cholesterol and low-density lipoprotein- (LDL)-cholesterol, and higher ratios of LDL-cholesterol to high-density lipoprotein- (HDL)-cholesterol, each of which is associated with an increased risk of coronary heart disease. There was no information about the amount or type of other foods eaten by the breastfed and bottle-fed babies, nor about the breastfeeding mothers' diets. The types, amounts and proportions of individual fatty acids and their major groups (saturated, monounsaturated, and omega–3 and omega–6 polyunsaturated, including essential fatty acids) differ in formula and breast milk. Breast milk's fatty acids reflect those in a breastfeeding woman's diet. The fatty acid composition of breast milk and formula influences a baby's cholesterol level and LDL–HDL cholesterol ratio.

The importance, if any, of breast milk's relatively high cholesterol level isn't clear. The cholesterol level in babies relates much more closely to their diet than it does in older children and adults, and breastfed babies have higher cholesterol levels than do bottle-fed ones. However, breastfed babies deal with cholesterol differently, partly because of differences in their production of bile acids (which partly depends on their different population of gut microorganisms) and partly because of hormones and growth factors in breast milk. It has been suggested that breastfed babies use cholesterol more efficiently and develop cholesterol-regulating mechanisms which allow them to deal better with diets high in cholesterol and saturated fats throughout life. This idea is supported by animal work (in the Texan baboons, see above) but comparisons between humans who were breastfed and bottle-fed have failed to show a consistent effect.

Cows' milk protein antibodies

Some susceptible bottle-fed (and a few breastfed) babies are sensitized by cows' milk and develop antibodies to cows' milk protein.

Immune complexes

Cows' milk protein antibodies can mop up molecules of cows' milk protein and form 'immune complexes' (also known as antigen-antibody complexes).

— Belgian research published in *Nature* (1978) found that all bottle-fed babies have circulating immune complexes in their blood. Breastfed babies, in contrast, have none. In adults, these immune complexes can damage joints, kidneys and arteries. Not only do they reduce immunity but they also make blood stickier and thrombosis (blood clots) in blood vessels more likely. Thrombosis in a coronary artery can lead to a heart attack; thrombosis in a brain artery to a stroke. The paper in *Nature* suggested that immune complexes may sow the seeds for heart and other arterial disease in later life by damaging artery linings and making them more likely to attract fatty deposits and the gradual build-up of atheroma.

— A British study (1974) found that men under sixty who'd had a heart attack had higher than normal levels of cows' milk antibodies in their blood.

— It has also been found that a heart attack is three times more likely to kill a man if he has any cows' milk antibodies at all.

Although breastfed babies can develop cows' milk antibodies if they drink cows' milk (or formula) later, there's evidence that these antibody levels are lower than in people who were bottle-fed cows' milk formula as infants. This may be because bottle-fed babies are exposed to such a large amount of foreign protein in the form of cows' milk protein in formula.

As far as we know, there has been no research into whether people who suffer from strokes are more likely to have been bottle-fed. Nor have there been any investigations into whether the clots in veins which lead to deep-vein thrombosis and pulmonary embolism are at all related to how the sufferer was fed as a baby.

The tendency to make cows' milk antibodies may be inherited: members of one family with a great deal of heart disease had cows' milk antibody levels eight times higher than average.

Clearly breastfeeding doesn't prevent heart attacks completely. Heart disease is so complex, and the factors involved so numerous, that even if bottle-feeding is a factor, it certainly isn't the only one. Smoking, high blood pressure, a lack of regular exercise, very high levels of blood fats, and being overweight are known to be very important and preventable risk factors.

LESS NAPPY RASH?

One survey showed that bottle-fed babies were twice as likely to suffer from nappy rash as were breastfed ones.

FEWER INGUINAL HERNIAS?

— A 1995 study found that babies with an inguinal hernia (a 'rupture' or weakness in their groin) were much more likely never to have been breastfed when compared with other babies. The researchers suggest that hormones in breast milk (such as gonadotropin-releasing hormone) may help prevent inguinal hernias.

LESS JUVENILE RHEUMATOID ARTHRITIS?

Studies which have looked at how children with rheumatoid arthritis were fed as babies, including one in 1995, suggest that breastfeeding may help protect a child from developing juvenile rheumatoid arthritis.

LESS MULTIPLE SCLEROSIS?

Several researchers have suggested a link between bottle-feeding with formula and the later development of multiple sclerosis (MS). Two studies failed to show a link between infant feeding and MS, but didn't consider how long breastfeeding had continued.

— However, Italian researchers reported (1994) that (regardless of their parents' socio-economic group) ninety-three adults with MS were not only less likely than those in a control group to have been breastfed at all but if they were breastfed, it was for a shorter time. They were breastfed for an average of 8.4 months, whereas the control group were breastfed for 12.5 months – nearly half as long again. Such a 'dose' finding is perhaps even more important than an 'all-or-nothing' finding. The reseachers suggest several reasons why prolonged breastfeeding may be protective. Breast milk and formula differ in their amounts and proportions of polyunsaturated fatty acids, including essential fatty acids.

— Other research reported in the *Lancet* (1992) found that the grey matter in the brains of bottle-fed babies has different proportions of fatty acids compared with that of breastfed ones.

It's possible, *though completely unproven*, that the fatty acid composition of bottle-fed babies' brains could allow easier viral damage, or make the fatty myelin in nerve coverings age faster. Breastfeeding is also known to influence the developing immune system and it's possible that this could affect the risk of MS.

LESS SCHIZOPHRENIA?

One in three people with schizophrenia has low levels of two polyunsaturated fatty acids, arachidonic acid (AA) and docosahexaenoic acid (DHA). Researchers don't yet know whether they fail to absorb these fatty acids from their food or whether they eat the 'wrong' foods, but three studies suggest that diet is a key factor, and that schizophrenia is much more common in people on a poor diet.

Schizophrenia appears to be less common in people who were breastfed as babies. Breast milk, as we've seen, contains more AA and DHA than formula.

OTHER FINDINGS

In 1994, Dutch researchers reported that at nine years of age, children who had been exclusively breastfed as babies had half the number of minor neurological problems as children who had received any formula. The researchers believe that the various polyunsaturated fats in breast milk (particularly arachidonic and docosahexaenoic acids) account for this difference.

So much for all the advantages of breastfeeding to your baby. It's quite a list! Let's now look at the other side of the coin. Are there any disadvantages to breastfeeding from a baby's point of view? The answer is that there can be.

DISADVANTAGES OF BREASTFEEDING TO A BABY

Lack of vitamin B_1 in babies of mothers with beri-beri

Women in some countries eat large amounts of polished rice lacking vitamin B_1 (thiamine) and, as a result, develop beri-beri. Their breastfed babies can become acutely ill with infantile beri-beri. The solution is for rice to be eaten unpolished, as brown rice. Polishing brown rice in order to produce white rice removes the outer layers of each rice grain. Unfortunately, vitamin B_1 is lost at the same time.

Lack of vitamin B$_{12}$ in the babies of some vegan mothers

Some strictly vegetarian or vegan women have too little vitamin B$_{12}$ in their milk and their babies develop symptoms of deficiency. This is sometimes because the women have not grown up in a vegetarian or vegan family with reliable knowledge passed from one generation to another about how to choose and prepare nutritious foods. Expert advice about what to eat, together with extra vitamin B$_{12}$ for vegan mothers, soon puts this right.

Malnourishment

If a woman is severely malnourished for some time and her diet is grossly deficient in protein and fat, her baby is liable to go short as well. The answer is to give the mother more food. The World Health Organization recently decided to concentrate famine relief monies on food for breastfeeding mothers rather than on formula for babies. This is because in famine circumstances bottle-fed babies have a much greater risk of dying, owing to the enormous risk of gastroenteritis from unsterilized bottles and water. Their mothers are also likely to give them dilute feeds in order to save milk powder in case they can't get or can't afford any the next day.

Frustration and hunger suffered by the baby whose mother is well-nourished but has insufficient milk

Babies who don't get enough milk can become very ill and unless someone notices and does something about it, they can actually starve. The problem of insufficient milk is usually easily overcome (see Chapter 10). However, in order to thrive a few babies need formula in addition to – or instead of – breast milk.

Learning to cope with stress by eating?

Frequent feeds are important for young babies. However, as infants grow they may not always want the breast every time they fidget or cry.

The only time it's ever sensible to cut down on breastfeeds is if you are giving very frequent feeds and letting your milk down well, but are getting into the habit of misinterpreting restlessness or cries as signs that your baby wants the breast, when he really needs attention of other kinds (for example, to be talked to, listened to, played with, or simply accompanied through a time of feeling grumpy). A crying or fidgeting baby will probably have a feed even if he isn't hungry, simply to get attention. However, if it isn't really milk that he wants, this could turn out to be a lesson in how to use food as a tranquillizer at times of stress.

Those of us who work with distressed and/or overweight adults know that many turn to food as a comforter for stress or emotional pain that frankly has little or nothing to do with being hungry for food, and that would be better met in other more specific ways. A baby's experiences certainly affect behaviour in adult life and it is possible (though unproven) that early experiences at the breast could lead to eating disorders and other attempts to find solutions to emotional distress in later life.

So the question is, how best can we help our babies grow up believing that the world is a good place and that they can get their needs met?

If a woman offers her baby the breast whenever he seems to need it, it's an excellent way of making him feel cared for. If he's hungry or thirsty or needs the non-specific comfort of sucking and being intimately close to his mother, then continuing to breastfeed is a good idea.

But if he doesn't seem very interested in the breast and you think he might need something else, interrupt the feed and see if you can find out what this might be. In this way you'll teach him a variety of methods of dealing with emotional situations such as being bored, lonely, angry, frustrated and so on. The sort of mothering that meets a baby's needs this precisely takes more thought and effort than simply pacifying him by indiscriminate breastfeeding but it will probably pay dividends over a child's lifetime.

Obviously many factors other than early feeding experiences influence the way a child learns to deal with emotional distress as he grows up. And, of course, what most breastfeeding women do is to combine both these behaviour styles. It would be naive to suggest that the breast isn't a very effective pacifier, and crazy to deny baby and mother the pleasure breastfeeding brings at times of stress. As with most things to do with breastfeeding, though, it's largely a matter of balance.

Breast-milk colitis

A baby who has blood-stained bowel motions, perhaps with colic, may have breast-milk colitis. This rare condition is diagnosed only after careful investigation. The cause is not clear, though it may be something to do with a sensitivity to one of the proteins in breast milk – and possibly to whole molecules of protein from foods the mother has eaten and that instead of being digested have 'leaked' in their entirety through the mother's gut into her blood and thence into her breast milk. Until researchers are more certain about what to do, the usual pathway at present is to stop breastfeeding. The symptoms then resolve within about seven to ten days, but recur if the baby again has breast milk.

More intussusception?

This is an infrequent emergency situation in which part of a baby's bowel telescopes into itself and requires surgery.

— An Italian study (1993) reported that intussusception was most common in exclusively breastfed babies, slightly less common in partially breastfed babies, and least common in bottle-fed babies.

Overall, breastfeeding is clearly best for almost all babies and, statistically speaking, breastfeds are healthier than bottle-feds.

FIVE

Best for you?

We've seen how breastfeeding benefits babies but it also has many advantages to mothers. Before we look at these, it may be helpful to consider a woman's reproductive life and put it in a biological perspective.

THE BIOLOGICAL PERSPECTIVE

Human females develop breasts when they are very young. Most mammals develop their mammary glands only in time to feed their offspring but human breasts, which are well developed several years before childbearing begins (even in hunter–gatherer and other traditional-living peoples), clearly serve other purposes too. The chief among these is as a source of sexual arousal.

The human race has probably been on the face of the earth for about five million years and until 10,000 years ago, when man started living in agricultural settlements, lived the life of hunter–gatherers and ate a vegetarian diet. It seems, from the evidence of historical remains and from the study of the few hunter–gatherer tribes remaining today, that their reproductive life is very different from that of people living in developed countries and indeed from that of most people in the developing world too.

Perhaps the best-studied present-day hunter–gatherers are the !Kung of Botswana and Namibia who live as our ancestors did for millions of years. !Kung women start to menstruate at about seventeen to eighteen, which is late by Western standards. They also have an earlier menopause (at about thirty-eight). So their female reproductive span is only about twenty years, whereas ours (from thirteen to fifty) is about thirty-seven. An average woman in a culture like this has six or seven children, some of whom may die young, leaving her with a family of three or four. Because she breastfeeds on an unrestricted basis for several years, she doesn't menstruate for much of her reproductive life. Women who live like this become fertile, menstruate a few times, have their first child, breastfeed for several years and then, when they ovulate again as they breastfeed less often, become pregnant again and then repeat the cycle. To such women menstruation is not a regular monthly event but an uncommon one.

So hunter–gatherer women are either pregnant or breastfeeding for most of their reproductive lives and have only twenty to thirty menstrual cycles. This was the picture for all women until a mere 10,000 years ago, which is very recent indeed in evolutionary terms.

Biologically we are akin to these hunter–gatherers, yet over the past 200 years of industrialization we have dramatically changed our way of life. Changes have, of course, been occurring gradually over thousands of years but our modern life-style has accelerated the rate of change considerably. The average modern Western woman has a totally different experience to a hunter–gatherer woman. As a girl she eats more and has a higher body weight, so she starts menstruating much earlier. She also has very few pregnancies and breastfeeds for only a few months, if at all. This means that in total she has as many as 400–450 monthly menstrual cycles with their accompanying surges of hormones until the menopause intervenes when she's about fifty-one. Just what effects this dramatic change in experience has on modern women we're not yet sure. However, it looks as if our modern way of life, with women menstruating early and spending only a very few months of their entire lives pregnant and breastfeeding, may cause us some problems.

But, we can hear you say, hunter–gatherers must have a child every three or four years, spaced only by the contraceptive effect of breastfeeding. I don't want a child every three years, so how is this relevant to me? Obviously this is a valid objection. Today in the West, where the vast majority of children survive, having so many pregnancies would result in families larger than society would consider acceptable.

So what has all this to do with breastfeeding? Simply that the breast is an integral part of a woman's reproductive system. Her breasts are linked into the same hormonal cycles that operate during orgasm, childbirth, breastfeeding and her menstrual cycle. We may not have many children nowadays, but we can breastfeed the ones we do have. Obviously a few months or even years of breastfeeding won't transform a modern woman into a hunter–gatherer but there are provable benefits, many of which are greatly underplayed. Our experience shows us that almost all women choose breastfeeding because they believe it is best for their baby. Just imagine how many more would breastfeed if they knew how good it could be for them too. Let's now look at some of these advantages.

LESS BREAST CANCER?

Several things can make breast cancer more likely and the question here is whether never having breastfed is one. In other words, can you reduce your risk of breast cancer if you breastfeed? Several studies have suggested that breastfeeding for a long time (estimated by totalling the number of months or years you feed each child) may help protect some women from pre-menopausal cancer – the less common type of breast cancer. However, not all studies agree, so there's no clear-cut answer. Let's look at some history.

Breast cancer is the commonest women's cancer in developed countries and worldwide it's the second most common. It is more common in the UK than anywhere else (five times commoner than in Japan and three times commoner than in Mediterranean Europe), with one woman in twelve developing breast cancer at some time in her life. It has also become more common over the last 200 years and it's been estimated that one in twenty women will die from breast cancer in the West today. In those parts of the world where women spend many years in total breastfeeding several babies, this cancer is rare.

Two out of three of the seventeen breast cancer studies before 1985 that looked at breastfeeding showed that *ever* having breastfed helped protect women from breast cancer. However, when looking at the various studies, it's important to realize that not all researchers define their terms in the same way, which makes their results difficult to compare. Some studies class women as long-term breastfeeders if they breastfed only one baby for a long time, whereas others add up the total number of months of breastfeeding in a woman's life and only then label her as a long-term breastfeeder or not. And 'long-term' in itself means different things to different researchers.

Several studies since 1985 have looked at how many babies a woman breastfed and for how long, and differentiated breast cancer before the menopause from that occurring afterwards. Their conclusions are largely in favour of a protective effect of breastfeeding. The US National Academy of Sciences reviewed all this evidence in 1991 and concluded that 'most epidemiological evaluations suggest that breastfeeding may be protective against breast cancer, but there is conflicting evidence'.

Let's take as an example three studies which found a protective effect:

— A US study (1994) found that breastfeeding was associated with a significantly lower incidence of pre-menopausal breast cancer. This protective effect increased as the total number of months of breastfeeding in a woman's life went up. The researchers calculated that if all women in the US breastfed their babies for a combined total of two years or longer, the amount of breast cancer could be cut by nearly 25 per cent. Another startling finding was that women who breastfed for the first time when they were young had an even lower risk of breast cancer. If a woman was twenty or younger and fed her

children for a combined total of six months, she had only half the cancer risk of a woman who had never breastfed.
— The UK National Case Control Study Group (1993) concluded that breastfeeding can help protect women from pre-menopausal breast cancer. Breastfeeding for at least three months cut the risk of early cancer by half.
— A Chinese study (1988) from Shanghai found that women who had breastfed for a total of six years or more had an extremely low relative risk of breast cancer.

Now let's look at three studies which did *not* find a protective effect:

— A US study (1996) of over 89,000 women (in the US Nurses' Health Study) found that there was no important overall association between breastfeeding and those who developed breast cancer. However, among women who gave birth only once, women who breastfed were less likely to get breast cancer. The authors concluded that it remains unclear whether there is an association between breastfeeding and a (reduced) risk of breast cancer, and called for further studies.
— A Swedish/Norwegian study (1990) found no association between lack of breastfeeding and breast cancer in women under forty-five.
— A Japanese study (1992) suggested that there was either no protective effect from breastfeeding or only a marginally protective one.

What does all this mean? Clearly the effect on a woman's breasts from breastfeeding one or two babies for a few hours, days, weeks or months is very different from feeding one or two babies for many months or even years, and different again from feeding more children for two, three, four or more years each.

As we've seen, women in developed countries treat their bodies in a very different way from their ancestors – a way so recent in evolutionary terms that they may not yet have adapted. Today most women in the West breastfeed very little, if at all. By turning their backs on breastfeeding, they rob their breasts of their main function. Let's look more closely at what happens in our bodies.

When a woman is neither pregnant not breastfeeding, her body prepares itself each month to welcome a fertilized egg. Her breasts, womb and ovaries undergo profound changes, many involving new cell growth and the stimulation of genetic material (RNA) in cells. However, in one sense it's a short step biologically from the repeated monthly multiplication of normal breast cells to abnormal overgrowth in the form of a cancer.

Most women in developed countries have 400–450 monthly cycles in their lives yet have only one or two babies or none at all. Their bodies' hormonal preparations for pregnancy each month are repeatedly frustrated, month after month, year after year. One theory is that the repeated monthly multiplication of breast cells may be one reason behind the high levels of breast cancer in developed countries.

There are two other theories on how breastfeeding may help protect against some breast cancers. If correct, these may act together or separately; however, as yet there isn't enough con-firmatory evidence.

1 – Milk left stagnant in the breast (because a woman lets it dry up because she's going to bottle-feed) may increase both the usual breast cell multiplication rate and the numbers of atypical cells, causing a state not far removed from that required for cancer to begin. This is because stagnant milk is slightly less acidic than recently produced milk from frequently emptied breasts. This slight decrease in acidity may be important as test tube studies show that cells are more likely to multiply rapidly and become abnormal in a relatively less acidic environment. Interestingly, the Tanka boat-women of Hong Kong who feed only from their right breast are more likely to get cancer in the left one.

2 – Milk production and the removal of milk from the breast by breastfeeding may flush out foreign chemicals which are poten-tially carcinogenic (cancer-causing). Once some of these chemicals have entered the breast (for example, from food we eat), they can

remain in the glands or ducts unless removed by being flushed out.

Given the current concern about breast cancer in Westernized countries, what should we do? Let's look at the risk factors you may be able to influence:

Breast cancer risk factors you may be able to influence

- Physical activity in adolescence and young adult life seems to lower the risk of breast cancer before and after the menopause.
- Having a first baby under twenty reduces the risk of breast cancer.
- Breastfeeding for the first time under twenty may be associated with a lower risk of breast cancer.
- One unconfirmed study suggests that an abortion may increase the risk of breast cancer by 50 per cent. An abortion before eighteen may increase the risk by 150 per cent; after thirty, by 110 per cent.
- Breastfeeding on an unrestricted basis, not giving solids for four to six months, and breastfeeding longer than currently fashionable usually prevent ovulation for many months, so delaying the monthly disruption of breast cells. Some women go a year or more without ovulating. Together with pregnancy, this gives at least two years free from monthly breast disruption with each baby. There's some evidence that this may reduce the risk of breast cancer, although not all studies agree.
- A healthy diet with plenty of vegetables, salads and fruit provides a good supply of anti-oxidants (including vitamins C and E, beta-carotene, selenium and flavonoids) which may help the body resist cancer.
- Other protective nutrients include plant hormones (for example in soy beans and soy bean products) which act as weak oestrogens. These seem to have an affinity for oestrogen-receptors in the breast and so block the action of other, potentially cancer-causing oestrogens.
- A large study to confirm whether a reduced-fat diet could protect against breast cancer is under way. Two omega–3 polyunsaturated fatty acids, DHA and EPA, found in fatty fish (such as herrings and salmon) suppress breast cancer cell multiplication. Until we know

more, it's wise to eat less fat in total, and especially less saturated fat, but to have some fatty fish two or three times a week.

- Being very overweight after the menopause increases the risk, so it's worth eating a healthy weight-reducing diet, exercising regularly and maintaining the weight loss.
- Drinking too much alcohol increases the risk of breast cancer by 50 per cent.
- Some researchers suggest that vitamin D may help control multiplying breast cells, so it may be wise to get some daylight on the skin each day as this is our main source of vitamin D.

— One study (1991) found an association between severe life events and breast cancer. Other researchers (1995) suggested that reacting to stress (caused by problems such as bereavement and other serious adverse life events) by confronting problems, and focusing on them by working out a plan of action, may raise the risk of breast cancer. They pointed out that active confrontation in a situation over which you have little control may not be beneficial. It uses up a person's resources and this, they suggest, may increase their risk of cancer (presumably by decreasing their physical resistance and immunity). The researchers postulate that women faced with severe life events might do better to 'withdraw' or 'disengage' rather than confront the issue.

Cancer cells are sometimes detectable under the microscope five years or more before cancer is detectable by feeling a lump. So it isn't only recent serious adverse life events which may be significant. A breastfeeding woman's high prolactin and endorphin levels are known to have a calming action, so here is yet another possible benefit of breastfeeding.

— One study suggests that women whose work exposes their breasts to high electro-magnetic fields have a higher risk of breast cancer. The women studied were industrial sewing machinists.

Pharmaceutical companies are working on synthetic hormones that mimic those produced by pregnant and breastfeeding women. Hormones in the Pill prevent ovulation but statistics show that the Pill doesn't prevent breast cancer and may in some circumstances be a contributory factor to breast cancer occurring in women under forty-five.

Hormone replacement therapy (HRT) taken for more than five years is associated with a slightly increased risk of breast cancer and, for more than ten years, with a markedly increased risk. However, although women who take it for longer than five years get more breast cancer, they are less likely to die from it than are those women who don't take HRT, possibly because regular breast-checks make early treatment more likely.

LESS OVARY AND WOMB CANCER?

Cancer of the ovary is more common in industrialized countries and kills more women than any other women's cancer. The factors which increase the risk are similar in many ways to those for breast cancer. For example, repeated monthly ovulation year in, year out, seems to make this cancer more likely. However, the more children a woman has, and the longer she breastfeeds each one, the lower is her risk. The sort of breastfeeding most likely to suppress ovulation is outlined later. Recent evidence (1995) suggests that long-term breastfeeding makes womb cancer below the age of fifty-five less likely.

NATURAL

Breast milk is the food nature intended for a baby. Each mother's milk is custom-made for her baby.

CLOSER RELATIONSHIP WITH YOUR BABY?

According to one large British survey, one in four women planning to breastfeed their first babies believed it would give them a closer bond with their baby.

SATISFACTION

There's something wonderful about being able to nourish your baby yourself, body to body. Being able to give him the pleasure of being at the breast is rewarding too, as is the ability to comfort a crying baby almost immediately. Women who breastfeed successfully for as long as they want report being very satisfied even if they are unaware of the health advantages to their babies.

Many mothers say they feel a tremendous sense of loss when they give their baby the last breastfeed. Perhaps this is partly because breastfed babies are more dependent upon their mothers for food than are bottle-fed ones, and many women enjoy feeling needed.

A survey of recently delivered women found that those who were 'greatly pleased' with their babies were much more successful at breastfeeding than those who were 'indifferent'.

— In a survey (1987) of 152 highly educated, 'long-term' (ten months or more) breastfeeding American and Canadian women, 98 per cent considered that the benefits of breastfeeding to their babies were emotional security, happiness and the earlier development of independence (presumably through the babies being allowed to be as dependent as they needed in the early years). They also commented that breastfeeding enhanced the love of mother and child for each other.

ENJOYMENT

One of the advantages people often forget is that, overall, most breastfeeding women enjoy it. There's something very special about the experience of having a baby at your breast staring up into your eyes and perhaps stopping sucking every now and then to break into a gummy smile. And the sight of a baby's tiny, dimpled, star-shaped hand resting on the breast as he feeds is one of the precious moments of mothering.

Many women enjoy talking to their baby, especially towards the end of a feed when he isn't concentrating so hard on drinking. And breastfeeding mothers around the world love speaking in baby talk. Researchers note that their voices all have a similar lilting, adagio rhythm. Feeds are delightful interludes when the level of endorphins (natural 'feel-good' chemicals in the blood) is almost certainly high, but that of stress hormones (such as adrenaline and cortisone) low.

FULFILMENT

Another feeling often expressed is that breastfeeding is one of the things only a woman can do. In today's world of sexual equality and unisex this feminine fulfilment is valued not only by the naturally maternal but also by the career woman who sees her enjoyment of breastfeeding as symbolic of her womanhood. The oneness many breastfeeding women feel with their babies is often quoted as the major advantage to breastfeeding mothers. Certainly they often seem very at ease with their babies.

EMPOWERMENT

A woman who breastfeeds as long as she or her baby wants gains in confidence and self-esteem.

— A US study (1993) found that women of poor economic means who breastfeed have more confidence in their skills as mothers and in their ability to meet their children's needs. This confidence lasts well beyond the time they are breastfeeding.
— Another US study (1988) found that young (average age sixteen) pregnant women from poor socio-economic backgrounds thought that breastfeeding would make them feel important.

GETTING YOUR FIGURE BACK

Three months after her baby is born a breastfeeding woman is more likely to be losing weight without dieting than one who is bottle-feeding. Breastfeeding uses up some of the fat stored in pregnancy and naturally helps a woman get back to her pre-pregnancy shape and weight, provided she isn't overeating. If her breasts change shape, they probably do so because of pregnancy, not breastfeeding. Women report that their breasts are variously either smaller, larger or droopier after breastfeeding but there is no general trend. However, breasts tend to return to their pre-pregnancy shape and size about six months after weaning.

CONVENIENCE

A big practical bonus is that breastfeeding is more convenient not only at home, with no bottles and teats to wash and sterilize and no feeds to prepare, but also when you go out as you'll have no equipment to get ready and take with you. Holidays and indeed all forms of travel become a much more practical proposition. Not for you the cooling of a bottle of hot milk by holding it out of the car window while travelling at great speed! And no spilt milk powder over car-seat upholstery.

A breastfeeding woman needs only her baby and a clean nappy to go anywhere and it takes only a little ingenuity and forethought to breastfeed in public without embarrassment to you or anyone else.

Another thing is that it's nearly always possible to comfort an infant with the breast easily and quickly, anywhere and any time, without overfeeding, whereas bottle-fed babies often aren't com-forted by sucking on a bottle of water or a dummy yet may get too much milk if allowed to suck ad lib at a bottle. This means a breastfed baby may be more contented than a bottle-fed baby.

CHEAPER

Breastfeeding is cheaper than bottle-feeding. However, the relatively more expensive cost of bottle-feeding isn't usually very important in developed countries, where a few pennies here or there don't influence the average woman either way. When working out the cost of bottle-feeding you need to add in the cost of formula, bottles, teats, and sterilizing tablets or fuel to boil the equipment.

A breastfeeding woman needs to consider the cost of any extra food she may need (see page 236). Experts suggest that some women need an extra 400–600 calories a day over and above their normal intake. The baby takes more than this but the difference is made up by calories from fat stores laid down in pregnancy. However, we now know that breastfeeding women use the energy from their food more efficiently than do bottle-feeding women, and may not need very much extra at all. Obviously the cost of any extra food depends on a woman's preferences – if she takes her extra calories as best steak it's more expensive than if she eats sandwiches. If she simply eats a little more of everything that she would normally eat, the cost of her extra food will be lower than the cost of bottle-feeding. This is especially important in developing countries where some mothers can't afford enough formula but can afford extra food for themselves.

BIRTH CONTROL

The contraceptive effect of breastfeeding used to be dismissed as an old wives' tale. This is trebly amazing as it can be just as efficient as better-known contraceptive methods such as the Pill; it's the only contraception available to many of the world's women; and in developing countries it has two vitally important effects.

1 Breastfeeding spaces children more widely apart. Research shows that in most of the world a child born less than two years after an older brother or sister has over twice the risk of dying young compared with one born after a longer gap.

2 Breastfeeding does more to contain the global population explosion than any other sort of contraception.

Using data gathered from over 4000 women in more than fifteen countries, an international group of experts stated in December 1995 that the contraceptive effect of breastfeeding in certain circumstances – when used as part of the lactational amenorrhoea method (LAM, see below) – is very safe and more than 98 per cent effective.

No popular method of contraception is 100 per cent reliable but the contraceptive effect of LAM is the same as that of the Pill and the condom and it's very useful as a temporary family-planning method after childbirth.

So what exactly is LAM and what are the circumstances that make breastfeeding such a safe contraceptive?

The lactational amenorrhoea method (LAM)

If a woman breastfeeds fully (that is, exclusively) or nearly fully (with at least six and preferably many more feeds well spaced throughout the twenty-four hours), and has not yet had her first period after giving birth, she has a better than 98 per cent chance of avoiding pregnancy. In other words, LAM depends on

• Your baby being under six months old.
• You breastfeeding exclusively (giving your baby no other drinks or food) or nearly exclusively.
• Feeding frequently, with no long gaps between feeds (NB, feeding very infrequently, with fewer than six feeds a day, allows the prolactin level to fall to levels seen when women are ovulating, see below).
• Your periods not yet having returned.

Scientists aren't completely clear why conception is less likely during the sort of breastfeeding necessary for LAM but know that the hormone prolactin is involved, as is some combination of vigorous sucking and milking by the baby and frequent breastfeeds with no long gaps night or day. There isn't a direct relationship between prolactin and the absence of periods. However, LAM helps prevent the prolactin level dipping low enough to allow ovulation. A high prolactin level seems to prevent ovulation by discouraging the ovarian response to follicle-stimulating hormone, a hormone which, in non-pregnant, non-breastfeeding women, allows an egg to ripen each month.

As time passes, a breastfeeding woman's prolactin level falls until eventually it's no longer high enough to prevent ovulation. In **exclusively breast-feeding women** this doesn't happen until the tenth week after childbirth at the very earliest, and only one breastfeeding woman in twenty ovulates before the eighteenth week. The contraceptive effect of breastfeeding differs from woman to woman even if they breastfeed in similar ways. But the type of breastfeeding makes a very big difference to the return of fertility. The average time before the first period in women who breastfeed exclusively and on an unrestricted basis for six to eight months, then introduce solids but continue to breastfeed frequently for drinks and comfort, is *over fourteen months!* A woman breastfeeding like this can expect an average gap between babies of two to three years, which means that ovulation returns, on average, after fifteen to twenty-seven months, the exact timing depending on personal factors.

In contrast, **bottle-feeding women** ovulate *on average* eight to ten weeks after giving birth, which means one in two risks becoming pregnant before her baby is eight to ten weeks old unless she uses some sort of contraception.

Partially-breastfeeding women ovulate on average later than bottle-feeding women but before exclusively breastfeeding women.

If a breastfeeding woman menstruates in the first six months after delivery, her menstrual cycles are likely to be anovular, which is why most women can rely on LAM until their first period after childbirth (but remember LAM is only for women with babies up to six months). *However, this certainly doesn't mean you can't become pregnant while using LAM – just that you have only a 2 per cent chance of doing so.*

As the months pass after delivery, ovulation before the first period becomes increasingly likely. One woman in twenty ovulates before her first period, which is one reason why LAM isn't 100 per cent effective. However, there are several ways of discovering when you're about to ovulate (see below under 'Other contraception').

Many studies suggest that breastfeeding's contraceptive effect is more powerful and lasts longer in developing countries. There are several possible reasons, including poor nourishment and taboos against sex with lactating women. But undoubtedly the main reason is that many of them breastfeed in an unrestricted way, with frequent feeds day and night, whereas in developed countries women tend to breastfeed only five or six times in twenty-four hours, with very few or no feeds at night.

Women in developing countries also tend to allow more non-nutritive suckling, putting their babies to the breast for comfort and pleasure as well as 'proper' feeds. This means that even if their babies have solids or bottle-feeds, they still spend a lot of time at the breast, which helps prevent ovulation.

The first eight weeks – If using LAM, you need no other contraception. It's *exceedingly* unlikely even for bottle-feeding women to ovulate now.

After eight weeks – Consider three questions:

1 Are you content with 98 per cent reliable contraception from LAM (which is better than most women settle for most of the time)?
2 Are you breastfeeding exclusively or nearly exclusively?
3 And are you still without periods (defined as either a recognizable period or two consecutive days of bleeding or spotting)?

If you answer 'no' to any of these questions, breastfeeding alone will give you nowhere near 98 per cent reliability and you'll need another contraceptive method.

But if you answer 'yes' to all three, LAM can be your only contraceptive method until your baby is six months old or until such time as your answers change.

However, if you feel strongly that you don't want to get pregnant again quickly, then because you just could be one of the one in twenty breastfeeding women who ovulates before her first period after childbirth, you may like to take one or two other precautions. These include:

- 'Extra-safe' LAM.
- An additional method of contraception compatible with breast-feeding and recent childbirth.

Extra-safe LAM – You can delay ovulation and help detect the unlikely event of ovulation occurring *before* your first period by stimulating your milk supply more. Do this by:

- Breastfeeding frequently, with no long gaps by day or night.
- Checking that your baby is well-positioned at the breast.
- Allowing non-nutritive suckling as well as 'proper' feeds.
- Avoiding a dummy.
- Delaying solids or bottles of formula, juice or water until your baby is four to six months old. Once a baby starts solids, the reliability of LAM falls from 98.5 to 96 per cent.

If you or your baby don't want to or can't breastfeed frequently (for example, if your baby is unwell or disinterested, or if you're not with each other) you can mimic the effect of breastfeeding to some extent by hand-expressing (or pumping) a little milk every two to three hours by day and every four hours or so at night.

— A study (1992) found that once periods had returned, frequent breastfeeding (an average nine feeds in twenty-four hours) prevented ovulation in seven out of ten women, whereas less frequent feeds (an average of six in twenty-four hours) prevented ovulation in only three out of ten women. The more frequent feeders had a higher average prolactin level.

Other contraception compatible with breastfeeding and recent childbirth

When you resume having sex, you could use a **condom** with spermicidal jelly, or a **diaphragm**. If you've used a diaphragm before, you'll need to be refitted after having a baby because you'll be a different size inside. This can be done at your six weeks post-natal visit to your doctor. Another idea is to have an **IUCD** (intra-uterine contraceptive device) fitted. As for the Pill, researchers say that while the combined Pill is inadvisable (because it decreases breast-milk production, see page 395) the **progestogen-only Pill** does not interfere with breastfeeding or affect the breastfed baby.

According to the World Health Organization, the disadvantages of monthly hormonal **contraceptive injections** for breast-feeding women during the first six weeks after delivery outweigh the advantages. Indeed, some doctors in India discovered that women who had contraceptive injections lost minerals from their bones, leading to lower bone density. They suggest these injections are unsafe for breastfeeding women.

The **sympto-thermal method** is a 'natural' form of birth control. An analysis of five studies showed that when carefully used it is 96.8 per cent effective. (When used imperfectly it is only 86.4 per cent effective). It involves:

* Being aware of the bodily changes (including those in the amount and nature of vaginal mucus and in the body temperature) which herald impending ovulation and the fertile days in your cycle. The average woman ovulates on the twelfth day of her cycle, counting the first day of her period as day one. However, ovulation may occur any time between the tenth and fourteenth day or, in a few women, even outside these times. Most women are especially fertile for the six days before – and on the day of – ovulation.
* Avoiding sex (or using a condom or diaphragm) if you recognize you're entering a fertile time.

The sympto-thermal method can help you recognize the unlikely event of ovulation before your first period after childbirth. It can also help identify whether or not newly returned periods are associated with ovulation. It becomes even easier as the months pass and you settle back into having ovulatory menstrual cycles.

However, it's wise to get expert help if you want reliable contraception from a combination of breastfeeding and the sympto-thermal method, as many women find that the signs indicating their fertile time are less clear while breastfeeding. When using the sympto-thermal method, a simple, small **saliva microscope** (see page 452) can help you identify the fern-like pattern in your saliva that precedes your fertile time. **Fertility test kits** (see page 452) which test hormone levels in a few drops of urine are another useful aid.

BETTER FOR BONES (see also page 244)

Two pieces of research suggest that breastfeeding helps protect against the long-term risk of osteoporosis.

— Australian researchers reported (1993) that among 311 women over sixty-five in their study, those who'd had a baby but had never breastfed had twice the risk of hip fracture of women who had breastfed. They also found that the longer a woman breastfed each baby, the lower was her risk of hip fracture in later life. Breastfeeding each baby for more than nine months lowered a woman's risk of hip fracture to a quarter of the risk of those who had never breastfed.

— A South African study (1992) showed that women who breastfeed have a higher bone mineral density in later life than those who bottle-feed. *Women who develop osteoporosis are much less likely to have been breastfeeders* than other women (in fact, four times less likely).

However, it's possible that if breastfeeding does protect against osteoporosis, as these studies suggest, it does so only if done for a cumulatively large number of months or even years. Long-term breastfeeding delays the onset of ovulation after each baby. This means that a woman's life-long supply of eggs in her ovaries lasts longer. She can then go on ovulating longer into middle age. The longer she has menstrual cycles, giving her high levels of oestrogen and progesterone, the later is her menopause and the further away the time when low hormone levels will make osteoporosis more likely.

LESS RHEUMATOID ARTHRITIS?

— Norwegian research (1995) looked at the records of 63,090 women, 355 of whom had died from rheumatoid arthritis (RA). They found an association between the total time a woman had breastfed and her chance of dying from RA. Women who breastfed for a total of twenty months or more had a particularly low risk of dying from RA. This was the first report of a possible association.
— However, North American researchers (1994) reported that in a small group of susceptible women, breastfeeding *increased* the risk of developing RA; they are currently investigating whether there is a genetic basis for this. One theory is that prolactin may in certain circumstances provoke the immune system to turn against the joint linings.

SOME POSSIBLE DISADVANTAGES

Many women decide not to breastfeed and it would be foolish to pretend there are no drawbacks. However, many perceived disadvantages can be overcome and other concerns often disappear when well aired.

Embarrassment?

Breasts have become equated with sex in our society and some people think that women who reveal their breasts while breastfeeding are immodest – or worse! At the beginning of the century no one turned a hair at the sight of a woman breastfeeding in public. Now, though, it must be done with more than a passing thought for modesty and causing offence to others or a woman runs the risk of people staring or even being overtly unpleasant. This fear of embarrassment is a great deterrent to many women who are anxious not only at the thought of feeding in front of strangers but also in front of relatives.

Most women who breastfeed do so very discreetly in public, partly for personal reasons and partly to avoid upsetting other people. With practice a woman can learn the knack of feeding her baby perfectly well without exposing her breast.

The swing back to breastfeeding in the early 1970s started with better-educated, freer-thinking women who realized that breast-feeding offered advantages to them and to their babies which far outweighed any difficulties in feeding away from home. Breast-feeding in public is slowly becoming more acceptable again and perhaps when TV and film directors start casting breastfeeding actresses, this move towards acceptability will speed up.

Being tied?

Some women choose not to breastfeed because they don't want to be tied. Certainly if a woman is to breastfeed successfully and exclusively for at least four to six months, she'll find it far easier if she's with her baby. However, some women learn the knack of expressing enough milk for someone else to give (by feeding cup, spoon or bottle) when they are out; and others give their babies the occasional bottle of formula. These occasional bottles of formula aren't a very good idea, however, especially before your milk supply is well established (see page 280).

Outings other than to people's homes may have to be limited in the first few weeks because very young babies can't last long between feeds. This can be overcome if you feed in the car, on a park bench, or in a café with helpful staff. Discreet breastfeeds are virtually unnoticeable unless you have a wonderfully noisy feeder who slurps, sucks loudly or 'glugs' with each swallow!

Some NCT and LLL groups have lists of shops and other public places which support breastfeeding. If no such list is available to you locally, why not consider compiling one and sending it to your local paper or baby clinic? It could be excellent publicity for supportive shops. Sainsbury's, the UK food retailer, recently declared that it provides facilities for breastfeeding customers.

Rather than worry about never being able to leave your baby, it helps to be positive about taking him with you when you go out. There are very few places you can't take a baby, especially a very young, eminently transportable one. Even a woman brought up to believe that anyone can take her place as a mother may decide to think of her baby as an extension of herself for a few months at least. A baby loves to be with his mother and once this becomes a reality to you, you may not want to leave him behind.

No one else can feed the baby

This isn't true. A breastfeeding woman can leave her milk for someone else to feed to her baby if she collects enough by expressing it after several feeds. However, a large survey in Great Britain showed in 1990 that nearly one in two pregnant women who planned to bottle-feed gave as one of their reasons the fact that other people would be able to feed their baby.

Expecting to return to work (see page 292)

One in twenty women said she planned to bottle-feed because she was expecting to return to work soon, according to a large survey in 1990 in Great Britain. However, very few women actually do return to work when their babies are very young. And even if they do, they can continue breastfeeding.

Friends aren't doing it

Friends have a big influence on a woman's choice of how she feeds her baby. If she has a lot of bottle-feeding friends she is more likely to bottle-feed herself, and vice versa. It can take courage to break out of the mould set by her contemporaries.

Pain?

Some women who have never breastfed imagine it will be painful. It's undeniable that many women occasionally have sore nipples and that a few have other painful breast conditions while breastfeeding.

In a study in Blackburn, Lancashire, nearly one woman in six who stopped breastfeeding did so because her nipples were sore. However, sore nipples are temporary, most are to some extent avoidable, and there's a lot you can do to make them better. We now know that the Blackburn women stopped breastfeeding unnecessarily. Their nipple soreness would have disappeared spontaneously in time, and help and encouragement would probably have made all the difference.

Can't see how much he's getting

We live in a society which has a near-obsession with measuring things. Indeed, we tend to view with suspicion anything that can't be measured. A midwife once asked us why nature didn't provide women with transparent breasts. We replied, why don't bottle-manufacturers make their products from opaque material?

We've all been brainwashed into thinking it's important to know exactly how much milk a baby takes but it very rarely is important, especially if breastfeeding is properly managed and the baby is healthy and thriving. No two infants are alike and each needs different amounts at different times of day. Properly managed breastfeeding is a perfectly balanced demand-and-supply system with the emphasis on the supply – the more and better you stimulate your breasts by breastfeeding (or expressing or pumping), with no long gaps and with the baby feeding well, the more milk you'll make (see page 17).

If ever you fall into the trap of test-weighing your baby to find out how much he's getting, remember that breastfed babies thrive on smaller volumes of breast milk than you would expect from knowing how much cows' milk formula bottle-fed babies take. This is partly because breast milk is perfectly digested. There's so much waste with formula that a bottle-fed baby needs a bigger volume than a breastfed baby to get enough nourishment.

Unfashionable?

To a certain extent humans have a herd instinct and like to copy each other's behaviour. Midwives often remark that if one mother is breastfeeding successfully, other women tend to copy her. If she fails, they're likely to stop breastfeeding too!

When bottle-feeding first became fashionable, only the relatively wealthy could afford to do it, but gradually the habit spread, with the middle classes leading the way. Today, women in low-earning families and with the least education are the ones most likely to bottle-feed.

In many hospitals now the majority of women start breastfeeding. Once back at home, though, many stop within a few weeks. Bottle-feeding has now become almost the norm – the accepted and modern way of feeding babies in the West. Most breastfed babies are soon given a bottle, although there's no need for this to happen.

Unsexy? (see also page 422)

Some women imagine breastfeeding will make them less sexy both in their own eyes and in those of their husband or partner. The cult of the breast as a sex object has undoubtedly helped speed the decline of breastfeeding. The up-pointed, conical breast of the

1950s and 1960s seemed to be there solely to attract men. Very few babies ever got a look in!

Perhaps the more recent trend towards more self-confidence and towards natural living, with many young women doing without tight bras and make-up and relying more on their inborn femininity to attract men, will encompass and encourage breast-feeding too.

Disgusting?

A few women feel disgusted by breastfeeding and either refuse to breastfeed or give up after a day or two because it seems too animal-like. It's unlikely that anything will make such women change their minds but one good way to help prevent girls growing up with such deep-rooted feelings is to introduce school lessons mentioning breastfeeding along with other aspects of child-care. Some education authorities already encourage such lessons as part of the school curriculum, and in mixed schools there's the added advantage that boys can discuss it too. In some areas local health educators take a woman and her breastfeeding baby along to these classes so that the children can watch and ask questions directly.

Risk of failure?

Many women are so afraid they'll fail to breastfeed that the whole thing becomes a self-fulfilling prophecy and they do. They then feel deeply disappointed. Some health workers don't like to use terms such as 'failure', but the fact is that many women themselves see it as a failure. So great can this feeling be that some doctors and nurses refuse to tell women about the benefits of breastfeeding for fear they'll be unable to breastfeed and then feel guilty. This is tragic because babies are denied their natural food and women their natural right – and all for nothing, because failure rarely needs to occur.

If a woman starts by breastfeeding for ten minutes a side every four hours or so during the day and once or even not at all at night, because this is what she's been told to do, she is, in effect, breastfeeding only in a token way. With token breastfeeding her breasts don't get enough stimulation (see Chapter 10) and it isn't surprising that her milk supply soon dwindles. When she realizes her baby isn't getting enough to eat she goes out and buys a bottle.

However, nearly every woman *can* breastfeed for as long as she wants if she understands how to make enough milk and has enough help. Taking steps to increase the milk supply generally works within a few days. But having said this, there are a very, very few women who are unable to breastfeed whatever they do. Rather than castigate themselves and allow their baby to go without adequate nourishment, it's essential that they put their pride to one side and give the baby some formula as well as their breast milk.

Broken sleep

Breastfed babies tend to sleep rather less on average than bottle-fed ones as well as tending to take shorter naps, especially if they sleep in bed with their mothers and feed at night. However, breastfeeding helps babies get off to sleep, which balances the picture.

Quite apart from the advantages to babies outlined in Chapter 4, breastfeeding has many very real advantages for women too.

In the next chapter we'll look at how you can prepare for your baby – and for breastfeeding – while you are pregnant.

SIX

Preparation and pregnancy

You can do a great deal during pregnancy to prepare for breastfeeding.

LOOKING AFTER YOURSELF

Looking after yourself is important both for your sake and that of your family, because you'll be spending a large part of a year carrying and nourishing your baby. It's a good idea to:

- Eat sensibly so that you maintain your health, prepare your body for breastfeeding and nourish your developing baby without robbing your body of its nutrients.
- Choose the best place to have your baby.
- Get informed advice about breastfeeding.
- Think about breastfeeding and discuss it with your partner.
- Get in touch with people who can help with breastfeeding if you have any problems.
- Prepare yourself and your household so that things run as smoothly as possible when your baby arrives.

EATING IN PREGNANCY

The weight you gain in pregnancy is made up of the baby, the placenta, the amniotic fluid and the increased weight of your womb and breasts, together with stored fat and an increased volume of blood and other body fluids. Controversy rages over the amount of weight-gain considered desirable.

The average woman eating what she wants gains 7–18kg (15–40lb), of which about 2–3kg (4–6lb) is fat. If she bottle-feeds, she may have trouble losing this fat. However, if she breastfeeds, her stored fat contributes nourishment to the baby via her breast milk and should gradually disappear. Research suggests that her fat stores provide up to 300 calories via her milk each day for three or four months. It's been said that a baby needs 600–800 calories a day. However, fat stores can provide between a third and a half of her baby's requirements and she'll need to eat only 300–500 extra calories a day at most to make milk without robbing her body.

— Interestingly, research from the US (1989) shows that healthy breastfed babies need fewer calories than previously thought. They also need fewer calories than bottle-fed babies, because they absorb more energy from breast milk than bottle-fed babies do from the same volume of formula.

You don't have to store fat during pregnancy to breastfeed successfully. However, a breastfeeding woman who doesn't gain enough weight in pregnancy to lay down much in the way of fat stores may have to eat more than 300–500 calories a day extra to make up for the lack of contribution from stored fat. Millions of women in developing countries lay down no fat yet breastfeed successfully for very long periods, provided they have enough to eat.

Too high a weight-gain in pregnancy can make a woman more likely to have swollen ankles, varicose veins, backache and heartburn, so, if you're going to breastfeed, don't imagine that the more weight you put on, the better!

Attempts to correlate breastfeeding success with pregnancy weight-gain have yielded conflicting results, one showing that the less body fat women stored, the more milk they made, and another showing that women who put on very little weight had difficulty breastfeeding!

What should you eat?

What you eat when you're pregnant is important for breastfeeding. This is partly because you're unlikely to change your eating habits quickly once your baby is born and also because a healthy balanced diet is good both when pregnant and breastfeeding. If you need to improve your diet, now is a good time to do so.

Eat a healthy diet with wholegrain foods and five helpings of fruit and vegetables every day, as well as plenty to drink. This way you'll probably avoid constipation – a common problem in pregnancy.

Most women eat no more food than usual during the early months of pregnancy and only about 100 calories a day more in the last few weeks. However, if you are a very active person and remain so during pregnancy, you may want and need to eat more. And if you go into pregnancy underweight, you may need more too. If you suffer from pregnancy sickness you may feel like eating less than usual, although later your appetite should increase.

Alcohol?

Experts can't say exactly how much, if any, alcohol is safe in pregnancy. Official guidelines in some countries, including the US, Australia and New Zealand, are to have none. If you drink, it's probably sensible to have no more than a glass of wine or its equivalent (half a pint of beer, a quarter of a pint of strong lager, a small glass of sherry or a measure of spirits) a day. It's important not to binge on alcohol.

Vegetarians

If you're a vegetarian, make sure you eat enough foods rich in iron (egg yolk, peas, beans, lentils, nuts, green vegetables, wholemeal bread and other wholegrain foods); calcium (milk, yoghurt, cheese, green leafy vegetables, wholegrain foods, peas, beans and lentils, nuts, seeds); zinc (nuts, wholegrains, peas, beans, root vegetables, garlic); and vitamin B_{12} (eggs, milk, cheese, Marmite, fortified and fermented foods, seaweeds), or take a vitamin B_{12} supplement. If you're a new vegetarian, or the first in your family, you need to take special care (see page 238).

Some special notes

Folic acid, calcium and iron need special mention, as well as certain foods that are best avoided in pregnancy.

Folic acid – Experts advise eating more foods rich in folic acid (a B vitamin) as surveys show that having enough around the time of conception and in early pregnancy makes several types of congenital deformity (including spina bifida and cleft palate) less likely. Folic acid-rich foods include most vegetables (especially dark green leafy ones), fruit, eggs, wholegrain cereals, beans, peas, lentils, fish, nuts, and yeast or beef extract. Some breakfast cereals and white breads are supplemented with folic acid – check on the packets.

As an extra precaution, many experts advise a supplement of folic acid for women who want to become, or who are, pregnant. The recommended amount is 0.4mg (400 micrograms) a day, starting before conception and continuing for the first three months of pregnancy. This is twice the amount in the average woman's diet. Some experts say that only women who eat an unhealthy diet should take a supplement, although of course it would be better if they could improve their diet as well.

If you've had a baby with a neural tube problem or cleft palate, you'll need a bigger folic acid supplement – 4mg (4000 micrograms) each day, starting before conception and continuing for the first three months of pregnancy.

Calcium – A baby needs calcium for bone development and if you don't eat enough calcium-containing foods your baby may rob your bones. It's important to get this in perspective, though, by looking at many parts of the world where pregnant women don't increase their calcium intake yet have normal babies and stay healthy themselves.

Calcium-containing foods include peas, beans and lentils, wholemeal bread and other wholegrain foods, cabbage, watercress, fish, milk, yoghurt and cheese. Soups made with well-boiled bone stock containing a little vinegar are another good source of calcium, as are the soft bones of tinned sardines. When you're pregnant you automatically absorb more calcium from the foods you eat.

Many people believe that milk is essential for a pregnant woman but provided she has enough calcium from other foods and eats a healthy diet, this isn't so. In any case, some women can't drink milk without getting tummy-ache, bloating, wind and diarrhoea. They have a condition called lactose intolerance, caused by a deficiency of lactase – the enzyme that normally breaks down milk sugar (lactose) in the gut. Lactose intolerance affects around one in twenty people of Northern European descent and up to nine out of ten people of Afro-Caribbean, Chinese, Mediterranean and Middle Eastern descent. If you are lactose-intolerant yet would like to drink more milk, you can buy lactase from pharmacies and add it to milk to pre-digest the lactose.

Eating too much animal protein (such as meat and eggs) can drain calcium from your body.

Iron – To guard against anaemia you'll need enough foods containing iron (meat, egg yolks, dark green leafy vegetables, peas, beans, lentils, wholemeal bread and other wholegrain foods, apricots, raisins and prunes) and folic acid (see page 140). Eating foods rich in vitamin C (citrus and other fruit, fruit juice and vegetables) at the same time as wholegrain cereal foods, beans, nuts and green leafy vegetables will help you absorb iron from them. However, it's better not to drink tea with your meals as tannins in tea can reduce iron absorption. About one in ten pregnant women has iron-deficiency anaemia and this is almost always due to a poor diet.

Most doctors no longer recommend routine iron supplements to prevent anaemia in healthy pregnant women who are eating a healthy diet. Also, the World Health Organization recommends that there's no need for women in developed countries to take iron provided they eat well. Many women don't take routinely pre-scribed iron anyway as its side-effects (such as constipation) can be such a nuisance. Routine blood tests (usually at the first ante-natal clinic visit and at thirty-two weeks) detect anaemia early enough for treatment before the baby is born. If your doctor prescribes iron there's almost certainly a very good reason but you should ask what it is.

Listeria – Many experts recommend avoiding soft cheeses (such as Camembert and Brie), blue cheeses, unpasteurized cheeses and insufficiently reheated cook-chilled foods in pregnancy because of the risk of them containing an overgrowth of *Listeria* bacteria. These bacteria are normally harmless but in certain circumstances can cause a flu-like infection in a pregnant woman and damage her unborn baby.

Liver and liver pâté – These are best avoided because of their high levels of vitamin A which have been known to damage unborn babies.

There's more information about healthy eating for breastfeeding women in Chapter 9.

GOING OUTSIDE

It's wise to get into the habit of spending some time out of doors each day. Having daylight directly on your skin enables your body to make a significant amount of vitamin D. Regular exposure to daylight will help keep your bones strong when you are breast-feeding and will supply your baby with vitamin D too.

CHOOSING WHERE TO HAVE YOUR BABY

One of the first things to do once you know you are pregnant is to book into a hospital for your delivery – that is, if you plan to give birth in hospital rather than at home. The good news, according to a large UK survey in 1990, is that hospital practices to encourage and support breastfeeding are slowly improving. However, choose carefully because some hospitals are very much more helpful than others with breastfeeding. This checklist may help you decide:

- Ask your doctor whether the practices in your local hospitals match up to the globally acknowledged criteria set out by the World Health Organization and UNICEF. In other words, how 'Baby-Friendly' is your hospital ? (See below.)
- If your doctor doesn't know, ask friends and other women locally whether the staff in the hospital they went to were helpful with breastfeeding.
- Ask each hospital you are considering for a copy of its breastfeeding policy.
- Persevere until you find a hospital in which most women who want to breastfeed manage to do so without using bottles of formula or giving up sooner than they wished.
- Try to find a hospital which encourages rooming-in (where babies and mothers stay together day and night). Rooming-in makes breast-feeding easier.
- Ask whether you'll be allowed – and, preferably, encouraged – to labour in an upright position if you want to. More and more midwives encourage women to give birth upright, rather than lying flat, as being upright can speed up labour, make contractions less arduous and increase a baby's oxygen supply. Labouring in an upright position in the first and second stages tends to make labour easier and quicker, episiotomies less likely, and birth safer. And because both mother and baby are more likely to feel well after-wards, breastfeeding is more likely to get off to a good start.

With the right information, support and help if necessary, being in hospital need not load the dice against successful breastfeeding, even though feeding a baby in hospital is a somewhat unnatural affair and experience shows that breastfeeding is more likely to be successful at home. The stress of being in hospital, after all, does little to encourage the establishment of the let-down (see page 19). One newly delivered American woman logged the number of people who came into her private hospital room each day: it came to between fifty and seventy. This couldn't have been relaxing! The good news is that some hospitals employ midwives whose main job is to encourage and advise breastfeeding mothers.

BABY-FRIENDLY HOSPITALS

More and more hospitals around the world are changing their policies to become eligible to apply for Baby-Friendly Hospital status, awarded by UNICEF. To date over 1000 hospitals have applied and met the standards required, which still leaves an enormous number that may or may not be good enoungh!

Baby-Friendly Hospitals have a ten-point code of practice – otherwise known as the Ten Steps to Successful Breastfeeding. This means they:

1 – Have a written breastfeeding policy that is routinely communicated to all health staff.

2 – Train all health-care staff in skills necessary to implement this policy.

3 – Inform all pregnant women about the benefits and management of breastfeeding.

4 – Help mothers initiate breastfeeding within half an hour of birth.

5 – Show mothers how to breastfeed and how to maintain lactation even if they should be separated from their infants.

6 – Give newborn infants no food or drink other than breast milk, unless *medically* indicated.

7 – Practise rooming-in (allow mothers and infants to remain together) twenty-four hours a day.

8 – Encourage breastfeeding on demand.

9 – Give no artificial teats or pacifiers (dummies or soothers) to breastfeeding infants.

10 – Foster the establishment of breastfeeding support groups and refer mothers to them on discharge from the hospital or clinic.

In the UK, because so many hospitals are such a long way from meeting the Baby-Friendly criteria, three awards can be made:

- The Certificate of Commitment, given in recognition that a hospital has adopted Steps 1, 7 and 10 and is actively working towards achieving the remaining Steps.
- The Standard Award, given in recognition that a hospital has adopted the Ten Steps, has at least one in two women breastfeeding when they leave, and is working towards continued improvements.
- The Global Award, given in recognition that a hospital has adopted the Ten Steps and has at least three out of four women breastfeeding when they leave.

Any hospital working towards an award, or already having an award, has to report its statistics to the UK Baby-Friendly Office every year and agree to regular re-assessment.

In May 1995 the Royal Bournemouth Hospital became the UK's first Baby-Friendly Hospital. By January 1995 Canada had five Baby-Friendly Hospitals, all in Ontario; Japan had four; Australia two and the US none. In contrast, in 1995 China had 947, Africa 128 and India 376!

- A hospital in the UK which wishes to apply for one of the stages of Baby-Friendly status can contact the UK Baby-Friendly Initiative, 20 Guilford Street, London WC1N 1DZ.

- Other hospitals can write to UNICEF Baby-Friendly Hospital Initiative, Palais des Nations, CH–1211, Geneva 10, Switzerland.

MAKING A BIRTH PLAN

You may wish to draw up a birth plan, or your midwife or ante-natal teacher may suggest this. A birth plan generally covers a woman's ideas of the way she would like to give birth and should ideally be discussed and agreed with the hospital staff before you have your baby. However, there's every reason to include in your plan your ideas, wishes and hopes for how you would like to breastfeed and care for your baby. For example, you might say you would like to hold your newborn baby immediately after birth and offer the first feed when the baby is ready. This is also the time to pont out that you want your baby to have *only* breast milk and not be given bottles without your personal permission. And you could say that you would prefer not to have pain-relieving drugs, such as pethidine, too close to the actual birth, as these might make your baby too sleepy to feed well at first.

PLANNING FOR WHEN YOU GET HOME

If you and your baby are well, you'll probably be better off arranging to stay in hospital for only a short time, returning home as soon as you can. The quiet, loving, constant emotional support and encouragement you need at this time can best be supplied by family and friends. Your community midwife and, later, your health visitor, can help you at home with their professional skills if necessary. Women who arrange to leave hospital within forty-eight hours are more likely to breastfeed successfully than those who stay in longer. This is scarcely surprising as most relax better in their own environment and are thus likely to let their milk down more reliably.

If you've been unlucky enough to give birth in a hospital where babies are kept in nurseries at night, you'll be able to have your baby with you all the time when you get home. This means you can breastfeed on an unrestricted basis by day and night, which will help you get off to a good start.

Well ahead of time, arrange for a relative, friend or paid help to come and do some domestic jobs when you return after the birth. This will help you get the rest you need, give you time to enjoy your baby and help you get breastfeeding off to the best possible start.

INVOLVING YOUR PARTNER

During your pregnancy discuss with your partner what breast-feeding is going to mean to him. Tell him what you know about the advantages of breastfeeding and suggest he goes to the fathers' nights at your ante-natal class, where he can discuss any doubts and queries he may have. He might be interested in reading parts of this book, especially Chapter 14 for fathers and Chapter 15 about sex.

He'll probably be only too pleased to support your decision to breastfeed once he understands how important breastfeeding is and how valuable he can be as protector and encourager of you and your breastfeeding baby.

— A North American study (1992) reported that her man's attitude is the single most important influence on a woman's decision about how to feed her baby. Partners of women who plan to bottle-feed are likely not to know about the health benefits of breastfeeding; they also tend to imagine, wrongly, that breastfeeding makes a woman's breasts sag and will spoil their sex life. The researchers concluded that fathers shouldn't be left out of the educational process when it comes to learning about breastfeeding.

Discuss mundane but important matters, such as how he'll get home from work if you usually pick him up but happen to be breastfeeding at the time; how he can cook supper sometimes, or how, if you cook it, you can have meals at flexible times; and how it'll mean more sleep for you both if the baby sleeps in bed with you or by your bed so that you can feed easily at night without waking your man.

Some women choose to bottle-feed so that their partners can sometimes enjoy giving the baby a bottle of formula. But breastfeeding is nature's way of giving a baby milk, so no mother needs to feel guilty of depriving a man of this experience! He can enjoy cuddling his baby as much as he likes any time other than during a breastfeed.

CHOOSING HOW TO FEED YOUR BABY

Many factors influence women as they decide how to feed their baby.

— A survey of expectant mothers in the UK in 1990 discovered some interesting ideas underlying their choice of feeding:

What's so fascinating about these findings is that the women who chose bottle-feeding all gave reasons *against breast-feeding*, not *for bottle-feeding*. In contrast, the women who chose breastfeeding were positively *for* breastfeeding, not against bottle-feeding. In other words, the bottle-feeders gave negative reasons and the breastfeeders positive ones.

So perhaps a more thorough discussion in ante-natal classes of the imagined disadvantages of breastfeeding, preferably with the help of a successfully breastfeeding woman, might go a long way to help women who would have chosen bottle-feeding decide to overcome the perceived negatives and choose breastfeeding instead. Also, as the number one choice breastfeeders give for breastfeeding is that it's best for babies, this fact must obviously be well aired and not hushed up for the sake of allaying guilt in

%	Reasons for planning to breastfeed first babies
88	Breastfeeding is best for the baby
35	Breastfeeding is more convenient
24	Closer bond between mother and baby
18	Breastfeeding is cheaper
16	Breastfeeding is natural
8	Breastfeeding is best for mother
3	Influenced by medical personnel
2	Influenced by friends or relatives

(Percentages don't add up to 100 as some women gave more than one reason.)

%	Reasons for planning to bottle-feed first babies
74	Other people can feed baby with bottle
28	Didn't like idea of breastfeeding
10	Would be embarrassed to breastfeed
8	Can see how much baby has had
8	Expecting to return to work soon
6	Other reasons
4	No particular reason
3	Persuaded by other people
2	Medical reasons for not breastfeeding

(Percentages don't add up to 100 as some women gave more than one reason.)

(Both tables from *Infant Feeding*, 1990, HMSO)

those who don't want to breastfeed and in the very few who really can't.

Underlying many of these reasons, however, may be a woman's feelings about breastfeeding.

Your feelings about breastfeeding

Some people have strong feelings for or against breastfeeding; others are undecided. If you feel strongly that you don't like the idea of breastfeeding, you may like to do a little emotional spadework to discover why; the information on page 250 may help.

Getting to the bottom of your feelings may:

• Allow you to leave ancient emotional clutter behind.
• Create greater personal awareness.
• Enable you to make a much freer choice about how to feed your baby.

SOURCES OF INFORMATION ABOUT BREASTFEEDING

Find out as much as you can about breastfeeding before you actually start to do it. Even if you have breastfed before – and successfully – read about it or discuss it because all babies are different and the way they feed is different too. Later there'll be all too little time and you may not be satisfied with other people's advice. If you understand how breastfeeding works, you'll know roughly what to expect, you'll be more confident and you'll know where to get help for any problems that crop up.

Ante-natal classes

These are usually valuable and with any luck the session on baby feeding will focus on breastfeeding. By making friends with other women who want to breastfeed you can encourage each other face to face or on the phone when you've had your babies. They will be your 'bosom buddies', encouraging you, perhaps pointing you in the right direction if you need extra information or advice, laughing (or crying) with you, and sometimes even caring for you.

— A North American study (1984) reported that ante-natal education about breastfeeding made successful breastfeeding more likely. Giving information about breastfeeding and the care of a newborn baby – including an idea of the large number of feeds and nappy changes, the lack of a predictable schedule, and possible setbacks – gave pregnant women a more realistic idea of their future role as breastfeeding mothers. The researchers pointed out that women who hadn't been taught about breastfeeding tended to blame the baby for any problems instead of blaming factors under their own control, and suggested that their less positive perceptions of their babies could, theoretically, interfere with their parenting and affect their child's development.

— A 1970s study found that when classes included talks or discussions on infant feeding, only two out of three women thought the person running the class was in favour of breastfeeding. These women were more likely to plan to breastfeed than the one in three who thought no preference was expressed. It seems obvious that people running these classes should not only talk about feeding but also make it clear that they think breastfeeding is best.

Information pamphlets

Be vigilant about the source of booklets and leaflets about pregnancy and baby feeding, such as the ones available in many clinics and surgeries. The way information about breastfeeding is put across in booklets sponsored by milk formula companies may be very different in tone from that in booklets sponsored by non-commercial bodies.

— Canadian researchers (1993) reported that 80 per cent of pamphlets produced by non-profit sources were rated very positive about breastfeeding, compared with only 8 per cent of those produced by commercial sources. What's more, 80 per cent of the non-profit materials scored a good degree of accuracy about breastfeeding, compared with only 20 per cent of commercial ones. Interestingly, one pamphlet sponsored by a large milk formula company had a photograph of a woman breastfeeding with her sweater pulled *down* over her breast, leaving her breast totally exposed. No successfully breastfeeding woman would do this – she would pull her sweater *up* over her breast, so it still covered the top of it. Given that the idea of exposing their breasts while breastfeeding so embarrasses many women that it puts them off the whole idea, this photo must make one seriously question the motives of the formula company. Could it be that at some level, conscious or unconscious, the company wished to put women off breastfeeding? This would certainly please the shareholders!

Health professionals

If you live in the UK you may meet your health visitor at the ante-natal classes. She will be your official breastfeeding adviser once you part company with your community midwife four weeks after the birth and her support and advice may be invaluable when you are at home. You can contact her either at your baby clinic in person or by phone. Ask acquaintances expecting second babies whether her breastfeeding advice is good. If she has the reputation for advising formula at the drop of a hat, get in touch with an NCT breastfeeding counsellor, an LLL leader or a lactation consultant as well (see page 453).

Learning together – Some health professionals are wonderful in that they are willing to go on learning about successful breast-feeding alongside women who are doing it. The very best helpers know they can always learn more.

Some breastfeeding women are willing and confident enough to learn about successful breastfeeding independently and to teach and encourage their midwife, doctor (and, in the UK, their health visitor) as they learn themselves. This requires eagerness to learn, as well as intellectual humility, on the part of the health pro-fessional, but some brave breastfeeding women and helpers have teamed up with excellent and mutually rewarding results. Such helpers have subsequently gone on to help a great many women. People who work together with this generosity of spirit light the way for others and deserve warm congratulations and gratitude.

There's a special word for health professionals on page 454.

The National Childbirth Trust (NCT)

In the UK the NCT organizes courses of ante-natal classes. An NCT breastfeeding counsellor usually gives a talk during one of these courses and you can contact her when you've had your baby if you need help with breastfeeding. These counsellors are volunteers who are well trained in helping with breastfeeding problems; they have, almost without exception, breastfed babies themselves; and can discuss things on a mother-to-mother basis. Some NCT branches arrange post-natal meetings and support groups too.

La Leche League (LLL)

This is part of a worldwide organization of women who are breastfeeding or have breastfed and want to encourage and help each other and anyone else with breastfeeding. Anyone interested in breastfeeding is welcome to attend local LLL branch meetings. Your nearest LLL leader will give you her telephone number so you can contact her at any time if you need help. League leaders are volunteers with an excellent training in assisting and encouraging breastfeeding women; they have all breastfed babies successfully for long periods; and they can discuss things on a mother-to-mother basis. LLL group meetings are open to anyone, whether they are pregnant, breastfeeding or neither.

BRAS

When your breasts start growing, from about the fifth month of pregnancy or even before, you'll need a bigger bra. The NCT Maternity Sales catalogue sells simple bra extenders to increase the chest size of existing bras (see page 453).

Buying bras ready for breastfeeding

You'll need several bras suitable for breastfeeding, because they'll require frequent washing, especially early on when you're bound to leak. Some people think cotton 'breathes' better than synthetic fabrics. It's important to wear a bra which supports and fits you well yet doesn't squash your breasts or nipples.

Some women wear an ordinary bra and undo it or pull it up or down to breastfeed; only 40 per cent of breastfeeding women have a special bra. However, ordinary bras can create problems – for example, it's difficult to do a back-fastening bra up quickly if the doorbell goes when you're feeding, though if you simply pull the cup up or down, you don't need to undo it at all. But be careful to avoid pressure under your breast from the pulled-down cup, as this could lead to a blocked duct. If you have small breasts, you may not need to wear a bra at all.

Whatever your breast size, you may prefer to get a special nursing bra.

Nursing bras – there are two main types, one with drop-down cups, the other with zipped cups. The NCT Maternity Sales catalogue has a good selection, including one going up to an HH cup size. In the UK women can also be measured and order their bras from local NCT branch bra agents.

A bra at night?

Pregnancy is the time to be especially careful about looking after your breasts. It's sensible to wear a bra in bed during the last three months of pregnancy to support your increasingly heavy breasts and help prevent your skin from stretching. Maternity bras sold as sleep bras are usually too insubstantial to provide much support.

CLOTHES

Good clothes to have ready for breastfeeding include T-shirts, sweat-shirts, jumpers, blouses and almost anything that pulls up from the waist. Not only do these make for easy breastfeeding but they allow you to feed in public without showing everything. Clothes that do up in front are fine for breastfeeding at home when you don't need to be discreet. If you're wearing a blouse when you're out, pull it up to feed rather than undoing the buttons.

Some women alter existing clothes to make them more suitable. Make sure you have several changes of clothes to wear over the weeks or months of breastfeeding because nothing is more depressing than being in the same things day after day. There are lots of pretty nighties which undo in front.

Anything new should be easily washable because, apart from your milk leaking, your baby may bring up small amounts of milk and dry-cleaning bills can mount up quickly with a new baby in the house.

FURNITURE AND EQUIPMENT

You'll probably want your baby near you so that you can hear him, so you'll need a crib, a cot on wheels, a carrycot or a pram to use downstairs. Similarly, if you want your baby by your bed at night for easy feeding, it's a good idea to have a readily movable cot. You can now buy a cot with a removable side so that the level of the baby's mattress is level with your bed. This makes it easy to slip him into your bed for a feed and back again (see page 451). Babies sleep anywhere if they are tired, warm and have a full tummy, and in the early days, well before they are old enough to roll over or wriggle and fall, they can sleep on a sofa or easy chair. However, this isn't always a good idea. Your baby may sick up some milk on to the upholstery; someone may accidentally sit on him; a pet is more likely to interfere with him; and the day will come when he'll be able to roll for the first time. Some sort of cot is safer for the times when he isn't sleeping in your arms.

Some baby books talk about buying a special nursing chair. You may think this sounds like a waste of money. However, a comfortable place to breastfeed is a very real help, as it's all too easy to end up after a feed with aching shoulders and arms if you aren't relaxed. The chair needs to be low so your lap is flat to support the baby and you'll find it more comfortable if your elbows are well supported, for example by cushions at the right height. Experiment before you have the baby. A rocking chair is often pleasant and many women find that they are most comfortable sitting on a sofa or bed with their feet up. Lying down to feed is the most relaxing of all!

SHOPPING AND HOUSEWORK

Store as much food as you can before you have your baby. Stock up with tinned and dried food and if you have a freezer fill it with prepared meals so you and your partner can rustle something up quickly if you are too tired to cook. Convenience food is a great help early on although of course it's better to eat fresh food when possible.

If you can afford it, buy stocks of things such as washing powder, disposable nappies or terry-nappy sterilizing solution, and ordinary household goods. Shopping with a very young baby can be a headache as he may want feeding so often that there isn't much time to be out for long. You might like to find out whether any local shops deliver, though this seems to be a dying service these days. Your partner could go late-night shopping, or a relative or neighbour might do some shopping for you until your baby is old enough to last longer between feeds.

A great revelation to first-time mothers is the amount of laundry one small baby generates. It's worth preparing for this well in advance. If you don't have a washing machine, see if you can possibly afford one now as it'll make all the difference, especially if you use terry nappies. Otherwise think about sending bed linen, towels and other big things to a laundry for the first few weeks. This is especially important if you come home after forty-eight hours as you may soil bed linen in the first few days. Washing nappies without a machine will tire you in the early days, so buy a few boxes of disposable ones for this time, even if you intend eventually to use terry ones. You may find they're too expensive to use after the first week or so but they'll give you an easy start.

HELP AT HOME

When you're back home with your new baby, you'll need to take things easily for a few weeks. This will be much simpler if you have someone to help you in the house. This is even more helpful with a second or third baby because there's more work with a family of this size. If you haven't any willing relatives nearby, you might want to pay for the luxury of domestic help for an hour or two each day. Many husbands (or partners) take a week or two off work to help out, especially if there are other children. Whatever happens, you'll need time if you are to breastfeed successfully, especially at first when the baby needs very frequent feeds, so don't put yourself in the role of superwoman.

NIPPLE AND BREAST CARE

The advice often given to expectant mothers about how to care for their breasts and nipples has done a lot to put many off the whole business of breastfeeding. The average modern woman doesn't want to push and poke her breasts and nipples about for months before the baby's even born!

There's no convincing evidence from surveys that any ante-natal preparation – such as rolling nipples, rubbing them with a rough towel, putting on lanolin, cream or alcohol, expressing colostrum, and so on – does any good at all! For example, rolling nipples doesn't increase breastfeeding success. The only reason for doing it might be to make your nipples less sensitive but that will happen anyway once your baby starts feeding. It can also be useful if you are one of those women who are not used to having their breasts handled. We look at this more in Chapter 15.

Some women go without their bra or cut a small hole in the centre of each bra cup to allow their nipples to rub against their clothing and become less sensitive. Rubbing nipples with a rough towel after a bath not only seems rather hard on them but also hasn't been shown to do any good.

Having said this, some women are so squeamish and unfamiliar with their breasts that were it not for some sort of breast prep-aration they might not breastfeed because of their reluctance to handle their breasts. In this case familiarizing themselves with their breasts by ante-natal preparation might 'decondition' them and thus enable them to breastfeed.

However, three things *are* worth talking about:

1. Nipple shape

Some women's nipples don't stick out but are **flat** or **inverted** (turned inwards). This is because the milk ducts are short and tether the nipples down. Some ante-natal clinic staff routinely look at pregnant women's nipples to see if they are poorly shaped. However, if nipples are flat or inverted it's no good just looking – they must do the **pinch test** for their advice to be worthwhile.

You can do this test yourself. Pinch your areola between your finger and thumb to see if the nipple comes out. If it does, it's unlikely your baby will have any difficulty. Also, if your nipples usually come out when you feel cold or sexy, you shouldn't have a problem.

Between 7 and 10 per cent of pregnant women who want to breastfeed have either truly inverted nipples (ones that won't come out at all) or **poorly protractile** nipples (which don't come out much). However, nipple shape and protractility often improve spontaneously in pregnancy, probably because of the action of oestrogens on the tissues behind the nipple.

Some women with poorly protractile nipples have a problem breastfeeding and inverted or poorly protractile nipples are said to hinder one woman in twenty feeding her first baby, one in fifty feeding a second, and none who have fed two or more. However, a great many manage perfectly well, especially if a skilled carer helps them position their babies and reminds them not to limit the number or length of breastfeeds, or give bottles of formula.

— A study in 1995 looked at 463 pregnant women in England and Canada who intended to breastfeed and had inverted or 'non-protractile' (not protruding half a centimetre with the pinch test) nipples. The women were divided into four groups: one doing Hoffman's nipple exercises twice a day, one wearing breast shells each day, one using both exercises and shells, and one using neither. The researchers found that 45 per cent of the women in each group were still breastfeeding at six weeks after childbirth. There was no evidence that either doing nipple exercises or wearing breast shells was certain to increase the chances of breastfeeding at six weeks. Worryingly, many of the women reported that their advisers had actively discouraged them from breastfeeding. Health professionals should certainly encourage women with inverted nipples to breast-feed if they wish, as the results in this study underline.

Some people think **breast shells** help inverted or poorly protrac-tile nipples, though no studies so far have shown that they do. Breast shells are hollow, made of plastic or glass, and saucer-shaped, with a circular hole on the inner surface for the nipple to come through. Wearing shells inside a bra is supposed to press the nipples through the holes and gradually improve their shape.

If your doctor or nurse advises breast shells, wear them if you want, though nipples which improve with shells probably would have done well on their own in pregnancy anyway.

When ordering or buying breast shells, you may have to ask for *breast shields*. We call them breast shells to differentiate them clearly from nipple shields, and they are widely known as shells. Even more confusingly, some people in the US call them 'milk cups'. Also in the US you can buy a different sort of breast shell (made by Medela) – one with numerous openings on the rounded dome to allow more air to circulate around the skin.

Breast shells are probably more useful after a baby is born, when using them for a short while before a feed helps poorly protractile nipples protrude enough for him to get a good mouthful. After a few seconds the nipple returns to its original shape, so the baby has to catch hold fairly quickly. The disadvantage is that the pressure of the shell can obstruct milk ducts and increase the risk of engorgement. Also, the skin under the shell can become moist and swollen and more liable to soreness and cracks.

Avent Niplettes (see page 449) are relatively new suction devices which look like little clear plastic thimbles. Devised by a plastic surgeon, they are said to help bring out inverted or flat nipples by encouraging short milk ducts to lengthen.

If you have inverted or poorly protractile nipples and would like to try Niplettes, you hold one on your nipple, then use the syringe (which you've already attached to a valve on the Niplette) to suck out some of the air between nipple and Niplette and make a vacuum. When the nipple comes out, you let go of the Niplette and remove the syringe. You can leave the Niplette on all day under loose clothing, and overnight if you wish – either as well as during the day or instead. When your nipples fill the Niplettes, you can gradually stop wearing them. Two to three months of use should lead to a permanent result. Niplettes are designed to be used during pregnancy, not while breastfeeding.

— A small trial found that each of nineteen women with inverted nipples (six of them pregnant) who used Niplettes had normal-looking nipples after two weeks' use. They all found them easy to use. These figures look good, though more research is needed before Niplettes can be recommended with confidence.

2. Nipple cleanliness

The tiny protuberances called Montgomery's tubercles around the areola secrete an oily fluid which keeps the areola and nipple supple and kills bacteria. If you wash this away with soap, your skin is much more likely to become sore when you breastfeed. Avoid using soap for the last few weeks of pregnancy and wash your nipples only with warm water.

There's no need to use any ointment or cream on your nipples to prepare for breastfeeding because nature's own lubrication is best. Similarly, there's no need to remove the yellowish grains of dried secretions you may see on them. A simple water splash is enough.

3. Expressing milk

There's no need to express milk ante-natally to remove colostrum or 'clear the ducts', as was once advised. However, it may be worth learning the technique of expressing now, because it could be useful later (see page 189 for details).

So, in summary, all you need do when you're pregnant is wash your nipples with water; practise the technique of expression to save you learning later; and, if your nipples are poorly protractile, consider using breast shells.

With everything prepared for breastfeeding you can look forward to your baby's birth. The next chapter will show you how to manage from the very first few minutes after birth.

SEVEN

The early days

This chapter is about breastfeeding your newborn baby, whether you've given birth in hospital or at home.

CHILDBIRTH

A good midwife or obstetrician is a reliable one who stands back while women labour and intervenes only if necessary.

There's mounting evidence that labour in an upright position is safer for babies and easier for women. Women are also less likely to need pain-killing drugs or an episiotomy.

Why is this important for breastfeeding? Because the better a woman feels after her labour, the easier it is for breastfeeding to get off to a good start.

Pain-killers in labour

If a woman has the pain-killing drug pethidine late in the second stage of her labour, it will tend to make her baby sleepy. This may interfere with breastfeeds for the first day or two. With a difficult feeder on their hands some women become dispirited and give up breastfeeding, but there are ways of coping (see page 332 for some ideas).

— Swedish researchers (1995) found that babies whose mothers had had pethidine didn't suck or root (search for the nipple) as quickly or as well as others. They pointed out that the babies may have been exhausted both by a difficult labour and by pethidine. And they recommended that such a baby needs longer than a non-pethidine-exposed baby to get going with the first breastfeed.

So if you need pain relief when your labour has progressed quite a long way, it's better from the point of view of making a good start with breastfeeding if you choose one or more other methods of pain relief. These include breathing gas and air, having mild electro-stimulation of the lower back with a TeNS (transcutaneous electrical nerve stimulation) machine, and a light, rapid 'butterfly' massage towards the bottom of your spine by your birth companion.

THE FIRST FEW MINUTES

The moment of birth comes after nine months' waiting and preparation and possibly many hours of hard labour. Not surprisingly, most women are relieved, excited and tired. Pride in having produced a baby that a few hours ago was nothing more than a wriggling bump mingles with fatigue, curiosity and elation. A few are so exhausted that all they can think of is having a rest.

If all is well, you'll be able to hold your baby for a time before the routine weighing, washing and labelling. While you're having a cuddle, the staff will stand by while your placenta is delivered, and do any necessary stitching. It takes a single-minded woman to put her baby to the breast amidst all this but it's a good idea if you can. Some women find that immediate suckling seems the most natural thing to do. Others are not really sure and feel awkward if the baby seems disinterested, as some are at first.

WHY EARLY SUCKLING IS A GOOD IDEA

The oxytocin a woman produces when she puts her baby to the breast the first time makes her womb contract, which helps to expel the placenta and reduce bleeding. Early suckling means you may not need a routine injection of Syntometrine (oxytocin plus ergometrine) to make your womb contract, dislodge the placenta and push it out. Some doctors suspect that the ergometrine in Syntometrine sometimes reduces a woman's milk supply.

— A study in Singapore (1994) found that breastfeeding immediately after birth makes the womb contract nearly as much as an oxytocin injection would.

If you put your baby to the breast before the cord is cut, your womb contractions give the baby an extra helping of blood and increase his iron stores. Your midwife or doctor need not cut the cord until the placenta has separated.

Another good reason for early suckling is that a baby's sucking reflex is strongest in the first thirty minutes after birth. After this many babies become tired and disinterested for forty hours or so before they're keen to suck again.

Your placenta may take up to half an hour to come out and during this time you can be getting to know your baby. Many women aren't a bit sleepy and want to be with their baby. Most studies agree that being with her baby at this time makes a woman more likely to breastfeed successfully and for longer. A woman is more likely to sleep well later if she has time to cuddle and suckle her baby and isn't anxious about where he is and what's happening.

Have a good look at your baby and enjoy your first meeting. You may not feel an instant rush of motherly love – indeed, this often takes time to come – but you'll probably be curious to examine and touch your baby. Newborn babies have a very distinctive smell which many mothers find delightful.

PUTTING YOUR BABY TO THE BREAST THE FIRST TIME

Let your baby nuzzle your breast and feed if he wants to. Don't be discouraged if he isn't very interested. He doesn't know what to do yet but when he tastes the sweetness of your colostrum he'll probably be much keener!

Interestingly, some newborn babies left naked on their mother's naked tummy eventually somehow wriggle up to find the breast of their own accord.

Studies in France and England have found that a baby turns to a pad that has been placed next to his mother's breast in preference to a clean one which has no milk on it and has not been in contact with the breast. It is the contact of the pad with the breast that is most important because babies don't turn to pads soaked in their mother's expressed breast milk. Babies prefer the smell of their own mother's breast to that of other mothers. And one study showed that twenty-two out of thirty babies preferred the smell of their mother's breast when it hadn't been washed.

Just what it is on the mother's breast that produces this unique recognition isn't known but it could be the smell of natural hormone-like chemicals called pheromones known to be vital in animal recognition systems.

Sadly, bottle-fed babies like the smell of a pad soaked in breast milk from another mother better than that of a pad soaked in their usual milk formula.

If you're lying down

Roll on one side and lay your baby on his side by you so that his head faces the breast. Stroke his lower lip with your nipple until he opens his mouth wide and moves it towards the breast. This searching movement is called *rooting* and is a natural reflex in newborn babies. Don't hold or push his head or he'll turn towards the pressure of your hand.

Some babies get excited and lick the nipple, others just hold it in their mouths and don't suck until later. Many aren't in any hurry and simply want to gaze at their mothers.

If you're sitting up

Hold your baby in one arm with your hand under his bottom, making sure you're comfortable, preferably with your elbow supported. Tuck your baby's lower arm around your side to keep it out of the way if necessary, and hold your breast from underneath if it helps, but don't lift or squeeze it. Then stroke his lower lip with your nipple and continue as above.

Don't worry if you don't automatically know what to do. This is normal, especially if it's your first baby. Studies of animals show that they too need time and experience to become good mothers and some zoo animals need to be taught by male keepers!

So far we've talked about the average woman who's had a normal labour. This doesn't always happen though, and we'll talk about the mother who has had a Caesarean section or other problems in Chapter 13.

What happens next? Ideally, if you, your partner and baby are content, the staff will leave you together for half an hour or so. You can have a wash and put on some clean clothes afterwards. It won't be long before you can feed your baby again and start becoming expert.

MORE TIPS ON HOLDING YOUR BABY

Make yourselves comfortable because you'll be feeding for some time. Let your baby's head rest on your arm and try supporting his weight on a pillow on your lap, rather than taking the weight on your arm, which might make your back and shoulders ache. If you're relaxed you'll let your milk down more readily.

Position yourselves so it's as easy as possible for the baby to 'latch on' (take your nipple and some of the areola into his mouth). If you're sitting, it's easier if you're upright and perhaps leaning forward slightly. Your baby's chest and tummy should face your body so that he doesn't have to turn his head as he feeds. He may like something to hold – your finger will do – and he'll let go when he's had enough to drink.

Don't push your baby's mouth on to your breast or the rooting reflex will make the baby turn towards your hand instead. Continue stroking his bottom lip with your nipple until he opens his mouth really wide. (If you tickle his upper lip, he won't open his mouth as widely, and tickling both lips also seems to be confusing. Some babies show a strong rooting reflex even when a sheet or some clothing touches them near their mouth.)

Quickly offer your breast and if he latches on well his lips should splay out around a large mouthful of breast.

If your breast is very big you may have to hold it back so that it doesn't obstruct his nostrils, but be careful not to squeeze it too much in case you obstruct the underlying milk ducts. However, you don't need to hold your breast when your baby is feeding unless it's easier, in which case support it gently from underneath with the flat of your upturned hand, without lifting or squeezing as this might distort the milk ducts. If your breast is tense and full, express a little milk (see page 189) before you begin so as to soften it enough to make latching on easier.

LATCHING ON

Your baby needs to latch on not only to your nipple but also to some of your areola so that he can 'milk' the reservoirs under the areola by moving his tongue in strong muscular waves. If he takes only the nipple into his mouth, he'll 'nipple-suck', which means he'll get only the milk he can suck from the reservoirs or swallow when it's spurting or flowing fast. When he realizes he isn't getting enough he'll suck more strongly, which will make your nipple sore. Another problem with nipple-sucking is that it doesn't stimulate the breast well enough, which could mean you won't make enough milk.

If a baby is well positioned at the breast, someone standing by will be able to see more of your areola above the baby's upper lip than below his lower lip. In order to milk the breast efficiently, the baby's lower jaw needs to be tucked right in, well towards your chest. If it isn't, his lower jaw will be tipped away from the breast and an observer will see more of your areola below his lower lip, instead of more above his upper lip.

If he finds it difficult to latch on, try holding your breast between finger and thumb (or index and middle fingers) so as to make the nipple and areola a little easier to latch on to. Don't squeeze hard, though, or you'll obstruct the milk ducts, and release this hold as soon as he starts feeding well.

As he latches on, aim your nipple up towards his nose. This helps ensure it's high in his mouth and won't get hurt as he sucks.

WATCHING YOUR BABY FEED

You may notice your baby doesn't feed continuously, like a bottle-fed baby, but every so often takes short pauses between bouts of sucking. This is because let-down milk spurts into the ducts and from the nipple in an uneven flow. After several spurts there's a short pause before they begin again. Your baby is simply adapting to your milk flow.

Some babies suck on and off for long periods, perhaps falling asleep every few minutes, only starting to take more 'forced' feeds when they're older and much stronger.

One researcher noted that newborn infants 'write their signature with their sucking rhythm', showing a constant, individual pattern in the number of sucks and in the intervals between sucks per minute. This helps explain why some babies take longer over a feed than others.

Generally, 'nutritive' sucking (sucking to get milk) is slower (one suck per second) and stronger than 'non-nutritive', comfort sucking (when the baby sucks for comfort or pleasure and swallows very little). A baby sucks less strongly when doing non-nutritive sucking. However, both nutritive and non-nutritive sucking are important to stimulate milk production and further let-downs of milk.

TRYING DIFFERENT POSITIONS

You can breastfeed your baby comfortably while you are sitting, lying on one side, or standing (though this isn't as comfy as sitting because you have to support all his weight unless you're clever with a babysling). As you get used to breastfeeding, you can experiment at leisure and in private with different feeding positions (see also page 309).

WRAPPING YOUR BABY

If your baby goes to sleep after a feed and you want to put him down, wrap him snugly in a shawl or piece of soft material (though make sure he doesn't get too hot). This way he's less likely to wake with a start. Towards the end of pregnancy the walls of your womb held him fairly tightly; being snugly wrapped probably reminds him of the security of the womb. Certainly babies carried next to their mothers in the firm hold of a sling seem to like it.

RELAXING AND ENJOYING YOUR BABY

Relaxing as you feed helps you enjoy your baby. If you're happier with curtains drawn around your bed, ask someone to draw them. Be encouraged by positive comments, but if anyone says something negative about your breastfeeding, listen but tell them calmly that you've all the time in the world to learn.

Your newborn baby may stare at you fixedly from the breast from time to time, or even all the time. Having a baby gazing up at you is a wonderful feeling, so take time to admire and stroke him. It's all too easy to be so intent on doing everything 'properly' that you don't enjoy these early experiences of being so close.

You may sometimes like to hold your naked baby close to your naked body to feed him, with the room warm and nappies in strategic places to soak up leaks from both of you!

You may also like to cuddle, wash and even feed him while you are having a bath. Hold him securely and he'll probably like it much better than being in a baby bath. Make sure the room is warm and the water is at a suitable temperature and ask your partner to come and take him when you're ready.

Some women enjoy massaging their babies all over with warm oil and their babies enjoy it too, but remember it's safest to do it on a towel on the floor where your baby's oily body can't come to any harm if it slips between your fingers.

The important thing to remember is that there are no limits to the time you and your baby can spend together. Babies thrive on lots of body contact, love and attention.

WHAT'S YOUR BABY GETTING?

At first your baby gets only colostrum. A baby can safely go for the first few days without much to drink as nature intended him to have only small amounts. It's meant to be this way and even very small volumes are worth their weight in gold. So valuable is colostrum in protecting newborn babies against infection (among other things) that some experts believe every bottle-fed baby should have a 'colostrum cocktail'. Farmers have been giving them to their valuable calves for years. Don't doubt your ability to nourish your baby in these first few days. Your colostrum may not look much but cows' milk formula, in however large a volume, cannot compare for goodness.

Colostrum's higher protein level enables many new-born babies to last longer between feeds than they do when mature milk comes in. This may be nature's way of ensuring that newly delivered women have a chance to sleep.

Colostrum changes into mature milk during the first few days but there's no sudden alteration. The phrase 'the milk coming in' is misleading as it leads some people to think the breasts are empty until this happens – which, of course, they aren't. The more a baby feeds, the sooner the breasts produce large amounts of milk. When this happens it's known as the milk 'coming in'. Women who've had more than one baby find their milk comes in sooner than with their firstborns. A woman who feeds her baby frequently may find that her milk comes in on the second or third day. If she feeds infrequently, it may not come in for four or five days. The sooner your milk comes in, the sooner your baby will have plenty to drink.

When you express milk you may sometimes see different coloured drops at the nipple. Some are creamy-white, some thinner and bluish-white and some halfway between. This is because the composition of milk changes according to whether it's expressed early or late in a feed (see page 18). Different milk reservoirs under the areola are emptied at different rates, depending on the baby's position. Sometimes the milk in one reservoir is a different colour from that in other reservoirs, because the gland it drains may not have been completely emptied at the previous feed. This means that at the same time you may see drops of bluish-white, thin, low-fat fore-milk; thicker, creamy-white, high-fat hind-milk;

and milk which is somewhere between the two owing to mixing of the milk in the ducts and reservoirs.

Usually at the beginning of a feed most drops are of fore-milk, while towards the end most are hind-milk. If the breast wasn't emptied completely during a feed, then at the beginning of the next one you'll see drops containing hind-milk (remaining in the reservoirs since the previous feed), perhaps diluted slightly with fore-milk pushed into the elastic-walled reservoirs since the previous feed.

Yet another reason for different-coloured drops is that some of the fifteen to twenty milk ducts from the milk glands may merge within the nipple, so there may be fewer openings at the nipple than there are glands, ducts and reservoirs. If one gland was emptied more thoroughly than another at the last feed and if their ducts merge in the nipple, you may see milk coming from that duct halfway in colour between fore-milk and hind-milk.

HOW OFTEN SHOULD YOU FEED?

Feed your baby on an unrestricted basis – whenever he cries; when he seems to want feeding; when your breasts are full; and more often still if you want to (see below). *Don't* count how many feeds you give or feed on any sort of schedule. The more schedule-feeding there's been this century, the less successful breastfeeding there's been.

Studies strongly suggest that women who breastfeed in an unrestricted way not only produce more milk and continue breastfeeding for more months than schedule-feeding women, but are also less likely to develop sore nipples. Their babies put on more weight and are less likely to become jaundiced.

Breast milk is so well digested that it stays in the baby's stomach for a maximum of an hour and a half (compared with nearly two and a half hours for formula), which is partly why breastfed babies need frequent feeds, usually every one and a half to three hours.

Many people speak of breastfeeding on demand – when a baby 'demands' a feed by crying – but this isn't really a very useful term. Demand-feeding can work well but is sometimes a disaster. This is because some babies don't ask for enough feeds, so they don't give the breasts the stimulation they need to make milk. As a result the supply dwindles. Demand-feeding is better than schedule-feeding. But it isn't as good as the successful, natural way of breastfeeding which meets both mother's and baby's needs and desires (see below).

— A large UK survey (1990) found that one in ten mothers said they had to feed at set times in hospital. However, this is an improvement on the 19 per cent who had to feed at set times in 1985.

Women who feed on an unrestricted basis aren't concerned when their babies want more feeds some days than others – they simply give them what they want, trusting their baby to know what's best for him.

Some babies, though, need reminding that the breast is there before they ask for feeds. The smell of your skin and milk can help. Other feeding triggers are your body's sounds – your voice, heartbeat and tummy rumbles, as well as the sight and feel of you. A baby left alone in his cot has only his empty tummy to remind him of you and your breasts, which isn't always enough, especially if he was born early or is jaundiced, ill, or apathetic (for example, because you had pethidine in labour). Keep your baby with you as much as possible, either lying in your arms as you sit up, lying beside you as you sit or lie in bed, or held in your arms or a sling as you do things. The stimulation from being with you should encourage him to ask for more feeds and to be alert enough to take them.

Growth spurts (see also page 267)

Babies may suddenly want more feeds because they are entering a growth spurt – a time when they need more milk because they are growing faster. Common ages for growth spurts are three weeks, six weeks and three months, though they may occur at any time, depending on the individual baby. Don't think that because your baby suddenly seems dissatisfied this must mean you don't have enough milk. You may very temporarily not meet his needs but two or three days of extra feeds will boost your supply.

Lots of babies go through stages lasting anything from a day or two to several weeks when they prefer to spend what seems like much of their waking time at the breast. Sometimes this corresponds with a need to increase the milk supply, for example during a growth spurt, or after a cold or other illness when your milk supply may have fallen because of having fewer feeds.

Check you aren't putting him down immediately after each feed. If you do, he'll soon learn the only way to stay near you is to breastfeed. Try carrying him in a sling so he is lulled by being next to you – you can easily do things like shopping, housework and cooking with it on.

He'll be so very dependent on you only for a short part of his life. Whether you enjoy this dependency or hate it depends partly on your expectations and attitude. Experienced mothers and psychologists agree that babies given as much time as they want at the breast, and being cuddled or carried a lot, are more independent as toddlers and older children than babies whose mothers rationed their time and attention.

Carry out a time-and-motion analysis of your day and find more ways of playing with your baby. Women whose previous jobs were highly organized may find it difficult to relax and some come to enjoy their new profession of motherhood only with their second or third baby. Don't waste these early months with your first baby. Settle down, guilt-free, and run your new life as a proud mother, not someone who sees her baby as an encumbrance and a hindrance in life. So what if you never seem to finish what you're doing! Do it in several stages throughout the day instead, as millions of other women have learnt to do.

If you find feeding so frequently unpleasant, irritating or

intolerable, you may be able to persuade your baby to take fewer feeds (see page 336).

Successful breastfeeding

You'll be well on your way to breastfeeding successfully, for as long as you want, if you know you don't have to wait until your baby cries before you breastfeed him. You can feed him when:

- He seems ready (perhaps because he's fidgety or nuzzling your breast).
- Your breasts are full and you want the pressure relieved.
- You're about to go out.
- He's jaundiced, affected by drugs in labour, ill, pre-term, small-for-dates, or apathetic for some reason – and unlikely to ask for a feed.
- You want to.

The only time to watch the clock is if your baby doesn't ask for feeds very often. Even if he's sound asleep it's probably better not to leave a young baby unfed for more than three hours at the longest. Too many longer gaps could endanger your milk supply and mean he doesn't get enough. Some babies go four to five hours between some feeds but this isn't generally sensible in the early days until you are more confident with breastfeeding and your milk supply is well established.

Babies gain weight better with frequent feeds because these stimulate their mothers' breasts to produce more milk. Suckling also stimulates the development of prolactin receptors in the breast. These attract prolactin from the breast's blood supply and allow it to get to work making milk.

The number of feeds each day – This varies according to each mother-baby pair and depends on:

- A baby's preferences and needs.
- A woman's culture, lifestyle, preferences and needs.
- The maturity of the milk – in the first few days babies may not want many feeds, partly because colostrum's relatively high protein level

is very satisfying – but they need more frequent feeds of mature milk.

- The milk capacity of the breasts.
- Whether a baby gets enough hind-milk (if not, he'll be hungry sooner).
- Whether a baby is allowed to go to the breast for comfort (non-nutritive suckling) as well as for milk (nutritive suckling).
- How strongly a baby sucks and milks the breast. (The more vigorously he does so, the more prolactin – and therefore the more milk – his mother makes.) However, a baby who doesn't suck and milk very strongly may simply get what he needs by taking longer over each feed. The exception is a baby who is is small or poorly, doesn't have the energy to take long over a feed and so needs more frequent feeds instead.
- Whether he is well positioned at the breast so he can suck and milk the breast optimally (and therefore stimulate his mother's prolactin and milk supply well).

It isn't a good idea to compare yourself with other breastfeeding women because while it may be interesting to know how many feeds someone else gives, the danger is that you'll compete over whose baby lasts longest between feeds. This is one reason why many women breastfeed more successfully if they go home soon after delivery.

Some women feed their babies as many as thirty to forty times in twenty-four hours (in some cultures mainly in the evening and night), others as few as six. However, six times a day gives the breasts very little stimulation; five usually makes the milk supply fail; eight is probably the absolute minimum for young babies; and almost all young babies need more. One distinguished American paediatrician says that giving at least twelve feeds a day helps prevent jaundice.

Babies also need different numbers of feeds from day to day, depending on how they're feeling, how fast they're growing, and how well they are.

To help put frequent feeding into perspective, remember that until your baby was born he was 'fed' continuously by your placenta. In fact a breastfed baby of under nine months has been dubbed 'an extero-gestate fetus', implying that he is so immature that he has to rely on being virtually attached to his mother.

Women differ as to how much breast stimulation they need to make enough milk for their baby, but the vast majority find their milk supply increases if they feed more often (see also Chapter 12). Breastfeeding tends to be much more successful in cultures in which women feed frequently.

Frequent breastfeeding is good news for midwives too.

— Research in an Oxford hospital found the midwives' workload fell dramatically when they no longer misguidedly insisted on schedule-feeding.

Babies allowed completely unrestricted feeds – for example, those carried next to a naked breast all day in developing countries – don't have to cry before they are fed. These babies feed *very much more often* than most Western breastfed babies.

Anthropologists can predict how often any mammal's young need to be suckled by the amount of protein and fat in the milk. If there's a lot (as in cows' and rabbits' milk), the young need infrequent suckling – perhaps only once a day. However, if the milk is low in protein and fat, the young need frequent suckling. Human milk has very little protein and along with other mammals with low-protein milk we are grouped as *'continuous contact mammals'*. Human babies suck on and off much of the time, given the chance, which seems to be what nature intended. We automatically reduce the frequency of feeds our babies ask for by not carrying them next to our naked breasts all day and not sleeping naked next to them at night. But if we make feeds too infrequent, we run the risk of reducing our milk supply through too little breast stimulation. We also run the risk of separating our babies from ourselves so much that we can't give them enough physical and emotional comfort.

WAKING YOUR BABY

Some women worry about waking their baby for feeds during the day. But it's best to do so if it's a long time since a feed, or if your breasts feel full. If you don't wake your baby or express some milk, your breasts will become tense or engorged (badly swollen, see page 302) and your milk production will slow down. You should never go so long between feeds that your breasts feel tense and lumpy. Remember you're a nursing pair – sometimes you'll feed for your baby's benefit and sometimes for yours.

Mothers who breastfeed on an unrestricted basis are only half as likely to get sore nipples and engorged breasts as those of schedule-fed babies (see also pages 302 and 307).

ONE BREAST OR TWO?

When your baby has finished all he wants from the first breast and stops feeding, change to the second, either straight away or after a short break. Try to feed from both breasts in the early days or the unemptied one won't produce as much milk as it could. This is partly because of the pressure of the remaining milk on its milk-producing cells, and partly because there's an as yet un-named hormone in milk which reduces further milk production if some is left behind. (See also page 274.) When your baby finishes what he wants from the first breast, he'll almost certainly stop spontaneously. Don't stop him feeding at the first breast in order to give him the other breast. If you do, then neither breast will be well emptied and you are more likely to become engorged (see page 302).

WHICH BREAST TO START WITH

Don't forget to start the next feed with the breast you last fed from. It's important for the breasts to take turns at being emptied first (see also page 214). The let-down is more efficient early in a breastfeed and a baby sucks more strongly at the first breast. This means that the first breast is usually emptied better than the second.

Some women find that they or their babies prefer feeding from one side. This is often the left side. It has been suggested that the sound of the mother's heartbeat (which is on the left) soothes her baby. Most women have one breast which is bigger than the other. If the difference is mainly caused by fat, their babies may find it easier to feed from the smaller one, but if the difference is in the amount of glandular tissue, their babies may prefer the larger one. Some women only ever feed from one side – such as the Tanka boat-women in Hong Kong, mentioned in Chapter 5, who feed only from their right breast.

HOW LONG SHOULD FEEDS LAST?

Let your baby feed until he's had enough. Different babies feed for different times, depending on:

- How hungry they are.
- How strongly they suck and milk the breast.
- Whether they have one breast or two – and whether they have several goes at each.
- How much they need the comfort of being at the breast (non-nutritive suckling, page 169).
- How fast their mother's milk flows.

Any one baby takes different-length feeds at different times too. Babies, like adults, want different amounts of food from day to day and at different times of the day. Sometimes a baby wants a snack, at other times a feast. Research in southern Africa shows that a baby feeding on demand takes feeds of very different volumes at different times. Sometimes one feed is ten times as big as another. Some women's milk flows faster than others, and their babies tend to get what they need sooner. Some babies finish their feeds very quickly because they suck and milk the breast so enthusiastically and strongly, stimulate several let-downs in quick succession and quickly get the milk they need. Gentler or weaker babies may run out of steam sooner and have to wait a while before they have the energy to suck hard enough to stimulate another let-down of milk. You may be able to help by stimulating a let-down yourself by massaging your breasts as if you wanted to express some milk.

You may be told, wrongly, to feed your baby for a specified number of minutes each side and to increase this time each day until the fifth day when you'll be 'allowed' ten minutes a side!

This restriction of feed length is completely unnatural. It hinders milk from coming in; may not give your let-down reflex time to work and become established; prevents your baby from getting as much colostrum as he could; and makes sore nipples more likely.

This has all been known for years but a few hospitals still insist on out-of-date rules. If you're not the sort of person to question rules openly, especially when you've just had a baby, and as long as your nipples aren't sore (see page 307), go ahead and suckle as long as you and your baby want.

— UK researchers reported in 1981 that eighty out of 100 women who decided for themselves how long feeds should be were still breastfeeding at the end of the first week, compared with fifty-seven out of 100 women who'd been told how long to feed.

HOW TO TELL WHEN HE'S HAD ENOUGH

Many babies show they've had enough and are ready to stop a feed by falling asleep and coming off the breast; others come off while still awake. A baby nearing the end of a feed may relax his fists, smile, or arch his back. Accept your baby's judgement of how much he needs. After a while you'll get to know how much he's had by feeling your breasts. Lots of babies, especially in the evening or if they are pre-term, like to have frequent small feeds with short gaps of, for example, ten to fifteen minutes, or to doze on and off during a feed. This can make it difficult to know when they've had enough. See also page 264.

WHAT ABOUT STOPPING A FEED?

Some babies have to be gently removed from the breast or they'd be there all day. If your nipples are sore you may need to limit his time at the breast for a day or two. But don't do this for too long unless you express some milk after each feed to give your breasts more stimulation, or your milk supply will diminish.

Never pull your baby's mouth away from the breast while he's feeding as this could damage your nipple as it breaks the strong vacuum in the baby's mouth. It's better to put the tip of your little finger gently into the corner of his mouth and push the nipple sideways to allow some air in. Your baby will then come away easily without hurting you.

ROOMING-IN

It's best if your baby 'rooms-in' – stays by your bed day and night – and the good news in the UK is that increasing numbers of hospitals now facilitate this practice.

— Large surveys in the UK showed that rooming-in increased from 17 per cent of mother–baby pairs in 1980, to 47 per cent in 1985 and 63 per cent in 1990.

Most women sleep better and are more content with their babies beside them. Studies show that women who have their babies with them are twice as likely to breastfeed successfully as those whose babies go to a nursery at night.

It's wise to sleep with your baby in your bed only if you did not have pain-killing drugs in labour (as these might make you sleep too deeply to prevent you from rolling on him), if you're not a smoker, and if you can put your bed's 'cot sides' up or position a heavy chair by the side of your bed where your baby is lying so as to prevent him from falling out.

In general it's fair to say that no hospital can possibly have enough staff to give a baby the kind of love and care his mother can, so it's scarcely surprising that babies who room-in are more contented than those who stay in nurseries and visit their mothers only occasionally.

Even if you're in a large, open-plan ward, you can have your baby by you at night, provided you pick him up as soon as he needs a cuddle or feed to avoid waking other mothers. Rooming-in makes life easier for staff and pleasanter for mothers and babies, and leads to less noise because babies don't have to cry for long, if at all, to get attention. And women sleep better because they don't worry about whether their babies are crying unattended in the nursery or being given bottles.

Many women have described the agony they went through when they could hear crying yet weren't allowed to be with their babies. A woman doesn't know the sound of her own baby's voice this soon after birth and may worry that it's her baby every time any baby cries. She'll have far more peace of mind if she's with him. And her milk will come in far sooner if she picks him up for a feed not only whenever he cries but also whenever she wants to.

If you'd like your baby with you at night and there's no good reason for him not to be, but the hospital staff aren't keen and you're too tired to be assertive, ask your partner to have a word.

— In a very large survey (1990) as many as 37 per cent of mothers said they had been separated from their babies in hospitals. However, this was an improvement on the 1985 figure of 53 per cent.

— A Swedish survey (1984) found that at three months old, only 37 per cent of babies who had been separated from their mothers for between one and six days (because of jaundice or other usually minor problems) were being breastfed, compared with 72 per cent of those who had been with their mothers all the time.

BREAST MILK ONLY

If your baby has to be apart from you for some reason, make sure the staff know you want him brought to you for feeding as soon as he cries, and that you don't want him to be given anything to drink, even water or sugar water – except in the unlikely event of it being medically essential, for example, if your baby has a low blood-sugar which doesn't respond to frequent breastfeeding (see page 363).

Giving breastfed babies anything other than breast milk is unnecessary for the vast majority. It's also unacceptable as it can interfere with the establishment of successful breastfeeding. Don't be fobbed off with excuses. He's your baby and, as we explained earlier in this chapter, the best way to establish breastfeeding is to feed frequently and on an unrestricted basis. If he has anything else to drink he won't want to breastfeed as often as he otherwise would, and unless you express your milk frequently to make up for him wanting relatively few feeds, your milk supply will diminish.

Unfortunately, the staff and administrators of some hospital maternity units are so out of date that breastfeeding mothers are routinely given bottles of formula to 'top up' their babies after a feed.

— A large British survey (1990) found that as many as 45 per cent of breastfed babies received bottles of formula while in hospital! This is slightly better than the equivalent figure in 1985 of 50 per cent but it is still vastly higher than desirable or necessary. The stark reality is that mothers who give their breastfed babies bottles of formula are much more likely than others to give up breastfeeding before they are ready.

If someone asks why *your* baby is not allowed to drink formula, sugar water or boiled water at night, when other babies have it and seem all right, reply that there are many reasons why breast milk alone is best for almost every baby.

Here's a list of why breast milk alone is nearly always best

1 The more your baby feeds, the sooner your milk will come in.
2 Frequent breastfeeds help you make plenty of milk.
3 Colostrum gives your baby the nutrients he needs in the correct proportions, supplies him with protective antibodies and other substances not present in formula, and encourages his bowel to expel its sticky first motions (meconium).
4 Formula satiates a baby's appetite for several hours, making him less likely to want to breastfeed. This, in turn, reduces breast stimulation and may decrease the milk supply. Bottle-fed babies go longer between feeds than breastfed babies because it takes longer to digest formula.
5 Formula contains foreign proteins which (especially if your baby has an allergic family history) might sensitize him and increase his risk of allergic disease in later life.
6 Sugar water is nearly always unnecessary for full-term, healthy babies, because breast milk provides all the sugar and water they need. A high-calorie drink would satiate his appetite and make him less likely to want to breastfeed. A sudden slug of sugar is unnatural and best reserved for when medically essential.
7 Properly and exclusively breastfed babies don't need extra water. Breast milk provides enough even in the early days and in hot countries. Research at the University of Rochester in New York showed that breastfed babies given water or cows' milk formula

complements lost more weight in the first few days and were less likely to start gaining before they left hospital than exclusively breastfed babies. (The same went for bottle-fed babies.).

8 It's better for a young baby not to feed from a bottle. A bottle teat is easy to drink from and provides a strong stimulus to suck. A baby used to bottles has to work harder at the breast, which may put him off. If your baby can't breastfeed, or in the unlikely situation that he really needs something extra (for example, if he has a low blood-sugar level that doesn't respond rapidly to more frequent breastfeeds, or excessive weight-loss that doesn't respond to frequent breast-feeds), it's best for him to have whatever he's having from a feeding cup or spoon (or, if very premature, from a tube). Pre-term babies are more likely to have trouble breastfeeding if they've had bottles, as are other low-birth-weight babies, babies whose mothers had a diffi-cult labour, and babies who are unwell. Some women want a baby-sitter to give bottles of expressed breast milk (or formula), so are keen for their babies to get used to the bottle. However, giving occasional bottles (especially to young babies) can interfere with successful breastfeeding, so it's better to wait a few months. Most older babies readily get used to feeding from a cup, if not a bottle.

Some hospitals used to recommend water or sugar water as the first drink for all babies in case they had a congenital abnormality of the windpipe and gullet which made them inhale milk. How-ever, doctors now know that this precaution is unnecessary.

GIVING BOTTLE-FEEDS OF FORMULA AT HOME

The subject of giving your breastfed baby bottles of formula may come up again when you get home – either because you think it might be a good idea or because someone else suggests it.

However, *giving bottle-feeds of formula is nearly always bad news for breastfeeding women and their babies.* They reduce the supply of breast milk because a baby full of formula doesn't want frequent breastfeeds, yet breast stimulation is essential for milk production.

Women who want to breastfeed successfully should not allow

their babies to have formula. As one mother said, 'How can demand and supply work if you suppress half the demand?'

If bottles of formula are recommended because your baby doesn't seem to be thriving, you can almost certainly avoid them simply by increasing your milk supply – for example, by feeding your baby more often (see Chapter 10).

— A large survey in the UK (1990) found that 39 per cent of six-week-old breastfed babies had bottles of formula. In 1980, the figure was 28 per cent; and in 1985, 34 per cent. So as the years go by, more and more six-week-old breastfed babies are getting bottles of formula. Many of these babies undoubtedly have mothers who would have preferred to go on breastfeeding exclusively – which they could have done if only they had been told how and were given enough skilled support and encouragement.

Doctors and midwives may refer to drinks of formula as 'complements' or 'supplements'. Some people make no distinction between them; for others, a complement is a drink – in a bottle or cup – of formula given after a breastfeed; and a supplement is one given instead of a breastfeed.

SLEEPING AND NIGHT FEEDS

During your hospital stay it's best for your baby to be by you at night. It's worth mentally gearing up for night feeds because you'll be doing plenty of them. Night feeds may become less frequent from two months or so onwards but not necessarily so. Many babies continue to want night feeds for a long time.

Young babies have more periods of light, REM (rapid eye movement) sleep than older children and adults and are most likely to wake for a feed during these times. As your baby gets older, he will have longer periods of deeper sleep and wake up up less often.

Try to get as much sleep as you can between feeds, especially in the early days, as you'll probably be tired after giving birth and broken nights take their toll.

The midwives may suggest you rest on your tummy for an hour or so every day. If your breasts are at all full, you can make yourself comfy if you lie with your head on one pillow with another one below your breasts so as to make a sort of bridge.

You may be too excited to sleep much soon after you've had your baby. It's a common feeling to want to live through the birth experience over and over again in your mind, as though you were 'learning' it.

Some mothers dream very little in the first few days or weeks after the birth, probably because their sleep patterns are broken by their babies waking for feeds. Sleeping with your baby by your side means you soon get used to snoozing and resting during breastfeeds, even though you are not properly asleep.

If your baby goes into a nursery at night, make sure you tell the staff on duty each night that you are breastfeeding. Although they should know, it's easy for an inexperienced person, a new agency nurse, or a nurse who thinks she's doing you a favour, to give your baby a bottle of formula, sugar water, or water, along with all the other bottle-fed babies in the nursery. Some women tie a card on their baby's cot saying, 'I am breastfed, please take me to my mother when I cry.' This will probably make it easier for you to get what you want but isn't infallible.

NIPPLE CARE

In the old days the advice on preparing for a feed was so complicated that many women said it was more fiddly than preparing bottles – so they chose bottles. Nipple and breast care is in fact very simple.

There's no need to wash your breasts before a feed. There's no need to wash your breasts after a feed either, though you can rinse them with water if you really want to. When you have a bath, wash your nipples with water, *not* soap. If you put salt in the water to help heal an episiotomy, splash your breasts with plenty of plain water to remove the salt before you dry them. Don't soak your nipples in water as this will make them more likely to become sore and cracked. Nipples readily become soggy and liable to crack if left moist inside a bra. Avoid this by changing breast pads frequently and by leaving your bra off sometimes to give your nipples some air. This is easiest at night.

There's generally no need to put anything on your nipples. Lanolin, cocoa butter, vitamin E oil or special creams such as Mass cream are usually unnecessary as the Montgomery's tubercles around your areolae produce an oily liquid which is naturally protective. Avoid any cream containing peanut oil as this could trigger allergy in the baby. Your baby will prefer to taste you, not anything else. And the smell of your milk will attract your baby when you next put him to the breast. If he's a reluctant feeder, this could make all the difference to his desire to suck.

Many experienced breastfeeders say that expressing a little milk after a breastfeed and rubbing it gently into their nipples helps prevent nipple soreness.

This advice may still sound rather complicated but all you really need do is occasionally wash your breasts, avoid getting soap on your nipples and keep your nipples dry between feeds. That's all.

Nipple soreness and pain

Quite a few women have sore nipples at some time in the first week after giving birth or later. Unfortunately, poor advice – or no advice – on what to do to make it better and prevent it happening again leads many women to give up feeding their babies.

If you look after your nipples in the way we've described and feed naturally, taking care to position your baby well, you may be able to prevent soreness. But if you do get sore nipples, turn to page 307 for some ideas on what to do.

ENGORGEMENT

Your breasts will swell between the second and fifth day as you start making mature milk. Some degree of swelling is perfectly normal and you should carry on breastfeeding on an unrestricted basis to avoid getting painfully engorged breasts (see 'pathological engorgement', page 302). The most important thing is not to allow your breasts to become too full.

— Research shows that women feeding on a schedule are twice as likely to become engorged as those feeding more frequently.

Women who notice a large increase in the size of their breasts in the first week after delivery often think their milk supply must be failing when their breasts become smaller as the days go by. However, provided they are feeding frequently, this isn't so – it's just that breasts tend to get smaller once their milk supply matches up to the baby's demand.

EXPRESSING MILK

You may need to get rid of some milk in the first few days while your baby's needs catch up with your supply. Expression is a useful technique to learn, both for now and for later. If your breasts are tense, the angle between the breast and nipple tends to flatten, which may make it difficult for your baby to latch on. Expressing a little milk will soften the breasts just enough to make it possible. Mothers of pre-term babies who are as yet unable to take milk from the breast can provide their babies with milk and keep their milk supply going by expressing (see page 343). And if you develop a cracked nipple you can keep your breast empty yet allow the nipple to heal by regular expression.

To express milk, first wash your hands (and if you are in hospital, rinse with a disinfectant solution), then make yourself comfortable. Now hold your areola with your thumb above the nipple and your index finger below. Some women find it easier to use their left hand for both breasts and to collect the milk in a container held by the right hand. If you intend to store your milk in a fridge or freezer, sterilize the container first.

Move your hand firmly backwards towards your chest. Now move your hand away again, pressing your finger and thumb together, gently squeezing milk out of the reservoirs under the areola and to the nipple. Once your breasts fill with milk you may be able to feel the reservoirs as if they were bunches of little grapes under the areola. Some women can feel their milk ducts too.

Carry on expressing once the milk is let down even though there are intervals between sprays. Even when you're expressing, you still need to let down your hind-milk. Let-down milk comes in spurts with intervals between and you should go on expressing during these intervals.

Move the position of your hand from time to time to empty the other parts of the breast (using your other hand if necessary), and change to the other breast several times if the flow seems to be slowing. Many women start off by massaging their whole breast gently to encourage their milk to flow. Don't forget that when you let down your milk, it'll drip or spray from both breasts. If you're collecting milk for your baby and not just to relieve overfull breasts, you can catch the dripped (or 'drip') milk from the other breast as well as from the one you're expressing. Some women who donate milk to hospital milk banks for other people's babies collect only drip milk, however, drip milk is predominantly fore-milk, so it tends to have a low fat content.

It's easy to collect this in a sterilized breast shell worn inside your bra. Don't forget to position the shell with the tiny hole uppermost! Pour the collected drips into a sterile bottle or other container that you can cover.

Expressing often takes longer than breastfeeding but is easy once you have the knack. Don't worry if you can express only a small volume. Most successful breastfeeders never express more than one or two ounces at a go.

If you want to collect enough milk to leave for a minder to give your baby, you'll have to express after each feed for a couple of days. Leave the covered container in the fridge between times. But don't be put off by the very small volumes you get. The fractions of an ounce soon mount up. Expressed milk should be shaken or stirred before being given from a cup, spoon or bottle.

Pumps – Some mothers prefer to pump their milk; the different sorts of pump are covered in the Appendix (see page 443).

STORING MILK

Expressed breast milk contains many anti-infective factors and if you collect it in a clean (not sterilized) container and cover it, you can safely leave it at room temperature for several hours.

— A Nigerian study (1988) found no significant bacterial growth in expressed colostrum left at high room temperatures (27–32°C/ 80–86°F)for twelve hours. Mature breast milk was safe at room temperature for six hours.
— Another study in 1987 revealed that breast milk allowed to stand at room temperature had only minimal bacterial growth after ten hours – no more than immediately after it had been expressed or than samples stored in the fridge for ten hours.

You can store your expressed milk in the fridge or freezer. See page 349 if storing milk for a pre-term baby.

Fridge

Express your milk into a sterilized plastic container, cover and put into the fridge. Plastic is better than glass as some of the immunological components of milk stick to glass. If you wash your hands before you collect your milk, you can keep it in the fridge for up to three days (five days according to a study in 1987, and eight days according to a study in 1994). If you want to keep it for longer, freeze it immediately after you've expressed it. Your milk will separate into layers as it stands but these will soon disappear when you warm it up.

Freezer

You can freeze expressed milk if you want to keep it for longer than two or three days. Freezing has little effect on the milk's antibodies but harms its living cells, so don't freeze it unless you have to. However, frozen breast milk is better than formula.

Freeze only small amounts of milk because once thawed, it shouldn't be refrozen, so left-overs are wasted. You can always thaw more if necessary.

You can store your milk in a freezer for up to four months. However, use milk frozen in a frost-free freezer compartment within a fridge within two or three weeks, as the temperature inside will fluctuate a lot.

Thawing

Thaw frozen milk quickly by holding the container under running water – first cold, then gradually warmer until the milk is liquid.

Warming milk

Gently warm a container of expressed breast milk which has been refrigerated or frozen and thawed in a pan of water on the hob. Shake the container to get the milk to an even temperature. Milk at body temperature (slightly cool to your skin) is the most pleasant for a baby. Pre-term babies should never have cold milk.

Microwaving

On the whole, it's preferable not to thaw and warm expressed breast milk by microwaving.

— US researchers (1992) found that microwaving expressed breast milk at high temperatures (72–98° C) reduced its protective anti-infective properties, while microwaving at cooler temperatures (20–53° C) had no significant effect on the total amount of antibodies but reduced the amount of lysozyme and antibodies against certain *E. coli* (potentially harmful gut bacteria).

— Austrian researchers discovered that microwaving alters the structure of some of the amino acids, which might theoretically mean that a baby couldn't digest or use them properly. Don't microwave containers you use to store expressed milk or feed the baby. The temperatures reached aren't high enough reliably to kill any dangerous concentrations of bacteria.

COLLECTING DRIP MILK

Some breastfeeding women like to collect the milk that drips from the opposite breast to the one their baby is feeding from or they are expressing from. They do this either to keep themselves dry, in which case they discard it immediately, or they collect it so as to give it their babies later by cup or spoon (but preferably not by bottle). You can collect drip milk easily by putting a breast shell inside your bra. Make sure the hole or spout, if there is one, is uppermost!

VISITING

This can be a vexed subject. You'll feel left out if you don't have visitors when everyone else does; you'll want to show your baby to relatives and friends; you may feel shy about feeding in front of people yet don't want your baby to be hungry at visiting times; and an hour may be too much with some visitors but not enough with others.

There are several ways to cope. Try to choose a hospital that allows fairly unrestricted visiting and ask your partner to vet the people who want to come. If you wouldn't feel happy about feeding in front of them, ask him to put them off tactfully. When people visit you at home you can go to another room to feed if you're embarrassed or think they will be, but you can't do that in hospital.

NAPPY CHANGING

You may be advised to change your baby's nappy before a feed. This is all very well if he isn't crying for a feed but if he is, wait until afterwards, otherwise you may be so upset that you won't let down your milk. Your baby may also be so upset that he swallows a lot of air between sobs and then regurgitates much of his milk. Some babies don't feed well with a wet or dirty nappy and others are woken by being changed after a feed, which is why changing before a feed is suggested. But after a good feed many babies are so content and full that nothing wakes them, even a nappy change. Changing after a feed makes a lot of sense and saves nappies because babies often wet or fill their nappy during a feed. If you have a baby who won't feed with a dirty nappy on, you'll have to change it straight away. The good news if you have a baby who falls asleep halfway through a feed is that a nappy change may wake him enough to take the second breast.

YOUR BABY'S BOWELS

A breastfed baby's motions gradually change during the first week from the dark green meconium of the first day or so to bright yellow, liquid motions which may just leave a stain on the nappy. Young breastfed babies tend to pass bowel motions more often than do bottle-fed ones and in the early days of breastfeeding you may find that almost every nappy has a yellow stain. However, some breastfed babies pass very few motions. For example, we've heard of one perfectly healthy breastfed baby who passed no motions for twenty-seven days while between seven and eleven weeks old. When eventually passed, the motion was soft and vast!

WIND

Why haven't we mentioned winding yet? Because many breastfed babies don't need winding – they simply bring up any wind spontaneously or pass it out the other end. If you think your baby is windy, cuddle him after a feed in a fairly upright position, for instance against your shoulder, to let the wind come up. If you know he doesn't usually burp, lay him down to sleep immediately after a feed. Wind seems to have become an obsession with some people. But women in many countries, including some European ones, don't recognize it as a problem, so do nothing about it, with no obvious ill-effects.

Some babies are obviously uncomfortable after a feed but drop off to sleep when they've brought up some wind. Such babies sometimes frown or even go momentarily cross-eyed. The skin above a windy baby's upper lip may be slightly blue and he may cry or fidget. If you think your baby is windy and being upright doesn't do the trick, sit him on your lap with one of your hands rubbing his back gently and the other holding his chest. If you then bend him slightly in the middle, a bubble of air often comes up, perhaps with a little regurgitated milk. If at night you feed your baby lying down, he doesn't settle easily and you think he's windy, you may need to sit him up in bed to get rid of the swallowed air.

See also 'colic', page 199.

CRYING

There's an awful lot going on in the average maternity ward, what with trolley shops, paper rounds, meals, visitors, bed-making and room cleaning, to say nothing of doctors' and nurses' rounds, baths, talking to your neighbour in the next bed, letters to write, phone calls to make and, if you're lucky, flowers to arrange and letters and cards to open. In the midst of all this it's easy to let your baby come second and not feed him as soon as he cries (or even before).

At first you won't have any idea why your baby is crying because this is the only way he can communicate. As the weeks go by some women – but not all – learn to distinguish between hungry, tired, lonely, angry, dirty-bottom cries, and so on. Some babies cry very little, if at all, as their mothers are able to recognize, anticipate and meet their needs so well.

Causes of crying

However, some babies cry much more than others. Indeed, mid-wives and women who have had many children say that babies behave very differently and have different characters right from the start. Some are quieter, more placid and content, and easier to look after, whereas others make much more noise, are more demanding and less easily satisfied, and more challenging to care for! So, while every baby cries only for a good reason, some may cry more readily than others and be pacified less readily.

Babies cry for many different reasons. These include hunger, thirst, tiredness, loneliness, anger, tension, being too hot or cold, having a sore bottom, having something poking into or rubbing them, sensing their mother's anxiety or haste, a sudden noise, a reaction to something the mother has eaten, wind, smoke-filled air, colic and other medical reasons. Hunger and thirst are by far the most common reasons. However, your baby may need something else to pacify him. In this case, breastfeeding may comfort him for a while but not for long.

The first things to do

A mother can usually stop her baby crying by putting him to the breast and/or attending to his other needs as she perceives them. Babies who breastfeed successfully and on an unrestricted basis, who are carried around for much of the day, and who sleep with their mother at night, scarcely need to cry at all. And babies whose mothers respond to their needs promptly and feed them as often as they want tend to cry much less than other babies.

— A study in the US (1988) revealed that babies whose mothers breastfed them frequently and responded to their needs quickly cried less, both at two months old and at four months.

No woman likes to hear her baby cry because crying usually suggests unhappiness. Her baby's cries will probably upset her and the resulting anxiety may prevent her from letting down her milk (see page 20).

It's sensible to comfort a squalling newborn infant straight away as this will encourage him to think the world is a good place. You can't possibly spoil him like this. If you were left to yell for hours for your food you'd be dispirited or angry: babies are no different. Many mothers notice that babies who are fed and comforted at the breast whenever they cry grow up to be happy, independent, loving children – not demanding, unhappy and spoilt.

Being able to comfort a crying baby at the breast is one of the greatest rewards of breastfeeding. A woman who limits suckling time denies this pleasure both to herself and her baby. Breastfeeding is not only a means of getting milk: it's also a way of being close to a warm, soft, comforting mother.

If your baby cries at the beginning of a feed

He may be frustrated (or afraid or angry) because your milk takes time to let down. Try encouraging your milk to let down before you put him to the breast. It will help to wake him and/or offer the breast before he cries, so that he doesn't get so hungry he has to cry. If he does get so upset that he can't feed, though, try rocking him from side to side to see if this calms him enough to settle at the breast.

If your baby cries after a feed

In a young baby this probably means he's still hungry.

- Either he just hasn't had enough and needs to go back to the breast (see also 'How to increase your milk supply' in Chapter 10, see page 270).
- Or he may have had plenty of fore-milk but not enough satisfying fat-rich hind-milk, probably because you didn't let him stay at either the first or the second breast long enough.
- Try to calm him just enough to stop him crying temporarily, as crying makes a baby's tongue pull right back inside the mouth (just look and you'll see this happen), which could make it difficult to latch on properly. Then put him back to the breast and let him go on feeding until he drops off spontaneously.
- If your baby often cries in the evening and you think you may not have enough milk for him then, try expressing some after the first big morning feed the next day. Store this and give it to your baby in a cup (or in a supplementer, page 449), when he cries after a feed in the evening.

When your baby won't stop crying

Some babies go on and on crying. If you leave your baby crying for long he'll get tired out, because crying expends a lot of energy – just watch and you'll see why. After crying for a long time he probably won't feed well because he'll be too exhausted.

The commonest cause of continued crying is schedule-feeding. Exhaustion from long periods of crying is one reason why schedule-fed babies don't get enough milk and why their mothers often can't breastfeed successfully. A baby who wakes an hour 'early' and is left to cry until the clock says it's time for a feed may not be hungry when feed time arrives, just tired out and angry or frightened because his tummy hurts and he's all alone. Over a few days of this his mother's breasts don't get enough stimulation and her milk supply diminishes.

Could the crying be due to colic?

In medical terms colic is intermittent pain caused by muscle spasm of the walls of a hollow organ such as the bowel.

Many babies cry for long periods during their first three months, especially in the evenings, for no apparent cause. These bouts of crying are traditionally put down to colic, sometimes called 'evening colic' or 'three-month colic'. However, it's highly likely that such crying isn't caused by colic at all but by something else (see page 196 under 'Causes of crying'). Many people assume that crying results from air passing through the bowels, but there's no evidence to prove it. X-rays show that 'colicky' babies have no more air in their bowels than do other babies. Having said this, some babies cry less from 'colic' if they have a bowel-calming medicine.

The vast majority of studies show that whether a baby is breastfed or bottle-fed makes no difference to whether or not he has 'colic'. However, one study showed that 'colic' was more likely in babies who started solids before three months. And some women believe vitamin drops give their babies 'colic'.

Causes of actual colic

However, some babies do get real colic. There are several causes.

1 There may be too much lactose (milk sugar) in the gut. This can result from drinking too much low-fat fore-milk and not enough fat-

rich hind-milk, as happens if a mother takes her baby off the first breast before she's let down her hind-milk, then puts him to the other breast and does the same. The baby fills up quickly with a large volume of low-fat fore-milk. However, without the presence of fat-rich hind-milk, the fore-milk leaves the stomach and enters the gut quickly. The relatively large amont of lactose then ferments, producing gas, or wind, which causes colic. It may also cause a sore bottom. It is particularly likely to happen in a baby whose mother makes a large amount of milk and tries to curtail feeds (see page 290).

2 Breathing smoke-filled air or drinking nicotine-containing breast milk from a mother who smokes can cause colic.

3 A variety of medical conditions can cause colic, including food poisoning, food sensitivity, gastroenteritis and bowel obstruction. This is why if your baby cries a lot and you don't know why, if his cry is worryingly unusual, or if there are other abnormal signs, you should consult the doctor.

— A study from Sweden found that twelve out of nineteen colicky breastfed babies lost their colic when their mothers ate a diet free from cows' milk protein. The colic reappeared on at least two further 'challenges' (in the form of cows' milk for the mothers). At four months, only four of the babies reacted with colic when their mothers had cows' milk, which fits well with the observation that many babies lose their colic after three or four months anyway. We know that whole molecules of cows' milk protein (and other dietary proteins) can be present in breast milk, and we know colic is a well-recognized symptom of cows' milk protein intolerance, so the theory could be right. As yet, though, it's unproven and has been challenged by other researchers.

There's a suggestion that breastfed babies benefit from exposure to 'foreign' proteins and other dietary substances in breast milk because this gradually helps prepare their immune system for the switch to a mixed diet. However, certain babies, colicky ones included, are unable to cope with food traces in breast milk. This inability to cope is more likely if there is an allergic family history.

The latest research suggests that the breastfeeding mother of a child with an allergic family history, or just with colic, should vary her diet so as to avoid a large intake of any one food, particularly cows' milk and its products. Eggs, bananas, apples, oranges, strawberries, tomatoes, coffee and chocolate have also been associated with colic in breastfed babies whose mothers eat a lot of them.

Even a little of some foods in a woman's diet can make some babies have an acute bout of what seems to be tummy-ache lasting for a day. Beans, onions, garlic and rhubarb have all been observed to have this effect in some mother–baby pairs.

Colic nearly always improves after the first three months. Weaning a baby on to cows' milk formula is highly unlikely to make any difference.

Other reasons for continued crying include:

* The baby has swallowed too much air while trying to drink fast-flowing milk (see pages 195 and 290).
* The baby wants attention and cuddles at a time when his mother can't easily give them.
* The baby is sensitive to traces of foods (for example, alcohol, chocolate, spicy foods, peas, onions, citrus fruit or juice, cauliflower, broccoli, brussels sprouts, cabbage and cows' milk) his mother has eaten and passed into her milk.
* The baby hasn't had enough satisfying milk because his mother is waiting for her biggest meal of the day later in the evening.
* The baby is upset because he senses his mother is overwrought (perhaps with the evening rush of things to do). Family tension may also be a problem.
* The baby is reacting to his mother's stress. A Finnish study (1993) reported that women who suffered from stress and physical problems in pregnancy, or who were dissatisfied with their sexual relationship, or who had negative birth experiences, were more likely to have babies whose crying was put down to colic. They suggested it might be a good idea for pregnant women to learn stress-management and parenting skills.

Ten ways of caring for your crying baby and yourself:

1 – Feed him as much as he wants.

2 – Let him finish one breast before he goes to the other.

3 – Check simple things like a cold, wet or dirty nappy.

4 – Sit and cuddle him if he's happier like that – or get your partner to do the cuddling, as some colicky babies are calmer with someone else.

5 – Gently massage his tummy in a warm room, using a little warmed oil, circling his tummy with slow, rhythmic, clockwise movements.

6 – Check whether you've eaten anything known sometimes to upset babies (see page 201), and avoid it or eat less of it in future.

7 – Eat healthy, enjoyable, balanced meals regularly – and have something to eat between each feed.

8 – Try holding your baby in different positions after a feed, for example, with him leaning slightly forward and bending to the right, with your arm pressing against his abdomen. He'll assume this position if you hold him with his back to you, your arm round his right side and your right hand supporting his crotch.

9 – Consult your midwife, health visitor (in the UK), doctor or breastfeeding leader or counsellor.

10 – Last, but by no means least, look after yourself by relaxing and resting more and asking for help to ensure your needs are met.

REGURGITATION

Many babies, especially small ones, regurgitate milk during and after a feed, particularly if milk flows from the breast so fast that they swallow air as they gulp it down, or if they drink too much. Sometimes a baby brings up so much milk that he wants more.

There's no need to worry if your baby regurgitates as long as he's thriving. However, if your milk flows very fast early in a feed, you could try expressing some before he starts feeding so as to prevent him from having to swallow too much too quickly to keep up.

If the brought-up milk has been in your baby's tummy for some time, you'll notice that it's been changed into fine curds and whey.

AFTERPAINS

When you let your milk down, you may experience low tummy pains. These are caused by oxytocin making your womb contract. They also encourage the womb to return to its former size. Other signs that you're letting milk down are tingling in your breasts, dripping or spraying milk, the lessening of any nipple pain as milk reaches the baby, and the regular 'glug-glug' sounds of your baby swallowing (see also page 21).

A SORE PERINEUM

There's nothing like the nagging pain of a stitched episiotomy to put the dampers on the let-down reflex. Try something simple like a hot bath and ask the hospital staff for a rubber ring to sit on to take the weight off your most tender parts. If you still need a rubber ring when you get home, you should be able to buy or hire one from a surgical supplies shop. If these simple measures don't work, take some suitable pain-killers.

LEAKING (see also page 224)

You'll leak if you let your milk down before you put your baby to the breast but leaking can happen without the let-down if your breasts are full, especially if you're warm and if you lean forward. Leaking means that your breasts are full and ready for your baby. To relieve the pressure you can either suckle your baby or express a little milk. If in the first few weeks your breasts are full for too long, they're highly likely to become engorged (see page 302).

If you leak, don't immediately jump to the conclusion that you're producing too much milk and then decide to feed your baby less often, because leaking is perfectly normal, especially in the early days. And don't reduce your fluid intake either, as this won't prevent leaking. You can mop up leaking milk with breast pads (see below), soft material such as a hanky, an old terry nappy cut into squares, or a folded 'one-way' nappy liner tucked into your bra. To avoid soaking your nipple in soggy material while feeding from the first breast (which can make soreness and cracking much more likely), try uncovering the second breast and letting any leaking milk simply drip on to a terry nappy. A trick many women discover is to put the heel of one hand over the nipple and push it firmly towards the breast. This often stops leaking like magic.

WEARING A BRA AT NIGHT

When you're breastfeeding, you may want to wear a bra at night to prevent leaking over the bedclothes in the early days. A bra also makes heavy breasts more comfortable. However, going without a bra makes nipple soreness less likely as air can get to the nipples, and a terry nappy placed loosely over your breasts in bed soaks up any leaks. Also, it's much easier to put your baby to the breast at night if you're not wearing a bra!

BREAST PADS

You can tuck material or paper pads inside your bra to soak up any leaking milk. You can buy purpose-made paper nursing pads at chemists and babycare shops; cheaper ones are flat, the more expensive ones are cone-shaped. Don't use paper tissues or cotton wool because these dry on to the nipples and can be difficult to remove without washing. Some women use squares of soft absorbent material such as pieces cut from an old nappy or towel or a nappy roll. Plastic-backed pads sound like a good idea but prevent air from getting to the nipples and make the skin wet, soggy and more likely to become sore or cracked.

HOW YOU FEEL

Many newly delivered women feel weepy and emotional around the fourth day. This often coincides with their milk coming in and may result from changing hormone levels. It happens just as often, if not more, in bottle-feeding women. Unfortunately, if a woman is having any trouble feeding her baby, this temporary depression may be the last straw that makes her decide to give up and change to bottle-feeding. (See also page 252.)

Apart from hormonal changes, it isn't surprising that a newly delivered woman is emotional. Giving birth is both a crisis and a rite of passage in a woman's life and the accompanying loss of sleep and the excitement surrounding a new baby can disturb even the calmest person. It isn't uncommon for one mother in a ward to start crying and for all the others to follow suit. All the more reason, then, to learn how to cope with breastfeeding problems before you have your baby so that you won't have that to worry about.

Any hospital procedures that institutionalize and regiment

women – like insisting on scheduled breastfeeds – do little to help the fragile emotions of the new mother and depression is sometimes made worse by taking her baby away to a nursery. Kindness, encouragement and empathy on the part of the post-natal ward staff matter a great deal when you've just had a baby. Similarly, the slightest criticism can hurt a lot.

NORMAL WEIGHT-LOSS

A newborn baby's body contains extra fluid to tide him over the first few days when he's taking small volumes of colostrum. It's normal for a baby to lose weight as this fluid is lost. Most babies lose 6 per cent of their weight and some lose as much as 10 per cent.

WEIGHT-GAIN

The speed at which a breastfed baby regains his birth-weight depends to some extent on how often he is fed. Babies fed frequently tend not to lose much weight during the first week and then gain more rapidly than babies on a three-hourly schedule. And babies on a three-hourly schedule gain faster than those on a four-hourly one. Some babies take up to three weeks to regain their birth weight and a few perfectly healthy ones take even longer.

—One study found that 49 per cent of demand-fed babies and 36 per cent of four-hourly fed babies regained their birth weight by a week. However, the demand-fed babies had a restricted number of feeds for the first two days; had they had more frequent feeds, even more of them might have regained their birth-weight at one week.

But the speed at which birth-weight is regained is not usually very important. In the old days a woman wasn't allowed to take her baby home until it had regained its birth weight and this still sometimes happens today. However, provided a baby is fed on an unrestricted basis, seems contented, is healthy, is slowly gaining weight (or at least not losing any more), and produces enough wet nappies, and provided the mother's let-down reflex works, the rate of weight-gain is likely to be unimportant.

Enlightened hospital staff have stopped routine test-weighing (weighing before and after a feed to see how much milk was taken). In most cases test-weighing only worries people unnecessarily: it worries those staff who don't understand that breastfed babies don't need as much milk as bottle-fed babies, and it automatically makes some women doubt their ability to breastfeed. Test-weighing should be reserved for those very few babies who obviously aren't thriving in spite of excellent breastfeeding support and advice.

When you've negotiated the earliest days of breastfeeding, you're set to embark on the next stage as you feed your growing baby day by day.

EIGHT

Feeding day by day

COPING AT HOME

Taking your baby home is exciting but however tempting it is to rush around in hospital getting yourself and the baby ready, it's sensible not to overdo it because the last thing you want is to arrive home tired out.

Once home, sit down, have a drink and relax. Leave the washing-up, shopping and tidying to someone else for a few days if you can. You'll have your hands full with the baby. All too often a woman plunges back into her old routine and becomes exhausted. Then when her milk dwindles she's surprised and upset, which creates a vicious circle. For the next few weeks it's best to take things easy, eat nourishing meals and let the world go by as much as possible. This is all doubly important if you gave birth at home or have been discharged early from hospital.

Of course, not every baby is a first baby and you may have other children to look after. Hopefully, you and your partner will have arranged for a relative, friend or paid person to help for the first few weeks. Some men take time off to be at home. Your mother may be the best person to help but nowadays mothers often aren't close at hand.

A helper (or *doula*) is a very important member of society in those parts of the world such as India where successful breast-feeding is widely practised. Besides being of practical assistance, a good helper provides emotional support in the first crucial days. Her very presence makes things easier because on-the-spot reassurance from someone sympathetic is a godsend at this time.

Whatever help you think you'll need, discuss it with your helper before the baby is born so that you both know where you stand. Otherwise there may be a problem if the helper wants to take over the baby while you look after the house and other children. Clear this up as tactfully and quickly as possible.

How long do you need help? This is an individual decision, but remember that your milk supply may take several weeks to become properly established and that you'll need time to recover from the effort of pregnancy and labour. So don't rush things, especially if you have more than one child. Make the most of any help you have.

WHERE TO FEED

Although in theory you can feed your baby anywhere, you'll find it more pleasurable if you are comfortable. If you find you like cushions to support your arm, or the baby, make sure they are left in the chair you use. Having said this, though, there's absolutely no need to make a big thing about cushions, chair height and so on. One woman told us that she stopped breastfeeding because she couldn't bear all the fiddling with cushions! Many mothers find it more relaxing and enjoyable to feed their babies lying on a bed or sofa. If you perch on a hard chair to feed, with your shoulders aching from supporting the baby, and dreading the thought of a long stint with nothing to do other than look at him, it's unlikely that you'll relax or let your milk down and your baby will go hungry.

If you have a winter baby, keep the room warm. Cold air can make the muscle fibres in the areolae and nipples contract, which constricts the openings of the ducts at the nipple and delays the release of milk. This may frustrate your baby early in a feed. In practice, the warmth of his mouth warms the nipples and the let-down reflex makes the skin of the breasts feel warmer.

If you find you like something to do while you're feeding (and if you haven't got another young child), keep a book or magazine by your chair. One mother we know found a music stand invaluable for supporting her book, so leaving her hands free. You may find it relaxing to watch the TV or listen to the radio, though many women are quite happy just watching their baby feeding, especially if he stares up at them, as so many do. A lot depends on how long the feed takes – if your baby is a quick feeder, you won't get bored. Ideally, feeding can be a time to look forward to and enjoy. If you take care of your creature comforts, you'll relax, your baby will get the milk easily and everything should go well. In fact, many nursing mothers look forward to feed times as oases of peace in their day. Some babies like quiet feed times and refuse to feed well in noisy surroundings. Others, particularly older ones, are easily distracted.

You'll soon find you can breastfeed as you walk around. This means that you can fetch something you want during a feed or go to the phone without disturbing your baby.

Many women feel very thirsty when feeding, especially in the first few weeks (see 'What about drinks?' in Chapter 9, page 241). If you do, get yourself something to drink and put it by you before you start.

WHERE WILL YOUR BABY SLEEP DURING THE DAY?

If you put your baby in his room to sleep during the day, you run the risk of not hearing when he wakes. Try him sleeping in a carrycot in the room where you are, or at least well within earshot. This way you'll know when he wakes and will be able to feed or cuddle him as soon as he cries. Household noise is unlikely to keep him awake if he really wants to sleep, and if he doesn't it'll be more interesting for him to watch and listen to what's going on than lie in a quiet room gazing at the ceiling.

Having said this, you don't have to put your baby in a cot at all between feeds. Many enjoy being carried around in a sling or in their mother's arms, or sitting in a suitable baby chair.

HOW OFTEN TO FEED YOUR BABY
(see also pages 25 and 172)

More misleading advice has been given about this than anything else to do with breastfeeding. Such advice has done a lot of harm over the past fifty years or more.

Your baby is unlike any other – he's an individual, not just a stomach to be filled every so often. His only way of telling you he's hungry is to fidget or cry (given that in the West we don't carry our babies by our naked breasts so that they can feed when they want without asking). In the first few weeks all cries sound much the same to most new mothers, though some swear they can distinguish hungry cries, wet or dirty cries, bored cries and so on. Early on, the only way to decide whether his cry is a hungry one is to offer the breast. As young babies prefer frequent, small feeds, he'll almost certainly feed. Feeding on demand means interpreting any cry as a request for food until proven otherwise, even though sometimes you may feel sure your baby doesn't want a feed. You can also put him to the breast whenever he seems fidgety or restless, as that may well mean he's hungry. This way you'll pre-empt the need for him to cry.

— A study in Sri Lanka (1994) found that women fed their four- to-six-week-old babies anything between six and twenty times in each twenty-four-hour day; they gave between five and seventeen feeds during the day and between one and five during the night.
— In a study in North Carolina (1984) researchers observed twenty-four successfully breastfeeding women whose babies were betweeen five and sixteen months old and noted that the average number of 'suckling episodes' (feeds) during twenty-four-hours was fifteen.

Don't be concerned by the conflicting advice you'll get from friends, relatives, professionals, baby-feeding pamphlets sponsored by formula manufacturers, and baby books. Some sources still promote the old chestnuts about breastfeeding every four hours (2, 6 and 10 a.m., and 2, 6 and 10 p.m.). This advice is for the birds and bottle-fed babies, not you and your baby! A few women produce enough milk using such a routine but most find their milk supply slowly dwindles because six feeds a day simply don't give their breasts anywhere near enough stimulation. Women who *do not* produce enough milk with six feeds a day are the normal ones!

Once you accept that your baby may ask for feeds frequently and erratically you're halfway towards feeding successfully. You may seem to spend a large part of the day breastfeeding but it's worth deciding to accept and enjoy it rather than resent it as time wasted or time when your life seems to be out of control. And don't forget that your baby may want even more frequent feeds if he is unwell or upset.

Although many babies establish a routine after a time, not all do, so don't compare your baby with any other. The baby who has frequent feeds stimulates his mother's breasts (and hence her milk supply) better than one who asks for only five or six feeds a day. If your baby does ask for only five feeds a day, offer more, as five feeds are highly unlikely to be enough to keep up your milk supply for long. One researcher found that reducing the number of feeds to five a day led to an insufficiency of milk in one in three women.

We've found that many successfully breastfeeding mothers cannot say how many feeds they give in a day.

HOW LONG WILL FEEDS LAST?
(see also pages 179 and 272)

Again, let your baby guide you. The old rule of ten minutes a side was created because that was the average time babies needed for a *bottle*-feed. Few babies are average, anyway, and whereas some need much less than ten minutes a side, some want much more.

During the first few months there may sometimes be periods

when your baby wants to feed almost continuously for several hours. This is not unusual and is his way of increasing your milk supply. People may tell you that a baby gets most of the milk he needs in the first few minutes at each breast. There's some truth in this but studies show that not all get most of what they need so quickly. A lot depends on how vigorously and efficiently your baby sucks, how strong your let-down reflex is, how much milk is in your breasts and how long it takes you to let your milk down. Some babies like to play at the breast and feed sporadically while others go for speed above all else.

There's some evidence that two-month-old babies have a bigger (and so, possibly, longer) feed early in the morning if there's been a relatively long gap since their last feed. In other words, they have a big feed *after* a long gap. In contrast, six-month-olds who have a relatively long sleep at night tend to have their biggest feed in the evening, *before* that long gap.

Another point is that some babies enjoy sucking even once they have emptied the breast. There's no reason to stop unless you want to do something else or if you have sore nipples. This comfort sucking may be important for a baby's emotional development. A dummy or thumb is the bottle-fed baby's substitute for comfort-sucking at the breast. And all the time your baby is sucking for comfort he is also stimulating your breasts to make more milk.

Young primates suck whenever possible and by no means only when they are hungry. Human infants are no different in this respect. The main reason for the small number of short breastfeeds many babies in the West have each day is the relative inaccessibility of the breast and the reluctance of some women (because of cultural attitudes) to offer it for comfort. The large number of women whose milk dries up have invariably allowed their baby to suck only if he is 'certifiably' hungry. Babies don't like to suck only for food, fluid and comfort. They may also just enjoy being at the breast.

As your baby gets older, he'll finish his feeds more quickly unless he's tired, bored, ill or upset.

So what's the answer to how long feeds should be? There isn't one. When your baby seems to have finished one side – when he becomes less interested in feeding, or stops – change him to the other and let him carry on there as long as he wants to or for as long as you can. *And don't watch the clock.* The majority of people in developing countries don't have clocks, yet they feed their babies much more successfully than we do!

ONE BREAST OR TWO?

Many babies drink from only one breast during a feed. Provided that you alternate the breast you give at each feed, that he is satisfied, and that you express when necessary to prevent your unemptied breast from getting lumpy or tense between feeds, this is fine. Giving both breasts at each feed is a Western idea and often not done in those parts of the world where breastfeeding is more natural and schedules unknown. One breast at a time fits in well with the baby who wants frequent small feeds, as many prefer.

If you want, or if your baby is hungry or fussy, give both breasts, perhaps even changing sides several times during a feed, but let him go on feeding at the first breast until he's had enough of that side. If you don't, he runs the risk of getting only the low-calorie, low-fat fore-milk. This doesn't contain enough fat to slow down stomach-emptying and keep the milk in the stomach for a long time, so it quickly rushes into the baby's gut, where it ferments and may lead to wind, evening colic and a sore bottom. (See also page 274.)

YOUR BABY'S FEEDING PATTERN AND BEHAVIOUR
(see also page 331)

Although each baby is unique as far as his appetite, demand for the breast, sucking pattern and behaviour at the breast go, experienced observers group breastfeeding babies into several categories.

Which category yours falls into will depend on his personality, his past experience at the breast, how hungry he is, and on the way you let your milk down. Some babies always take a long time over feeds and enjoy spending what seems like all day (and night) at the breast, sucking on and off. Once you're sure your baby is thriving (plenty of wet nappies and putting on weight), you can stop a feeding session after half an hour or so if you want to do something else. Most of the time, though, relax and enjoy this special time with your young baby. Sooner or later he'll start taking his milk more quickly and may want to spend less time at the breast.

Other babies regurgitate several times throughout a feed and afterwards, sometimes bringing up most of the milk they've drunk. All you can do is to be patient and give him more if he wants. If all the stimulation from repeating feeds makes your milk gush fast, express some before putting him to the breast. (See also page 290.)

Many babies (especially if small, jaundiced or affected by your drugs in labour) snooze every so often during a feed. Don't make the mistake of thinking the feed is over the first time he snoozes. Just wait calmly and he'll wake again when he has more energy.

You may have the sort of baby who drinks in a very forthright, no-nonsense manner. Feeding him is over quickly. His behaviour is much more like that of older babies. You could say that in this respect he has grown up ahead of time.

Many babies behave differently at different times of the day and almost all alter their feeding behaviour as they grow older.

NIGHT FEEDS

Night feeds are essential for all young babies and many older ones and encourage milk production and successful breastfeeding. They can be very special, quiet times for you both to be together.

Understandably, most of us are so used to sleeping for hours on end at night that we like the thought of getting back to unbroken nights again. Some babies sleep through the night when a few months old – some even earlier. However, a great many perfectly normal, healthy babies don't. And a few wake for a feed most nights for some years.

Clearly you'll need to find ways of making night feeds as easy as possible, so here are some suggestions.

Keep the room dark

When your baby wakes, don't flood everywhere with bright light because this will wake you both up. Install a dimmer-switch on your bedside light, or a low-wattage bulb, or, if you have your baby in or by your bed, don't turn the light on at all unless you have to, for example if you have to change his nappy. There's less risk of him staying awake for long if the room is dark.

Keep everything quiet, calm and low-key

It's tempting to talk to your baby when you're both awake at night and everyone else is sleep. However, when your milk supply is well established, you may prefer to keep quiet. This way, feeds aren't so exciting, and if your baby doesn't need the milk, the time will come when he wakes less and less often.

Be prepared for nappy changes

Keep nappies to hand by the bed. However, your baby may go back to sleep quite happily without a nappy change. A one-way nappy liner will help keep his skin dry. Putting a pad inside his nappy provides more absorbency. Not changing the nappy is a problem only if he can't sleep without a clean, dry one; if he has a sore bottom; or if he gets cold.

Let your baby sleep in your room

Having your baby nearby makes getting up at night so much easier. It also means you may wake when he simply becomes restless, rather than when he's actually crying. This is less disturbing to everyone. Also, because he doesn't have to become thoroughly wide awake before a feed, he's more likely to go back to sleep soon afterwards.

Make things as easy as you can by keeping his cot near your bed, preferably so close that you don't even have to get out of bed to lift him into your bed when he cries. Most cot-sides don't drop low enough for this to be as easy as it could be. Hopefully, more cot manufacturers will start making them so the drop side can be lowered to the level of a standard bed. There's an excellent three-sided 'cot-bed' (the Bed-Side-Bed, see page 451) which you can put right by your bed. This means the baby is on the same level as you, and you can put an arm round him or slide him next to you for a feed, but he has his own mattress and bed-covers. You can convert it into an ordinary four-sided cot and, when your baby is older, into a bed without sides as well.

If you can't sleep with the baby in your room, or don't want to, then when he wakes, either bring him back into your bed to feed, where you'll both be warm and comfy, or put on something warm and feed him in his room. If he has a single bed instead of a cot in his room, you can lie by him to feed him.

Consider letting your baby sleep for some or all of the night in your bed

The easiest and most natural way of feeding a baby at night is to have him in your bed. This means you can feed him while you're lying down, which is more restful for you and disturbs both your sleep and your baby's much less. Also, there's no night-time crying to wake the rest of the household because you can feed as soon as he becomes restless. And you'll know he's safe and warm.

After a feed you can leave your sleeping baby lying by the breast. When he wakes for another feed, roll over with him in your arms so that he comes to lie by your other side at your full breast. Some women don't move their babies but manage to feed from the opposite breast by leaning over. You'll probably find it's comfortable to lie with your arm crooked round the top of his head. You can put one hand on his back to keep him in place at your breast.

Once he's old enough to roll over, put a chair-back against the side of the bed to stop him rolling out when you're asleep. In the early days your baby may be restless during or after a feed. If necessary you can wind him simply by sitting him up while you stay lying down. Don't forget to have something to drink by your bed – as previously mentioned, many women feel very thirsty while feeding.

Some people are horrified at the suggestion that very young babies should sleep with their parents. And some women fear they'll roll on or suffocate the baby. The chances of doing this are virtually nil (but see below). Millions of women the world over sleep with their babies and young children quite safely.

If you'd like the pleasure of sleeping with your baby, but don't want him to learn to depend on you lying by him to go off to sleep, there's a solution. When you give the last feed before you go to bed, don't let him go to sleep at the breast but when he seems sleepy lay him in his cot, so he gets used to going to sleep in his own bed without you lying by him. Then, when he wakes in the night, you can bring him into your bed for a feed, then take him back to his bed if you want. This means he'll be first in his bed, then in yours, then perhaps back in his again. Many families who use this approach go through a transitional phase of 'musical beds' for some months. The youngest child will probably enjoy sleeping with an older brother or sister when he's around two.

Some women feel guilty about having their baby in bed. They're uneasy at the thought of prolonged contact and some even feel it's incestuous. Some dads too are antagonistic to babies in bed, but it should be possible to sort out all of these issues between you if you both listen to one another lovingly.

* The only men and women who might be better advised not to have their baby in bed are the extremely overweight; those taking sleeping tablets or recreational drugs; those who are drunk, and those who smoke, because there's a link between bed-sharing with smoking parents and cot death (see page 84).

Look after yourself when you're giving night feeds

Broken nights may make you tired, so try to relax and catch up on some sleep in the day. Many mothers notice during the first few weeks of breastfeeding particularly, when their breasts are full, that they suddenly begin to feel hot and sweaty. This is especially likely at night. The longer full breasts are left unemptied, the more likely they are to become engorged – (see page 302), so either wake your baby up or express some milk.

When will your baby give up night feeds?

This is very much an individual matter. Every baby is an individual and will start to sleep through the night only when ready. Babies wake at night for many reasons: they may be hungry (or thirsty); they may want to snuggle up to the breast for reassurance and comfort; they may be cold; or they may wake for no reason other than that their level of sleep has become light (as it does every so often during the night) and a noise, light, smell or some other stimulus has woken them fully. Some breastfed babies sleep through the night after the first few weeks while others wake for many months or even years. Some babies wake several times, others just once after their parents have gone to bed.

Breastfed babies tend to go on waking at night for longer than bottle-fed ones, but both may go on wanting a night feed for months. (One consolation for the breastfeeder is that bottle-fed babies often take much longer to settle after a night feed than breastfed ones.) It isn't worth stopping breastfeeding in order to get unbroken nights, because many bottle-fed babies wake at night anyway. Giving solids makes no difference to whether or not a baby sleeps through the night.

Patterns of sleep can vary enormously in any one baby. Your baby may wake several times most nights but occasionally have a long stretch of sleep. Even if he is usually a heavy sleeper, he may still have a wakeful night from time to time, perhaps if you have eaten something that disagrees with him. If you drink a lot of caffeine-containing drinks (coffee, tea and cola), or if you smoke, cutting these habits out or at least down might help your baby sleep longer.

Your baby may give up night feeds early, in which case make sure you breastfeed often enough in the day to maintain your milk supply and prevent your breasts from becoming engorged. You may also have to express some milk before you go to bed or even during the night to prevent discomfort. If your baby has given up night feeds too early and your milk supply is dwindling, wake him for a feed just before you go to bed.

On the other hand, your baby may want to continue with one, two or more night feeds for many months or even longer. If he sleeps in a cot and wants more than one or two feeds, your partner can help by getting up and bringing him to you in bed, then putting him back in his cot after the feed. Put a thick nappy on your baby at the beginning of the night so that he stands a better chance of going through the night without a change. Babies often want frequent feeds, especially when very young and occasionally for the odd night or two when they're much older, so it's worth accepting and coping with them as best you can.

Sleep patterns change, sometimes with more waking, sometimes less, but young children grow up and night waking doesn't last for ever – though it often seems it will at the time! Try if you can to be positive about night feeds. They can become a special, quiet time to enjoy cuddling your baby. Some busy women enjoy the luxury of undisturbed time to think, relax or even pray. And if you like the light on, night feeds can be times for enjoying looking at your baby, or reading.

GETTING YOUR BABY OFF TO SLEEP

Don't make the mistake of imagining that your new baby will necessarily spend most of his time between feeds asleep, as some baby books would have you believe. Every infant is an individual and has his own sleep requirements. These change from day to day according to how he feels and what he's been doing, and also change as he grows older. In general, young babies sleep as much as they need, unlike some older children, who sometimes get more and more tired yet can't or won't go to sleep. While some babies go straight to sleep with a full tummy after a feed, others choose this time to stare at their mothers, to look around and, later, to smile and coo. Don't waste valuable opportunities for getting to know and love your baby by trying to get him to sleep if he's not ready.

You may be advised to put your baby in his cot after you've fed and winded him. If he doesn't go to sleep, the advice is usually to let him cry until he does. Eventually, it is hoped, the baby will develop his own resources for getting off to sleep without needing you there.

Going to sleep at the breast

The easiest way of helping a sleepy young baby get off to sleep is to let him stay at the breast until he nods off. If you want to bring up a bubble of wind, do so, then put him back to the breast. Some babies doze towards the end of a feed without actually letting go, waking every so often to nibble or lightly suck. If you gently remove your breast, he may drift into a deeper sleep. If you watch him, you'll notice he makes occasional sucking or mouthing movements as if still at the breast and, from time to time, a smile or a frown may flicker across his face as he dreams. You may see similar facial expressions just before he wakes. Once he is sound asleep and you've had enough time to enjoy cuddling him, put him somewhere warm, safe and within earshot to sleep.

Some people rightly point out that babies frequently allowed to go to sleep at the breast get into the habit of needing the breast to fall asleep, as if it were a dummy. This is sometimes true and some women prefer not to let their babies get into the habit of needing to be at the breast in order to sleep.

What you do about letting him fall asleep at the breast depends on:

1 Whether you enjoy getting him off to sleep at your breast.
2 Whether you are happy for him to rely on being at the breast to go to sleep.
3 Whether you want to be able to leave your baby with a minder (however, many babies who like to go to sleep at the breast settle without it when their mother isn't there, though some find it more difficult).
4 Whether you are content with the idea of training him to go to sleep without the breast if you change your mind as he grows older.

Other ways of getting off to sleep

Many babies happily go to sleep after a feed if put in a warm, comfortable, familiar place, preferably near their mother. Rocking your baby in your arms is a time-honoured way of inducing sleep if he's tired yet no longer wants the breast. And some babies regularly nod off in a car, pram or sling, lulled by the motion or noise.

You may find that how you get your baby off to sleep varies with the time of day, where you are and what you're doing. Many prefer to go to sleep in a familiar place, especially when they're older. However, just having their mothers there feeding them, cuddling them on their lap, or lying by them is enough to reassure them as they drop off.

There's nothing more pleasant than going to sleep yourself with your baby by you if you can find the time. You'll wake up feeling refreshed, especially if you've been having broken nights. You may find he sleeps extra well when you're there, perhaps because of the familiar and reassuring smell, feel and sound of your body. Many babies open their eyes several times as they go off to sleep as if to check that their mother is still there.

- A tip for mothers of babies who find it difficult to get off to sleep is to check how much coffee they drink. Coffee-drinking isn't usually a problem but some babies, particularly pre-term ones whose livers can't yet break caffeine down very well, have trouble sleeping if their mothers drink a lot of coffee or other caffeine-containing drinks, such as cola and tea.

HOW LONG WILL YOUR BABY SLEEP?

Your baby may fall into a pattern of sleeping for a certain length of time between some feeds, or he may be an irregular sleeper. Many young babies wake up soon after what their mothers thought was the end of a feed and want to go back to the breast. This is perfectly normal – especially in the evenings, and especially for babies who are unwell, very young or pre-term.

As long as you haven't planned on having an hour or two free, this doesn't matter at all. You can simply put the baby back to your other breast. However, it's worth checking that you are feeding with him well positioned at the breast (see page 167), so that he stimulates your milk to let down and is able to milk the reservoirs under the areola efficiently.

A few babies fuss and can't get off to sleep even though they need to, because they have drunk plenty of fore-milk but not enough of the satisfying, fat-rich hind-milk. This may be because they came off the first breast before they had any (or enough) hind-milk, and their mothers understandably thought they'd had enough of that breast and switched them to the other side, where they drank more fore-milk, filled their tummies up, but still hadn't had any (or enough) satisfying hind-milk. The way to check whether this is so is to put your baby back to the first breast. If it's empty, you'll soon know because he'll stop feeding and may cry.

Carrying an unsettled baby in a sling is one answer if you have to get on with essential jobs. You'll find it's easier to cook, clean, wash up, write and so on with the baby slung on your back rather than your front.

LEAKING (See also page 203)

The leaking seen in the first few weeks gradually becomes less of a problem, partly because your let-down reflex becomes more controlled as your milk supply becomes established and partly because the storage capacity of the milk ducts increases during the first few weeks so that they can hold more milk without letting it escape. You'll still leak from the opposite breast during a feed.

CRYING (see also page 196)

The sound of your baby's cry is designed to alert you so that you care for him. It's not the sort of sound that can easily be ignored, even by a stranger, and a baby that won't stop crying is very disturbing. If a baby seems to do nothing but cry for the first few days, weeks or even months, it's hardly surprising that his mother will feel something must be wrong with him or his food. Once the doctor reassures her that nothing is medically wrong, some women – and, unfortunately, their professional helpers – believe the next step is to change their feed. For a breastfeeding woman this means giving bottles of formula. Is this necessary? In almost every case the answer is no.

A crying baby's best interests are only rarely served by stopping breastfeeding and changing to a bottle.

The first thing to do is to breastfeed as nature intended, which means at least every time he cries (see pages 172 and 271). A baby breastfed according to a schedule will almost certainly cry a lot because not only will he sometimes be hungry before the clock says it's time for a feed but he'll also be denied comfort-sucking time because his mother thinks she must allow him only ten minutes at each breast.

Feeding your baby frequently, whenever he wants, for as long as he wants to feed, will almost certainly reduce or stop his crying.

— One study showed that frequently fed babies cried only about half as much at two months old as those fed less often. The difference, while slightly less, was still noticeable at four months.

Feeding your baby whenever he cries will also increase your milk supply, which is a good thing if he was crying because he was hungry. Research shows that breastfed babies fed on demand cry much less than schedule-breastfed babies. It's difficult to ascertain what the long-term psychological effects of prolonged periods of crying are, but they certainly cause unhappiness at the time.

Some babies cry because they're bored and need amusement. Others crave company and settle only when held. One way to cope if you're busy is to use a sling. Several types leave your hands free to get on with your work but keep the baby secure and contented as you walk around.

— A study in the USA (1986) found that when parents spent more time carrying their babies, the babies cried only half as much as they did before.

Other babies are pacified (as long as they aren't hungry) by a ride in a buggy or pram, or even in a car. Anything is worth trying but *always try suckling first*.

If all else fails, ask a friend, relative or neighbour to look after your baby for a time. If you are constantly worried about the crying, your milk supply will dwindle and that, in turn, will make him cry more. A change of face and scene often quietens a baby miraculously.

BREASTFEEDING THROUGHOUT THE DAY

As milk-producing cells constantly secrete milk, the amount in the breast will depend to some extent on the time since the last feed. If your baby doesn't wake and your breasts are uncomfortably full, either express some milk or wake him – after all, you'll sometimes need him to relieve you as much as he needs you at other times to relieve his hunger.

As he will hopefully have his longest break between feeds at night, your breasts will be especially full first thing in the morning. You may even wake up with your nightie and sheets or duvet cover drenched with milk. The early morning feed is often the most pleasant simply because of a very real sense of relief.

HOW YOU FEEL THROUGHOUT THE DAY

During the day your enjoyment from feeding will depend to some extent on how busy you are. If you slot feeds into a packed day, you may not feel calm and your baby will sense your tension and be more fussy than usual. Be careful not to get so tense that you don't let your milk down. If you don't experience the telltale signs (see page 21), try to slow down for the rest of the day and cut out a few jobs the next day.

Many women feel at their worst in the early evening. Not only may they have to feed other children and start getting them to bed but they may also want to tidy up, feed the baby and think about an evening meal for themselves and their family. The early evening is a physiologically low time for many people anyway.

If it's just too much for you and your let-down reflex, be your own time-and-motion expert and organize things so that they don't all happen at once. Meals can wait, as long as you and your family have something to eat to keep you going in the meantime; older children can be encouraged to help clear up their toys; and you could give them their tea and bath earlier. Do anything to avoid having lots of things to do at the very time of the day when you're beginning to feel tired anyway. Prepare food for the evening in the afternoon, make full use of your fridge and freezer, and cook dishes such as casseroles that you can prepare in advance.

YOUR BABY'S BOWELS

A totally breastfed baby's motions aren't foul-smelling like those of a bottle-fed one. They are liquid and passed very frequently at first but later perhaps only every few days. Their normal colour is bright yellow but occasionally they go green. Babies often open their bowels during a feed, so it's sensible to change the nappy after a feed, unless your baby is one of those who won't feed in a wet or dirty nappy.

SOME EVERYDAY CHALLENGES

A woman at home on her own will face many practical challenges when feeding her baby. For instance, what does she do if the doorbell rings? There are several ways round this. You can decide that nothing will be allowed to interrupt you when you are feeding, so you don't answer the bell. You can do up your clothes quickly and answer the door, either with your hungry baby crying in your arms or left safely somewhere. You can carry on feeding and answer the door anyway, perhaps with a shawl round you. Or you can make a little notice for the front door which says, 'I am busy, please ring only if it's important.'

What if passers-by – or the window-cleaner – can see in through the window? That's easier. Keep a nappy or shawl near you when feeding so you can do a hasty cover-up job if necessary. Practise first so that you can do it without annoying the baby. Or you could feed somewhere more private (which is a problem if the window-cleaner is going from window to window!).

The phone is more difficult because somehow it always seems such an urgent noise and many people find it difficult to steel themselves to leave it unanswered. One way round this is to take the phone off the hook while feeding. Another is to have the phone by you. This may need organizing with the phone company who will put a jack anywhere you want provided you pay for the alteration. A high-tech alternative is to have a remote handset which you can remove from its base and keep by you, or to have a mobile phone. You could also find an answerphone useful.

Whatever the disturbance, what you don't want is your let-down to be inhibited and the feed spoilt, so it's worth thinking about how you will cope with these practical things before you actually have to. You'll let your milk down better when you are calm and undisturbed.

FEEDING WITH OTHER CHILDREN AROUND

A new baby in the family is both a joy and a misery to the other children, especially if they are very young. The attractions of the new arrival are tempered by the fact that their mother now has a new interest which is central in her life and takes up much of her time.

A way round this is to be extra loving and attentive, especially to your youngest child, because it is probably he who will be most affected by the new baby. If he wants to have a feed, let him – he's only trying to compete for your attention and will soon get bored with the breast. Some mothers carry on breastfeeding throughout pregnancy and then feed their older child *and* the baby, which reduces jealousy.

Always try to bring your older children into the intimacy of the breastfeeding circle. Soon you'll be so adept at breastfeeding that you'll be able to sit reading to a toddler and feed the baby at the same time. If you can't, then keep an absorbing toy or game handy for when you're feeding and remember to spend some time later playing alone with the child who feels left out.

Your children will gain one huge advantage by watching you breastfeed – simply having the experience of observing breast-feeding in action. This will make a big difference to the likelihood of them breastfeeding (or, in the case of a boy, encouraging his partner to breastfeed) when they in turn have a baby. Surveys show that women who choose to breastfeed are more likely to have seen a baby breastfed than women who choose to bottle-feed.

BREASTFEEDING IN COMPANY

There are many ways of coping with this. Your decision will depend on you and your feelings and on who the other people are. You may always prefer to feed alone, in which case you'll miss hours of other people's company. If you do this, you can either send visitors to another room when you feed in the room you usually use, or you can go into another room yourself. Don't hurry the feed so as to get back to your friends. The baby will be much more likely to be in a good mood for being shown off if he's well fed and happy, and that means feeding him as you normally would.

If you are in someone else's house, make yourself warm and comfortable before you feed and ask for drinks, cushions or whatever you need. You may want to feed somewhere private for your own sake. If not, enquire tactfully how your hosts feel about your breastfeeding with them there. Some people are delighted to see a baby being breastfed and are not at all embarrassed. How-ever, others are embarrassed, sometimes simply because it's so unfamiliar, and a few are deeply disturbed. If you sense their embarrassment and let it get to you, you might not let your milk down.

Practical tips for feeding in company

- Sit at one end of the room so that you can join in the discussion but not be put off by the others.
- Wear clothes you can pull up just enough to feed in a way that reveals nothing.
- Drape yourself and your baby with a shawl to cover your breast.

A clever choice of clothing is useful when you are in a train, bus, park or restaurant – situations in which other people may be embarrassed or offended. If you pull up a T-shirt, sweat-shirt, jumper or blouse from the waist you can feed very discreetly and show almost none of your bare breast. Clothes that unbutton are more revealing. A practice feed in front of a mirror will give you confidence in what looks okay to you.

ENTERTAINING

If looking after people and cooking for them comes easily to you, you'll probably find breastfeeding no hindrance to entertaining. However, if you're the sort who worries for days about what to give friends to eat, think twice about entertaining. It's as simple as that. Whatever you cook, make sure it's something that won't be harmed by being left in a warm oven if you have to feed the baby before you eat. The calmer you are, the calmer he will be, as babies quickly pick up their mother's feelings and react to them. With a little practice it's usually possible to feed a baby at the dinner table in a way that doesn't reveal any bare breast, but be sensitive to the feelings of your guests.

CAR JOURNEYS AND HOLIDAYS

Breastfeeding is easy in a car – in fact it really comes into its own when you're travelling. Either stop and feed or, if someone else is driving, feed in the back seat for safety.

If you fly, it's not a bad idea to fly at night so that the baby will be sleepy, the aircraft dark for feeding and the chances of privacy increased because fewer passengers move about. Some airlines have a special seat that can be curtained off for a breastfeeding mother but the most practical answer is to feed discreetly in the main part of the aircraft.

If you travel with another adult, ask them to take care of the arrangements as much as possible or you could become tense and tired and not let your milk down so well.

Holidays are much simpler with a breastfed baby. There's no bottle-cleaning and sterilizing to worry about, no boiled water to organize, and the necessary equipment is always to hand!

GOING OUTSIDE

Try to get some daylight on your baby's skin every day, especially if he is dark-skinned or you live in northerly parts where the sun's rays are more oblique and less light gets through the atmosphere. The exposure must be outside in the open because window glass filters out a lot of this light. Daylight on the skin helps keep a baby's bones strong. Just twenty minutes of daylight each day on your baby's uncovered cheeks can provide enough vitamin D to protect against the bone-softening disease called rickets. Sun is important for you and your milk too. See pages 245 and 43.

GOING OUT WITH YOUR BABY

Most women prefer to take their baby with them whenever they go out. Once a baby has become used to his mother being there all the time, even a cup or bottle of breast milk may not comfort him.

You can take a breastfed baby almost anywhere, though it's better to put off going to the theatre, cinema, concerts and lectures simply because gurgles, glugs, goos, cries and so on are really not acceptable when other people have paid to be there and want to listen without disturbance. However, if you have the sort of baby you can rely on to let you know he wants a feed simply by wriggling quietly, and the sort that doesn't slurp or make other feeding noises, you might persuade yourself that you can sit at the back of the auditorium and leave immediately if necessary.

Restaurants are a different matter and increasing numbers now accept that mothers of breastfed babies may want to feed while they are there. Feed discreetly because although you could argue that other people shouldn't be upset, the fact is that many are. You'll do more to persuade them that breastfeeding is good if you do it discreetly than if you flaunt yourself. You may prefer not to go to upmarket restaurants with your breastfed baby, either because you may feel you won't let your milk down so well if you are concerned about disturbing other diners, or simply because it doesn't feel like the right environment for breastfeeding. If you do go to one, though, ask for a table in a corner to make breastfeeding and dealing with your baby easier for you.

You can easily take your baby with you if you go out to friends for the evening, even if you have a sitter for the older children. If he wants feeding, then it's a simple enough matter to pop upstairs if you would cause offence by staying with the other guests. Tell your hostess in advance that you would like to bring your breastfeeding baby, and this will give her a chance not to cook anything that might spoil if left in the oven a little longer.

If you have to go out without your baby you can leave a

container of expressed milk (see page 191) in the fridge for the sitter to warm when needed (see page 192) and give it from a feeding cup, spoon or even a bottle. If the baby is hungry, there should be no problem because the milk is his usual brew.

The difficulty with expressing, though, can be collecting enough. Try expressing after every feed for two whole days before you are due to go out. This way you should be able to collect enough to satisfy your baby for an evening.

Feeding a baby from day to day can be one of the most rewarding things a woman ever does. Yet it may not always be as easy as she thinks. Knowing what to do is half the battle. Knowing what can go wrong is the other. We'll look at some common problems in the next chapter.

NINE

Looking after yourself

WHY?

There are two very good reasons for looking after yourself when you've had a baby. First, as a mother you're probably the pivot of your home and if you are well and happy the chances are that the rest of the family will be too. If, like so many mothers, you become tired and run down with the pressures of home, husband, partner (or neither), other children and a baby to look after, your mood will reflect on those around you.

Second, a fit and healthy woman is far more likely to breastfeed her baby successfully than one who is permanently physically and emotionally exhausted. This isn't because the amount of milk produced is greater or the quality of the milk different, but because an exhausted woman's let-down reflex just isn't as reliable. Once the let-down becomes unreliable, her baby is frustrated, takes less and less milk, feels hungry, cries more and adds to his mother's exhaustion.

'Mothering the mother' is seen as a vital part of successful child-rearing in many cultures. These wise people know that a well-cared-for mother stands more chance of looking after her young children adequately. In our culture, it's unlikely that you'll have somebody to look after you for much of the time, so it's vital to look after yourself.

REST, RELAXATION AND SLEEP

If you have only one baby, you'll find it comparatively easy to make time for catnaps during the day when he sleeps. Indeed, if you are waking several times a night, which is highly likely, especially at first, you *must* make time for naps, even if you are the sort of person who would have turned her nose up at daytime sleeping before you had the baby.

For the mother who comes home after forty-eight hours in hospital, rest – and that means rest in bed – is *not* a luxury, it's a must. It's a pretty safe rule to say that you should aim to spend most of your day in and around your bed for the first week after the birth, whether you're in hospital or at home. This doesn't mean you should stay in bed *all* day – you certainly shouldn't. But it's sensible not to busy yourself around the house as if nothing had happened.

The temptation, especially for an efficient woman who held down a busy job before she had her baby, is to cram all sorts of household and other tasks into the baby's sleep time. But you have the rest of your life to be a superwoman – you don't have to be one now. If you are rested, cheerful and content, you'll be a far better mother than if you'd cleaned the oven, changed the sheets, kept in touch with the office and exhausted yourself! Keep your kitchen and bathroom clean, pick up obvious fluff and other mess and tidy up if neccessary – that's all you need to do to keep your home pleasant. Housework will always be there but you'll probably have a chance to mother a new baby only a couple of times in a lifetime, so make the most of them. To paraphrase the American saying, 'Kissin' don't last – cookery do', 'Babies don't last – housework does!'

Whenever you can, relax. Even if you don't sleep in the day, lie down and read or put the radio or TV on. Think about moving the TV into the bedroom. Try to relax when you're feeding the baby, peeling the vegetables, watching TV or driving the car. The secret is not to let undue muscle tension build up because this is tiring in itself.

Breastfeeding naturally, without schedules, helps ensure that newly delivered mothers sit down quietly for long periods.

At night, try to accept that it'll probably be a long time before you regularly have long, unbroken stretches of sleep. If you go back to sleep quickly when you've fed the baby, so much the better. If you can't, at least you can get some physical rest. If you keep your baby in bed with you, you'll be able to snooze during feeds.

A woman with more than one child has a harder task if she's to get enough rest. If your elder child still sleeps during the day, try to get the baby to sleep as well so that you can have a rest at the same time. If this is impossible, it's a good idea to lie down anyway with your baby. This is more relaxing than sitting in a chair. Sometimes you could ask a neighbour or a friend to help by taking your toddler off your hands for an hour or so while you sleep. He'll probably welcome the change too. An extension of this is to organize a group of local mothers so that you can help each other out.

YOUR FOOD

There's little evidence that any particular foods or drinks increase or decrease the milk supply (though see page 284), *provided you eat an adequate, well-balanced, nutritious diet*. If you eat a healthy diet, it's wise to eat according to your appetite. The woman who eats sensibly provides her baby with plenty of milk and ensures her own body isn't drained of nutrients.

Do you need to eat more?

Experts have been discussing this for years and have changed their recommendations on calorie allowances in the light of advances in knowledge. In the UK the Department of Health recommended in 1991 that breastfeeding women should have approximately 400–600 calories a day extra.

Indeed, some researchers have found that women who are breastfeeding successfully eat on average nearly 700 calories a day more than bottle-feeding women yet still manage to lose the pounds of fat they stored in pregnancy.

One survey found that stopping breastfeeding because of 'not having enough milk' was less likely in a group of mothers who had been actively encouraged to eat more compared with a group who had received no such advice. Not all breastfeeding mothers feel a need for extra food, though it's interesting that those who breastfeed for longer tend to have larger appetites compared with what used to be normal for them.

— A group of researchers reported (1993) that the healthy, successfully breastfeeding women they studied needed no more calories than non-breastfeeding women of the same weight. The breastfeeding women ate on average a total of 1666 calories a day (only 62 per cent of the 2700 calories recommended for breastfeeding women by the US National Research Council). The researchers note that other studies have shown that healthy, successfully breastfeeding women in developed countries eat a daily 1800–2300 calories, and in developing countries, a daily 1200–1750 calories – both less than the officially recommended amounts!

Breastfeeding women seem to be more efficient than non-lactating ones at using the food they eat to supply themselves with energy.

Researchers suggest that a woman's milk supply is more dependable if she spaces her food intake evenly throughout the day, rather than eating the bulk at one meal.

Should you eat more of anything in particular?

You need to eat more food – or more nutrient-dense food – to provide you with the necessary extra supplies of vitamins, minerals

and other 'micro-nutrients'. So, assuming you're already eating a
healthy diet, just eat slightly more of everything if you feel like it.
But if your diet is only marginally satisfactory, don't fill up with
'empty calories' from refined foods such as biscuits and crisps. You
need more healthy, nutrient-dense foods, otherwise although you'll
probably manage to supply your baby with enough nutrients, your
own body could go short.

Vegetarians

In many countries in which women breastfeed successfully, both
vegetarian and vegan diets are considered entirely normal. If you
are vegetarian, it's wise to check with a dietitian that you have
adequate food sources of vitamin B_{12}. This vitamin is essential for
the formation of red blood cells and the functioning of nerves.
Vegetarian sources include eggs, dairy products, some fermented
foods such as fermented soy beans (especially if these foods are
traditionally prepared by being fermented for long periods), Marmite, fortified foods and some seaweeds.

Vegans need to take particular care to consume plenty of
foods containing vitamin B_{12}. Low levels are most likely in 'first-
generation' vegans – people who eat no foods at all from animal
sources and are the first vegans in their family, so haven't had the
benefit of generations of traditional wisdom about preparing
nourishing vegan meals. They may, as a result, be in particular
danger of going short. If you think you may not be getting enough
vitamin B_{12}, you can improve your diet or take a supplement.
For a list of foods containing vitamin B_{12}, send an sae to the
Vegetarian Society, Parkdale, Dunham Road, Altrincham, Cheshire
WA14 4QG.

Vegans also need to eat plenty of foods containing calcium
(peas, beans, lentils, green vegetables, nuts, seeds), iron (peas,
beans, pulses, nuts, wholegrains, green vegetables, molasses, parsley, cocoa) and riboflavin (vitamin B_2 – in wholegrains and green
leafy vegetables).

— According to a study in 1992, vegans may also have low levels of zinc and magnesium and should consider eating more foods containing these nutrients or taking supplements. (Foods containing zinc include nuts, peas, beans, wholegrains, root vegetables, parsley, garlic and ginger; and magnesium: nuts, soybeans, wholegrains and green leafy vegetables.)

Is there anything you shouldn't eat?

Some spices like those in curry can flavour breast milk but have no harmful effect on babies. However, if you don't usually eat curry, your baby may be rather surprised by the taste when you do! The vast majority of foods seem to have little effect, even when traces enter the milk. No foods are forbidden, but if you find your baby reacts in an unusual way after you've eaten a certain food, simply avoid it until you stop breastfeeding. Some babies are more sensitive than others. Quite a few mothers report that onions, peas, cabbage, cauliflower and broccoli seem to make their babies fuss more. Chocolate gives some babies a rash, diarrhoea or constipation and can make them irritable. See also page 200.

It's wise not to eat any food that looks less than fresh and to avoid entirely foods past their sell-by dates as there's more chance of them being mouldy, even if you can't see this. Animal research shows that fungal by-products called aflatoxins have adverse effects on immunity, liver function, nutrition and survival. We don't yet know if this applies to human babies.

— Research (1988) from Ghana found aflatoxins in the milk of one in three women tested. The aflatoxins must have come from food contaminated by fungi and eaten by the women. Breast milk was more likely to contain aflatoxins in the wet season (when food was more liable to be damp and to start going mouldy).

Occasionally a breastfeeding woman and her baby have a spot of really bad luck.

— For example, researchers reported (1990) that a breastfeeding woman developed ciguatera fish toxicity from eating a ciguatera-affected kingfish. Ten hours after her baby had his first feed after his mother's kingfish meal, he became colicky and developed diarrhoea lasting for forty-eight hours, then a flat red rash appeared. He was unusually fussy but continued to breastfeed and was back to normal two weeks later.

What if you don't eat enough?

Severely malnourished, starving women in developing countries can feed their babies for three months before extra food for them is essential if their babies are to go on growing normally. However, these women breastfeed at the expense of their own bodies – for example, they become short of calcium and protein, and the more babies they have and feed, the poorer their physical state becomes. If they eat so little that their serum albumin (a protein in their blood) drops below 30g (1oz) per litre (1¾ pints), their milk supply may suddenly fall and, at worst, dry up completely. This situation is virtually never seen in developed countries where almost every woman has enough to eat. A great deal of research shows that malnourished women can produce very high volumes of good-quality milk and that milk production is extremely robust except in famine or near-famine conditions.

Slimming

Obviously, for both your sake and the baby's, you shouldn't go on a crash diet while you're breastfeeding. So if you are concerned about your weight and really want to lose weight now, ask your doctor to refer you to a dietitian for specialist help with a healthy, weight-reducing diet while breastfeeding, or go to a slimming club which offers sensible weight-loss diets approved for breastfeeding women. Remember that daily exercise can be a huge help in losing weight and keeping it off. Some women find the fat they put on when they were pregnant slowly disappears with breastfeeding. However, this isn't so for everyone.

— A Californian study (1994) found that women who breastfed for three to six months lost an average of 4.4 lb *more* weight than bottle-feeders, and that the fat stayed off for at least two years. They lost most fat from their tummy, hips and thighs. Women who breastfed longer than six months were more likely to be losing weight than were non-breastfeeding women. The researchers suggested that increased levels of prolactin produced while breastfeeding decrease the appetite.

— However, other researchers in Philadelphia (1983) suggested two possible reasons for breastfeeding women losing fat from their fat stores. The first was that the higher a woman's prolactin level, the lower are her oestrogen and progesterone levels. This is significant because progesterone encourages fat to be stored. They noted that women who gave more frequent breastfeeds had a higher prolactin level and lost more fat from their fat stores (estimated by measuring their upper arms) than women who breastfed less often. Their second suggestion was that maintaining a high prolactin level may reduce the activity of an enzyme (lipoprotein lipase) which encourages fat to be stored in fat stores other than the breast.

— Another US study (1994) found that women who went on a well-planned weight-loss diet (which provided 25 per cent fewer calories than breastfeeding women generally need) noticed no reduction of their milk supply. Dieting made no difference to the amount of fat and protein in their milk either.

What about drinks?

You'll find you're more thirsty than usual, which is scarcely surprising considering that a baby takes on average between 600 and 800 ml (more than a pint) of milk a day, depending on the individual baby, his age and weight. There's no need to force yourself to drink more – just drink as much as you want. Research shows that drinking more than thirst demands actually *reduces* the amount of milk. However, it isn't a good idea for you to become dehydrated.

Many nursing mothers feel most thirsty while actually feeding and like to keep a drink close at hand.

Milk? – Milk and other dairy foods are an important part of the
traditional diet in dairying countries. However, provided your diet
is well-balanced and contains the nutrients you would otherwise
get from milk, there's no need to drink a lot of milk. Indeed, if you
don't like it there's no need to drink any! You don't need cows'
milk to make breast milk. Cows don't drink milk but make plenty
of milk from their diet of grass. In fact no mammal needs to drink
milk to make milk. Some sources of dietary information for
pregnant and nursing mothers recommend one to two pints of
milk daily. But in the light of what they now know about allergy,
most experts consider it unwise for breastfeeding women to eat or
drink a large amount of any one food, especially if they have a
family history of allergic disorders. As cows' milk is so common
an allergen, you may want to consider avoiding a large intake
while breastfeeding, especially if there's allergy in your family.

Try to put cows' milk in perspective. It isn't a magic food but
simply one of many we can include in our daily diet. Its advantages
are that it's relatively cheap and contains a wide range of nutrients.
However, all these can be obtained from many other foods provided you eat a balanced diet. It's wise to check your diet if you
grew up in a family which ate and drank a lot of milk and other
dairy foods yet don't have much milk yourself, simply to make
sure you're choosing a healthy diet.

Alcohol? – Many breastfeeding women wonder whether or not
they should drink anything alcoholic. Drinking in moderation is
acceptable. Some alcohol passes into breast milk and if you drink
large amounts, correspondingly more gets to the baby. Drinking
alcohol raises the prolactin level in men and even more in women,
though studies to ascertain whether this is also true for lactating
women haven't been done.

Alcohol flavours breast milk and when a woman drinks it both
the intensity of the taste and the alcohol concentration in her milk
peak half to one hour later. Babies seem to want less milk when
their mother has had alcohol. The reason isn't yet clear but

suggestions are that the smell of the milk puts them off, or that the alcoholic breast milk somehow affects their behaviour, making them want smaller feeds. When babies drink alcohol-laden breast milk, they sleep the same amount but for more frequent, shorter lengths of time. Some babies are temporarily uncomfortable and irritable after their mother has had a drink. The type of drink seems to be important too. There's a report of an eight-day-old baby who became drunk after his mother had 750 ml (well over a pint) of port in twenty-four hours! Drinking enough to make you feel tipsy may harm your milk supply by affecting your oxytocin output, making your let-down reflex unreliable, or making you dehydrated – so go easy and remember to top yourself up with water or soft drinks.

Coffee? – When a woman has a caffeine-containing drink (coffee, tea, cola or other caffeinated soft drinks) the caffeine enters her milk within fifteen minutes and reaches peak levels within an hour. There's still some caffeine in the milk twelve hours later (and even longer in some women). In large enough amounts caffeine is a powerful drug. A young baby's liver breaks down caffeine very slowly and caffeine from a mother who has a moderately high intake (six to eight cups in twenty-four hours) can accumulate and cause abnormal activity and sleeplessness. However, this disappears when she avoids caffeine for a few days. Modest drinking of caffeine-containing drinks (such as one to three cups of average strength coffee a day) is unlikely to cause any problems. But if you drink more, you'd be wise to have your coffee or other caffeinated drink after you've finished feeding your baby, to give your milk's caffeine level time to come down from its one-hour high before you feed again. If you suspect you may be drinking too much caffeine, try cutting out tea and coffee for a week to see if this makes any difference to your baby. Smoking increases the effects of caffeine.

Vitamins?

The UK Department of Health recommends that all breastfeeding women take a vitamin supplement to ensure that their milk contains enough vitamins for their baby.

Mothers of pre-term babies should make sure they have enough foods rich in vitamin C (especially fresh vegetables and fruits). Pre-term babies have relatively low iron stores but the plentiful supplies of vitamin C in breast milk probably help them absorb iron better.

BREASTFEEDING AND BONES (see also page 129)

Breastfeeding may temporarily remove minerals, making your bones slightly less dense, but as long as you look after yourself (see below) they should soon catch up again.

— Research (1995) found that while the mineral content of women's bones decreased while they were breastfeeding, it returned to normal within six months of stopping.

— Research in the US (1993) monitored bone density in ninety-eight breastfeeding women for a year. The bones of those who breastfed for more than a month became temporarily less dense. But they returned to normal by a year in those who fed for up to nine months, and were on their way back to normal in those who did so for longer.

— Other US researchers found that women aged between thirty and thirty-five who had breastfed three or more babies for ten months or more each had more bone-loss than women who had breastfed less. This was in spite of eating the recommended amount of calcium-containing food.

— A report (1982) noted that young, teenage breastfeeding mothers lost more minerals from their bones than did older women. As far as we know this work was never followed up to see if their bones – like those of older women – recovered with time.

Whatever your age and whether or not you are breastfeeding, look after your bones by:

- Spending some time outside each day with daylight directly on your skin. Exposure to daylight enables your body to make meaningful amounts of vitamin D. This is especially important if you are dark-skinned or live in northerly parts where the sun's rays are more oblique and less light gets through the atmosphere. The exposure must be outside in the open because window glass filters out a lot of this light.
- Taking regular, moderate weight-bearing exercise (such as walking).
- Eating a healthy diet.
- Avoiding a crash, or otherwise inadequate, slimming diet.
- Not smoking.

There's no point in taking a calcium supplement as research shows that this makes no difference either to a breastfeeder's bone mineral density or to the amount of calcium in her milk.

If you are unlucky enough to have severe osteoporosis already, it's wise to take even more care of yourself while you are breastfeeding, and not to lift or carry your baby more than you need to as he gets heavier. However, as long as you look after yourself and your condition isn't getting worse, there seems to be no reason to stop breastfeeding.

EXERCISE

Regular, moderate exercise is good for us. It boosts our circulation, raises levels of natural 'feel-good' chemicals such as endorphins, and keeps muscles strong and flexible and our whole bodies fit. You owe it to yourself – and your family – to make time for exercise and to find ways to fit it into your life.

One study suggested that breast milk tasted unusual after exercise because of an increase in its lactic acid concentration and that this put babies off their next feed.

—However, a Californian survey (1994) found that breastfeeding women who exercised aerobically four to five times a week were measurably very much fitter and that their babies had no problems with feeding after they had exercised.

THE WAY YOU FEEL

Most women experience a mixture of heightened feelings after having a baby. Indeed, emotionally speaking, the whole of the first year may be like being on a roller-coaster. None of this is surprising because the changes in a woman's lifestyle after her baby is born are immense, particularly if it's her first. And when she becomes a mother she takes on a role of enormous practical and symbolic importance to her baby, herself, her baby's father and society.

Memories of being a baby

Simply being with her baby arouses many emotions in most mothers. This is a time when memories of her own experiences as a baby are stirred deep in her conscious – or unconscious – mind. Psychoanalysts believe that babies 'split' their impressions of their mother according to their experiences of how she meets their needs. This means that at first they may see her as virtually two different people, a 'good' mother and a 'bad' mother. So when a baby girl grows up to womanhood, becomes a mother and observes her own baby's reactions, distant recollections of joy and satisfaction at her hunger being satiated by her own 'good' mother may mingle with long-lost but still imprinted memories of frustration, fear, loneliness, anger, envy and despair over times when she was left alone, hungry and crying, by her 'bad' mother.

Being with her baby can evoke memories of any of these emotions. These echoes from the past are normal and their power in the here and now can be very strong. The astonishingly profound intimacy of breastfeeding can stir a woman's memories even more.

This is one reason behind so many women's ambivalence about breastfeeding.

Surprised by joy

A woman's delight at having her baby at the breast may stem as much from her own remembered bliss and experience of security at having her needs met at her mother's breast as from the pleasure of the present experience.

Indeed, breastfeeding is usually a very positive experience. Many women like it because of the satisfaction they get from knowing it's the best and most natural way of feeding their baby. They enjoy its convenience and believe it forges a closer bond with their child. And they realize it's best for them, quite apart from being cheaper than bottle-feeding. (See reasons for choosing to breastfeed, page 119.)

— This positive attitude is highlighted by a large British survey which found that the longer a woman continues to breastfeed, the more likely she is to plan on breastfeeding her next baby. Women who had breastfed a baby for more than six weeks were very much more likely than those who had breastfed for less than six weeks to want to breastfeed their next baby.

Percentage of women intending to breastfeed according to how they fed their first baby (OPCS, 1990):
Bottle-fed before – 22
Breastfed less than 6 weeks before – 45
Breastfed more than 6 weeks before – 88

Long-forgotten concerns

On the other side of the coin, a woman's fear that her baby might be under-fed, or her dismay at being woken yet again by her crying baby at night – not to mention her interpretation of her baby's feelings – may echo her own long-forgotten feelings as a hungry baby who feared the breast might never come. Sometimes feelings triggered by our own experience as babies can cause us problems. Difficult or painful feelings with which we never came to terms as children may be a problem when we become mothers ourselves.

New motherhood – a challenging time

Psychologists have called new motherhood 'the third childhood'. By this they mean that new mothers enter a sensitive time of far-reaching change – just as they did in childhood itself or in the 'second childhood' during their teenage years. This is a time in which deep feelings, some of them unresolved, are stirred up in every woman. It is also a reason why most couples find that their loving and sexual life is disrupted to some degree.

Long-forgotten girlhood fantasies about the sort of mother she would become mingle with remembered and shut-away feelings about the mothering the woman had as an infant. Her views about mothers in general, together with her hopes about the sort of mother she aspires to be, come face to face with her feelings about having this baby, with this man, at this time. Her attitude to babies in general and to this baby in particular may or may not match up with those of her partner. Her thoughts about her breasts (see page 423) and her body in general; the family messages she's received about breastfeeding and mothering; and, most importantly today, her work situation, all join to create a complex mixture of ideas and attitudes through which she has to sift. Some of this sorting is done consciously and rationally but a lot is not – it goes on unconsciously.

Some women look forward to motherhood and to breastfeeding as a way of answering some of their dilemmas in life; others fear mothering and breastfeeding in case they fail. A woman may 'choose' breastfeeding because someone else is pressurizing her to do it and she wants to please them – or get them off her back! She may have recognized or unrecognized fears about giving up work or going back to work – and, possibly, about knowing few people in her situation. Or she may be wary about both breastfeeding and its effect on her relationship with her partner. She may, of course, not have a partner and wonder how she'll cope with breastfeeding at all on her own. And some women are anxious about having to hand their baby over to someone else to look after when they return to work.

The baby may or may not have been wanted; and he may remind his mother of someone in the family – someone she likes or dislikes, perhaps. Some women feel totally unprepared to bé a mother, let alone to breastfeed.

Stirred-up emotions represent a challenge which can be seen as both a danger and an opportunity. A danger if the emotions are unresolved and we simply suppress them again. And an opportunity if we try to recognize them and find ways of dealing with them so we can grow in emotional maturity.

Personal growth

Personal growth in response to the challenge of being a mother can enrich our lives and make us more sensitive to our own needs and to those of our baby and other nearest and dearest.

Also, as babies we may never have learned that our mother was a normally imperfect human being. If it was too difficult and frightening for us to accept our anger or other painful feelings about her as a 'bad' mother who didn't respond to our needs and satisfy them soon enough, we may have suppressed these emotions. We were then aware only of our feelings about her as a 'good' mother. But seeing her only as a 'good' mother (instead of as a 'good enough' mother who met most of our needs most of the time) meant seeing her as if she were perfect – in other words, idealizing her.

If this happened to us, we may have internalized the image of the 'perfect' or 'ideal' mother and could well have trouble adjusting to being ordinary, 'good enough' mothers ourselves. We may set ourselves too high a standard, expect to cope with everything easily, and have a shock when the reality proves rather different.

A time of golden opportunity

So what can you do to help this time of mothering and breastfeeding your baby become a time of golden emotional opportunity? Here are just a few ideas:

1. Listen to your feelings

One way of making the most of this time is to become more sensitive to any difficult emotions by listening to your inner voice. Try simply looking at your feelings about breastfeeding first, because recognizing and naming them can be a great help to learning how to deal with them constructively:

When you're breastfeeding, ask yourself these questions:

1 Am I a good enough mother?
2 Do I know what I'm doing?
3 What will everyone think of me if I can't breastfeed?
4 Do I like breastfeeding?
5 Is my baby getting enough milk?
6 Will it be my fault if my baby doesn't get enough?
7 Will I feel guilty if I don't breastfeed?
8 Who's really in control if my baby feeds whenever he wants?
9 What will my health visitor think if I don't breastfeed?
10 Do I like the sexuality of breastfeeding?
11 Can I bear caring for this demanding baby who never seems to stop feeding?
12 Is my baby the only person who loves me?
13 *Does* my baby love me?
14 If my baby really loves me, why isn't he good all the time?

If any of these questions rings bells for you, ask yourself how it makes you feel. For example, questions 1, 2, 3, 5 and 13 make some women feel afraid; 5 makes some feel helpless too; 6 and 7 make some feel guilty or angry; 8, 11 and 14 make some feel angry; and 12 makes some feel a sense of desperate longing and neediness.

If these emotions aren't immediately familiar, either they don't apply to you or they may be there but lying suppressed in your unconscious mind. As we've seen, suppressed emotions frequently stem from unresolved experiences in our own infancy. We aren't aware of them because early on we erected one or more of a variety of defences to stop them hurting us. But anything that stirs up difficult emotions – and particularly being with a baby – can disturb these defences and thereby allow our difficult feelings out. Sometimes this throws up problems or, rather, challenges.

One relevant challenge for a woman might be feeling strongly that she doesn't want to breastfeed – or doesn't like breastfeeding – without being able to pinpoint why. Others might include depression, anxiety and compulsive behaviour (such as overeating, a history of promiscuous relationships, dependence on alcohol or drugs, or overwork). Becoming more self-aware and learning to deal with their feelings helps many women respond to these challenges, become more mature and care for their baby more effectively. Otherwise, their own neediness can interfere with their ability to respond to their baby and be 'good enough' mothers.

2. Share your feelings

If you'd like to come to terms with any difficult emotions triggered by becoming a mother, simple brain-power and a wish to change may not be enough. You may need to discuss things with a good and trusted friend or with others in a small group – perhaps, for example, at a post-natal class. If this sort of care isn't available to you, how about seeking the help of a professional counsellor or therapist?

3. Get encouragement and support

Dealing with your feelings about breastfeeding is one thing, finding ways of giving yourself encouragement and support is another. Boosting your self-esteem is a good way of doing this. Remember that you are a valuable person in your own right and as a mother you are caring for your child at a vitally important time in his life. Make time to:

- Recognize how valuable you are.
- Focus on the things you currently enjoy and do well (however small they seem) and affirm yourself. For example, you may love being with your baby (or at least like it some of the time); you may be pleased that you're enjoying the change in pace that accompanied leaving work to care for your baby; or you may be pleased that you've managed to get out to the shops and cook a meal. Spell out these positive frames of mind and achievements, take a justifiable pride in them and let them warm you. Spread the glow by telling other people.
- Ask your friends or loved ones – your midwife (in the UK, your health visitor), or your breastfeeding counsellor – for encouragement and support. They may not realize you need it unless you ask; in other words, you may need to give them permission to step into your emotional life in this way.

4. Look after yourself

Take extra special care to look after yourself as you begin to recognize and adjust to your feelings about being a mother.

FEELING LOW? (see also page 205)

If you feel low, or depressed in general, several things may help:

1 Tell the story of your labour and birth experiences as many times as necessary to make them 'concrete' and 'real'.
2 Confide in someone you trust and think will be supportive, such as your partner, mother, sister or other relative, friend or neighbour.
3 Ask for help and be specific about what you'd like done; you may simply want someone to stay with your baby for a couple of hours a day so that you can have a refreshing sleep or get out for an hour.
4 Check you're eating a healthy diet with plenty of fresh vegetables, fruit and complex carbohydrates (such as wholemeal bread and

other wholegrain foods, beans, peas and lentils) to provide nutrients essential for emotional and physical health. Supplements of vitamin B complex, magnesium and calcium may help if you're feeling low.

5 Get outside every day for at least half an hour (longer if it's very early or late in the day). Daylight on the skin helps prevent winter depression (SAD or seasonal affective disorder).

6 Take some exercise each day, whether it's a brisk walk (for example, with your baby in the buggy), a swim, an exercise class or working out at home to an exercise video.

7 Keep up with your friends, however tempting it may be to shut yourself away.

8 Make time every day to do something you enjoy.

9 Brush up your empathic listening skills and ask your closest ally (partner, friend or relative) to practise with you. Being able to recognize, name and, possibly, discuss or otherwise express difficult feelings (such as anger at being cooped up with a difficult baby, or sadness at losing your previously carefree and rewarding lifestyle) brings these feelings into the open and prevents trouble building up.

10 Realize that each baby is different. If, for example, you have a baby born at a lower weight than expected from your length of pregnancy, he may seem to spend most of his time having frequent small feeds, sleeping or crying. It may be some time before he matures enough to be alert for long and to respond well emotionally, both of which would be more rewarding for you.

11 Last, but by no means least, tell your doctor (or, in the UK, health visitor), who may suggest you see a counsellor, join a group of women in the same situation who are working with a trained facilitator or, if necessary, take anti-depressant drugs.

— A study (1989) found that whether a woman breastfed or bottle-fed made no difference to her risk of suffering from post-natal depression.

— However, an older study (1983) found that exclusively breast-feeding women were more likely to become depressed than partial breastfeeders. The researchers suggested that possible factors involved were tiredness, having a dependent baby, and experiencing difficulties with breastfeeding.

— Another study (1987) found that the stress of having a baby who cried for long periods, didn't respond well when their mothers tried to comfort them, disliked new people, food and routines, and had unpredictable patterns of sleep and hunger, increased a woman's risk of post-natal depression. Women who had a lot of support from their partners, parents or friends had more confidence as parents, were less likely to blame themselves, and were less likely to be depressed three months after delivery.

SMOKING

Most people know that smoking during pregnancy isn't a good idea, partly because smokers' babies tend to have lower birth-weights. Not so many women know that if they smoke during the time they breastfeed, their smoking may reduce their milk supply, because nicotine reduces prolactin levels. Smokers tend to wean their babies from the breast sooner than do non-smokers, and heavy smokers (more than twenty to thirty cigarettes a day) tend to wean earliest of all.

— In 1992, researchers reported that when mothers of pre-term babies had to pump their milk for several weeks, smokers were already producing less milk than non-smokers by two weeks; and by four weeks only 36 per cent of smokers were making enough milk for their babies, compared with 72 per cent of non-smokers. The smokers' milk contained on average only four-fifths of the fat of the non-smokers' milk. This would have made their milk less sustaining and satisfying for their babies.

Smoking also increases the effects of caffeine (see page 243). Large amounts of nicotine in breast milk can have several unpleasant effects on babies. The most common are nausea, vomiting, tummy cramps and diarrhoea.

It's a good idea to cut smoking out or at least down if you can, especially if you're a heavy smoker. There's a great deal of help available in the form of quit-smoking groups, telephone help-lines and so on. If you do decide to continue, at least consider cutting down the number of cigarettes you smoke while actually breast-feeding. Your baby will breathe in large amounts of second-hand smoke if you smoke near him (and especially if you blow smoke at his face). This also applies if other people smoke near him. Inhaling smoke increases his risk of getting respiratory disorders such as pneumonia and bronchitis and puts him at a greater risk of the sudden infant death syndrome (see page 84) and of leukaemia.

CONTRACEPTION (see also page 123)

Unless you don't mind getting pregnant again soon, you'll need to take contraceptive precautions from the first eight to ten weeks after delivery. You can choose from the lactational amenorrhoea method (LAM), a diaphragm, a condom, the progestogen-only Pill or, expertly used, the sympto-thermal method. An intra-uterine contraceptive device (IUD) is best left until later.

WHEN PERIODS RETURN (see also pages 56 and 439)

When you start having periods again, take special care of yourself a week before and a week after ovulation. (Most woman ovulate somewhere between the tenth and fourteenth days of their cycle, counting the first day of the period as day one.) You may need extra reserves of energy and patience then as there's a chance that your baby might find it difficult to settle. If this happens, it's probably because your milk tastes different.

> — Australian researchers reported (1983) that the amount of sugar and potassium in breast milk falls temporarily on the fifth or sixth day before ovulation, and on the sixth or seventh day afterwards, presumably making it taste less sweet. At the same times, the amount of sodium and chloride increases, so it could possibly taste saltier.

SHOPPING

If you normally travel some way to the shops you'll find that you have very little time between feeds to do the shopping in the early weeks. You could do a big weekly shop with your partner or try to find shops which will deliver. There's nothing worse than going shopping and having to wheel a hungry, crying baby home when you're tired and heavy-laden.

SEEING FRIENDS

While some women like their own company best, many others feel very lonely if they leave their jobs, have a baby and don't make new friends. A baby is a very good conversation-opener and you'll probably find it easier to make friends now than at any other time. Breastfeeding is absolutely no hindrance to seeing people – especially other mothers – during the day. It's best not to arrange set times for meetings at other people's places because you'll probably end up breaking appointments when your baby wants to spend long, unhurried times at the breast. If you ask friends to your home, remember to look after your baby first and foremost. They can make drinks and answer the front door for you if necessary and will probably enjoy being useful.

SINGLE MOTHERS

The number of single mothers is increasing in every western country. In Great Britain in 1985, 11 per cent of mothers of young babies did not live with a husband or partner, while in 1990 the figure had risen to 14 per cent. Single mothers are less likely to breastfeed. Every bottle-feeder has different reasons for not breast-feeding, and it can be an excellent idea to identify them in case this enables such a woman to change her mind. For example, if she believes that she won't have enough encouragement and support to breastfeed, she could ask a close ally – such as a relative, friend, health professional or other breastfeeding helper, or social worker – to give her the back-up she needs. She may, of course, not know exactly what she'll need until she's had her baby, and she may have to adapt her request for encouragement and support if she finds that her needs change.

In a sense single mothers are particularly special and valuable and need to look after themselves very well.

ASSERTIVENESS SKILLS

Practise being assertive without being aggressive or hostile. By doing this you recognize, name and state your own needs (as you see them) as a pregnant or breastfeeding woman. At the same time you acknowledge other people's needs and their motives (as you see them) for their behaviour or attitudes. Being assertive means getting your needs met without trampling over other people.

You can learn assertiveness (or 'assertion') skills by copying other people who are pleasant but firm and don't act as doormats. Or you could learn from a book or attend courses.

You'll find such skills useful in many areas of life – including, perhaps, dealing with people who try to put you off breastfeeding or who make things difficult for you in some way.

ONE LAST WORD

Don't expect to get back to feeling like your old self overnight. Having a baby is physically and emotionally challenging. Many women don't feel like their old selves for some time and some say it takes at least a year. The odds are, though, that even though you may feel like you used to in many ways, having a baby and breastfeeding will provide insights and experiences which will change and mature you in ways you could never have expected.

> Looking after yourself well should help you get the best out of your pleasure in mothering and help you make plenty of milk. Sometimes, though, other things can interfere with the milk supply. We'll look at these in the next chapter so that you can get breastfeeding off to the best possible start.

TEN

Your milk supply

NOT ENOUGH MILK – THE COMMONEST CHALLENGE

Many mothers easily supply the right amount of milk to match their babies' needs, but others find they have too much or too little, especially in the early weeks before their milk supply is properly established. Too much milk can be a nuisance but rarely stops a woman breastfeeding. Too little, however, is the commonest reason women give for stopping breastfeeding or for giving bottle-feeds as well in the first few weeks after delivery.

You might be tempted to think that women who stop breast-feeding in the first few months want to stop, but this usually isn't so (at least not at any conscious level). The vast majority don't stop breastfeeding by choice – they do so because they think they haven't enough milk. This is clearly shown in a large survey of mothers in Great Britain done by the Office of Population and Censuses and Surveys (OPCS), see overleaf.

The message from this study is very clear: when a woman stops breastfeeding, by far the most likely reason – unless she's decided she wants to stop – is believing that she doesn't have enough milk. This is more important than nipple soreness, far more important than going back to work, and beats breastfeeding being 'too tiring' by a long way.

Women's belief that they have insufficient milk is the main dis-order of breastfeeding both in the UK and the rest of Great Britain, not to mention in other developed countries too. Unfortunately, it is a reason women increasingly give in developing countries too.

Women's reasons for stopping breastfeeding	Stopped by 6 weeks %	Stopped between 3 and 4 months %	Stopped between 4 and 9 months %
Insufficient milk	65	56	30
Breastfeeding too tiring or taking too long	13	9	6
Painful breasts or nipples	8	1	2
Baby wouldn't suck or rejected breast	7	10	22
Going back to work	7	23	15
Mother ill	7	5	3
Breastfed long enough or as long as planned	3	9	42
Baby ill	3	3	2
Domestic reasons	2	3	2
Didn't like breastfeeding	0	1	0
Baby can't be fed by others	2	2	3
Embarrassment	2	0	0
Inverted nipples	1	0	0
Other reasons	2	4	7
Inconvenient or no place to feed	1	5	4

Yet what most women don't realize is that a poor milk supply is nearly always a preventable and/or treatable condition. A woman may not have enough milk today but the odds of her being able to make as much as her baby needs within a few days are stacked high in her favour – if she takes the right steps to increase her milk supply.

What is often needed, though, is a paradigm shift – a completely different way of thinking about breastfeeding. If you're willing to try this, you'll need to forget the clock and learn some new skills.

Almost every woman can breastfeed if she wants to and has enough information and skilled support. Just think how much sadness and disappointment would be spared if only this were understood.

Women with 'insufficient' milk are often advised to give complements of formula or to abandon breastfeeding altogether. This is wrong.

The advice they should have straight away is how to increase their milk supply. (Unless, of course, a baby is starving because of a lack of breast milk, in which case formula or, preferably, donated breast milk should be used to supplement his mother's milk while she concentrates on increasing her milk supply.)

Most women who fail to breastfeed one baby at all – or for as long as they want – manage very well next time if they have enough information about successful breastfeeding techniques and if they also have enough encouragement and support. If you couldn't feed your last baby but want to feed the next one, tell your midwife (or, in the UK, your health visitor), as well as your NCT breastfeeding counsellor, La Leche League leader or lactation consultant, what you want to do so they can give you the help you need.

Does every woman have enough milk?

Many women think they don't have enough milk – and some indeed may not, at any given moment – but almost every one can make enough if they know how. Every woman can increase her milk supply to her own full potential and there's every reason to suppose that almost every healthy, well-nourished woman can feed her baby adequately if she knows what to do. In fact, with the right breastfeeding techniques the vast majority of women are capable of supplying twice the volume of milk their baby needs, if not more! Most women can easily breastfeed twins once they know how (see page 357). However, just as with dairy cows, some women are naturally capable of making more milk than others. Even on a four-hourly breastfeeding schedule (still wrongly recommended by some authorities), a few women produce plenty of milk. These are the women who may unknowingly undermine the confidence of the majority who need to give their babies many more feeds than this to stimulate their milk supply sufficiently. The answer is not to take any notice of how much milk anyone else has but simply to do what you and your baby need in order for him to be happy and well nourished. This means that some need much more breast stimulation, attention to breastfeeding technique and skilled support than others to produce the same amount of milk. Research also shows that women differ markedly in their breasts' milk-storage capacity, which means that some women naturally have to feed more often than others. A few decide that they don't want to devote the time and effort it takes to produce enough milk. This is, of course, their choice. Only a tiny minority, though, are unable to increase their production.

No one knows how many women are actually incapable of breastfeeding successfully. In developed countries figures of up to 4 or 5 per cent are quoted. But even if we accept that possibly as many as one in twenty women has trouble supplying enough milk, this doesn't mean that she necessarily can't do so once she knows how. The problem rarely lies with a woman's breasts but simply that so many women lack good advice and information about successful breastfeeding and have poor levels of skilled support. Having said all this, the figure of up to 5 per cent of women being unable to breastfeed is almost certainly an over-estimate anyway, as the following studies show:

— Among nearly 4000 mothers studied in Nigeria and Zaire, including both poor women and the 'urban elite', NOT ONE was unable to produce milk.

— Among over 400 babies who survived their first two days in Guatemala, EVERY ONE was successfully breastfed.

— At the Farm Midwifery Center in Tennessee, midwives reported that ONLY ONE WOMAN IN ABOUT 800 had had trouble in producing enough milk.

— ALL twenty babies born in a prisoner-of-war camp in Singapore during the Second World War were satisfactorily breastfed for six months before 'supplementary feeding' was started. All the mothers continued to breastfeed until their babies were over a year old.

However, as things stand today, some babies undoubtedly don't get enough breast milk and it's very important to find out which they are so that their mothers can take steps to increase their milk supply and – if they can't – so that the baby can be adequately nourished in some other way.

One expert in the US has identified some useful pointers:

1 The mothers of these babies may have failed to produce enough milk for a previous baby. (However, this may in itself mean very little, because many of these women would have failed to produce enough for their previous baby simply because they were breastfeeding in a 'token' way and didn't know how to increase their supply.)

2 Their close female relatives may have failed to produce enough milk. (Again, however, this may in itself mean very little, because they may have failed to produce enough simply because they were feeding in a 'token' way and didn't know how to increase their milk supply.)

3 They may have noticed little increase in the size of their breasts during pregnancy and little or no fullness of their breasts a few days after delivery.

4 One breast may be very different in size from the other. (However, this may in itself mean very little because most women have different-sized breasts).

Your milk supply

IS YOUR BABY HAVING ENOUGH?

This question originates from the years when strict four-hourly schedules were enforced. Many breastfed babies in fact did *not* get enough milk then because the schedules didn't allow them to breastfeed often enough to give their mothers' breasts the stimulation they needed to make more milk.

It's also a loaded question and the very fact that it's asked at all worries some newly delivered women so much that their milk production diminishes. Anxiety can be detrimental to a healthy letdown of milk. When this happens, the presence of stagnant milk in a woman's breasts, together with its pressure on her milk-producing cells and the lack of stimulation from the baby being unable to empty her breasts, combine to reduce her milk production.

Most importantly, it's a question which wouldn't need to be asked at all if women were encouraged to breastfeed as nature intended.

However, as breastfeeding is so often mismanaged and as so many women today are still wrongly advised to restrict suckling time according to some sort of schedule or routine, it's a question that must be asked.

Signs that your baby is getting enough milk

You'll know your baby is getting enough when he:
- Sucks and milks the breast well.
- Feeds often – usually every one and a half to three hours and averaging at least eight to twelve feeds a day in the first few weeks.
- Is satisfied after a feed.
- Grows – in weight, length and head circumference. Your baby may lose up to 10 per cent of his birth-weight in the first few days. After that your milk will come in and he will probably start gaining 120–200g (4–7oz) each week, or 450g (1 lb) in four weeks. Make sure that you work out his weight-gain starting from his lowest weight, not his birth-weight!

- Thrives – that is, when he is healthy, has a good colour and firm skin, and is active and alert.
- Has six to eight really wet terry nappies, or five to six really wet disposables, each day from about the third day. However, in the first day or two after birth, your baby may have only one or two wet nappies a day. This is because he takes only small amounts of your valuable colostrum.
- Passes meconium (see page 194) on the first day or two, then begins passing at least two to five motions a day from about the third day. However, some healthy, thriving babies have extremely few motions (see page 195).

And when you:
- Know you're letting your milk down (see page 276).

Knowing what to expect

Many women are surprised to find that their baby doesn't spend all the time sleeping, feeding or cooing and gurgling. When he wants frequent feeds, day and night, or sometimes wants to go on sucking at the breast for ages, they worry that something is wrong. The most anxiety-provoking behaviour for the woman who doesn't know what to expect is often when her baby finishes his feed, has a cat nap, then wants to start all over again, repeating the pattern evening after evening. It's enough to make many a woman think she hasn't enough milk – that her baby is somehow dissatisfied – whereas in fact it's usually perfectly normal behaviour.

Much of the anxiety and false expectations come about because of a greater familiarity with bottle-feeding. A mother empties a bottle of formula into her baby and the only limiting factor is how quickly he accepts it. Breastfeeding, on the other hand, is a two-way dynamic process in which both partners give and take, with the baby partly responsible for the amount of milk his mother makes.

Sometimes, though, this unexpected behaviour so disturbs a woman – especially if it's her first baby – that she feels helpless, out of control and hopeless. Her baby wants mothering – and so does she. If this happens to you, don't be proud but ask for all the help and support you need from your doctor or midwife (or, in the UK, your health visitor), from lay breastfeeding helpers, or from family and friends.

Weighing your baby

In the first month after the initial weight loss following delivery, the average baby gains 120–200g (4–7oz) a week. From the second to fifth months, 175–225g (6–8oz) a week; and from the sixth to twelfth months, 50–75g (2–3oz) a week. An average breastfed baby tends to double his birth-weight by four months and triple it by a year. However, these are only averages and in any case may be based on bottle-fed (and sometimes overweight) babies. Some healthy, thriving babies regularly put on less than the average, and others more. Take little notice of his changes in weight from one week to another. A healthy, thriving baby sometimes gains no weight and may occasionally even lose some in any one week. The overall rate of gain, however, is usually fairly steady.

If your doctor or midwife (or, in the UK, your health visitor) suggests regular weighing, they'll keep an eye on the rate of weight-gain over the weeks as it's a reasonable guide to growth and health. If your baby isn't thriving because you aren't giving him enough milk, they'll spot this early and hopefully will advise you how to increase your milk supply.

Don't weigh your baby at home. Neurotic weighing is a sure way to work yourself up into a panic as soon as his weight-gain fails to live up to your, perhaps unrealistic, expectations. If your baby's weight consistently lags behind average weights for his age, yet he is well, don't be alarmed. Research shows that we are often foolish to judge a baby's health by his weight-gain in the early months. A study in southern Africa found that in communities in which babies gain weight and grow quickly, the population as a whole tends to die younger. Fast early growth may go hand in hand with early ageing.

Signs that your baby may not be getting enough

You may notice that your baby:

- Cries or fusses a lot.
- Often seems hungry after feeds.
- Happily drinks a bottle of formula after a breastfeed.
- Doesn't soak six to eight nappies a day.
- Isn't gaining weight.

And that:

- Your breasts never leak.
- Your breasts never feel full.

Remember that although you may temporarily not have enough milk, you can make more if you know what to do (see page 270).

Pitfalls

Two pitfalls may mislead you into thinking you can't make enough milk. These are, first, your baby's changing needs and, second, the disturbance of coming home from hospital.

1. Changing needs – It's easy enough to imagine that a baby will take the same amount of milk at each feed. But babies don't necessarily want the same amount from feed to feed, let alone from day to day. Sometimes your baby will want more than you've made, sometimes less. In this sense babies are just like older children and adults. However, when his appetite increases, your milk supply may not immediately be able to match his needs. Don't make the mistake of thinking you can't make enough milk just because he is fussy for a few days. Be guided by him, take steps to increase your milk supply and marvel at the way your body's demand-and-supply system works.

And don't forget that he may be entering a **'growth spurt'**.

If your baby has previously been satisfied but becomes edgy and miserable and you think he's still hungry after a feed, he may be showing signs of a growth spurt. Babies can have growth spurts at any age but they are especially common at around six weeks and three months (see also page 174).

— Researchers in the US very carefully measured babies each day and found that some grew half an inch in length in twenty-four hours! They noted that these babies were often restless and cried more before their growth spurt, but settled quietly afterwards.

The good news is that when your baby begins a growth spurt he'll automatically ask for more and/or longer feeds, as babies instinctively know that spending more time at the breast increases the milk supply. However, it'll take two to three days of increased breast stimulation for you to produce much more milk, so be prepared for him to be extra 'demanding' for this period. Let him suck for as long as he wants at each feed and give him as many feeds as he wants.

If you're already demand-feeding, give at least two extra feeds a day, and even more if you have time. The increased stimulation will soon increase your milk production, although it'll be several days before your supply catches up with your baby's demand.

It's easy for an inexperienced breastfeeder to panic if her baby seems unsatisfied. But a mismatch between demand and supply happens to almost every mother and baby from time to time.

2. **Coming home** – Another pitfall can occur when you return home from hospital, whether it's at two or ten days. Your milk supply is quite likely to dwindle temporarily, making your baby hungry and unsettled. This is because of the change, the excitement and the extra work you may have to do. Family doctors frequently receive calls from women just back home saying that their milk has gone. Of course it hasn't gone for good, and they can readily increase their supply, but many, especially first-time, mothers do not know this. If this happens to you, there's no need to give your baby a bottle or stop breastfeeding. Milk dries up in a well-nourished woman only if she doesn't have enough nipple stimula-

tion or if her breasts aren't well enough emptied. The early drying-up of milk is a problem caused purely by poor technique.

The reason underlying an inadequate milk supply may be that your baby isn't milking your breasts well enough. This means that your nipples aren't stimulated adequately and you don't produce enough milk, even though you could – and would have done from the beginning had your baby milked you well. All the time in the world spent with a baby who isn't performing optimally at the breast won't necessarily produce more milk. But it will certainly tire you both out. When your baby milks you well, you'll let your milk down more efficiently and your breasts will empty more completely. There are many reasons why this may not happen and correspondingly many ways of overcoming the problem (see pages 271 and 365).

'Happy-to-starve'?

A few seemingly contented, breastfed babies are actually starving. They have been dubbed 'happy-to-starve'. The danger is that they risk brain damage or other problems if no one realizes what's happening.

The commonest reason behind any breastfed baby failing to thrive is a restriction in the number and length of breastfeeds, including night feeds. The three-to-five-hourly, ten-minutes-a-side type of breastfeeding works only for those few women with a very plentiful milk supply. Most of us need to feed our babies much more frequently and for longer to get the breast stimulation and emptying we need to make enough milk.

If you and your professional advisers are concerned because your baby's weight-gain is small or non-existent for a few weeks, don't be put off breastfeeding but take immediate steps to increase your milk supply (see page 271). If complementary feeds with formula are advised, discuss whether it's possible to put them off for a few days while you increase your milk supply instead. If your doctor or midwife (or, in the UK, your health visitor) agrees that it's safe to wait while you increase your milk supply, it's highly likely that your baby won't need formula feeds at all. If he is so under-nourished that he needs formula fast, give it by cup after each breastfeed while you spend several days increasing your milk supply. Once you are making more milk you'll almost certainly be able to withdraw the formula.

If you don't feel confident, ask your local NCT breastfeeding counsellor, La Leche League leader or other breastfeeding helper (see page 453) for some skilled mother-to-mother support. She'll have helped many women with this problem before.

Don't forget that with our society's strange method of 'token' breastfeeding, even a solely breastfed baby can be underfed. Never be lulled into complacency just because you are breastfeeding but take heed of any warning, make sure your baby is safely nourished, and change to a more successful way of breastfeeding if necessary (see page 175).

Failure to thrive

If, despite taking steps to increase your milk supply, your baby still isn't growing well, something may be wrong (see page 374).

Now let's look at how you can increase your milk supply.

HOW TO INCREASE YOUR MILK SUPPLY

Never imagine that you are limited to the amount of milk you're currently making for your baby. Once you are aware of the many things that influence your milk supply you'll be able to do something about them.

TWENTY STEPS TO INCREASING YOUR MILK SUPPLY

1. Make sure your baby is positioned well (*see page 166*)

This allows him to suck and milk more effectively which, in turn, empties your breasts and stimulates milk production better.

- Your baby's chest and tummy should face yours so that he doesn't have to turn his head.
- Your breast should not be dragged down.
- Your baby's lips should splay out around a large mouthful of nipple *and* areola.
- Your baby's lower jaw should be well towards your chest. This means you'll see less of the areola beneath his mouth than above.
- Your nipple should point towards the roof of his mouth so that it touches his palate.
- Your breast shouldn't obstruct his nostrils.

2. Increase your total suckling time

Breastfeed your baby frequently for as long he wants to go on. The more chance he has to be at the breast, the more readily you'll let down your milk, the more milk he can take, the more prolactin you'll have and therefore the more milk you'll make. Breasts respond to the removal of milk by making just as much again, and feeding frequently will encourage them to make more – so there's absolutely no danger of 'using up' your milk by feeding frequently.

It's the total length of suckling time each day that's important. This in turn depends on the number and length of feeds, together with the time spent comfort-suckling (see page 169). It's best to avoid a long gap between feeds in the night hours while you're building up your milk supply in the early weeks.

Your baby will ask for a certain number of feeds. He may also want to carry on feeding when you think your milk is finished. Allow as much of this comfort-sucking as you can. You may also need to offer some unasked-for feeds to build up your supply if he's not getting enough.

Make sure you are feeding naturally and on an unrestricted basis. Breastfeeding today is sometimes only a token effort. It's governed by schedules and the restriction of suckling time and usually lasts for only a few weeks, during which time formula, juices or solids are added to the baby's diet. However, successful breastfeeding depends on the demand-and-supply principle, which allows a woman to produce the right amount of milk for her baby. With this there's no limitation of suckling time and no need for any other food or drink for the first four to six months at least.

If you are already feeding your baby on an unrestricted basis, you can do two further things:

First – Let him feed as long as he wants at each breast. Although some babies take all the hind-milk they need in ten minutes or so at each breast, many need very much longer. Indeed, many a successfully breastfeeding woman reports that her baby sometimes likes to stay at the breast for up to an hour or even as long as two or three hours, especially in the early evening, feeding, comfort-sucking, and having an occasional short nap. However, an inexperienced woman may panic and think something's wrong when her baby wants a long feeding session. Nothing is wrong with a baby wanting to stay at the breast – he's just behaving normally. If you want to increase your milk supply, keep him at the breast when he wants to be there, as this is a good way of increasing your breast-stimulation and hence your milk supply. If, on occasion, you haven't the time or inclination to sit with him, or have to pick older children up from school – no harm will come from curtailing a feed, but this should be occasional and as a general rule you should let your baby stop only when he wants to.

Second – Feed him more often by fitting in some extra feeds – perhaps even twice as many. This may mean waking him up by day and night. Try not to let more than two hours go between the beginning of one feed and the beginning of the next, except at night, when it's a good idea to wake yourself up so that no more than three or at the most four hours elapse between feeds.

If you increase your baby's suckling time by building up the number and length of his feeds, your milk supply will improve because you'll make more prolactin, get used to letting your milk down, and empty your breasts better and more frequently. This usually takes at least two to three days.

It may help not to think of the time your baby spends at the breast as a 'feed'. Of course breastfed babies feed from the breast but they also get comfort and pleasure. (What's more, their tongue, cheek and jaw movements stimulate optimal development of these areas.) It's interesting that members of one African tribe were flummoxed when asked by western researchers about their breastfed babies' feeding times. They apparently didn't equate the times their babies spent at the breast with them getting food at all! They simply put their babies to the breast because that was what made their infants happy!

Some babies diminish their mother's milk supply by sucking their thumbs or fingers instead of breastfeeding. This may be a sign that they've been denied comfort-sucking time at the breast in the past. A dummy has the same effect and is best discarded if you want to increase your milk supply.

— A study (1993) reported that babies of one month old who used a dummy tended to be weaned earlier than others.

Having solids or drinks of juice or water may reduce your baby's demand for the breast. No extra fluid is needed, so don't hesitate to cut them out if they interfere with your baby's desire to breastfeed.

Occasionally a woman's milk supply diminishes because she carries her baby around in a sling or carrier, or on a hip, and because he's lulled so well he doesn't ask for feeds. If this happens, put your baby to the breast much more often than he seems to want.

When you've increased your milk supply and are breast-feeding successfully, your baby may eventually want fewer feeds.

3. Feed from both breasts at each feed

You'll gradually produce less and less milk if you take your baby off the first breast before he has finished, if you don't let your milk down or let it down incompletely, or if your breasts are full long before he feeds. This is because:

- The tension from the build-up of milk reduces the blood supply to the milk glands, making the milk-producing cells less efficient.
- This tension harms the milk-producing cells, making them temporarily less able to produce milk.
- The tiny contractile cells can't contract so well around swollen milk glands, so you let your milk down less efficiently.

Whenever your breasts feel full or the slightest bit tense and uncomfortable, put your baby to the breast or express some milk. You can also boost your milk supply by expressing at other times too:

4. Express milk after and between feeds

Expressing all the remaining milk in the breasts four or five times a day for two or three days stimulates your breasts more, which in turn increases your milk supply. Express the milk about half an hour after each feed. Collect it and offer it to your baby in a cup after the next feed.

5. Make sure you let your milk down well (*see also page 19*)

You'll need to let your milk down if your baby is to empty the breast, drink high-calorie, fat-rich hind-milk, and thrive.

Factors such as fatigue, anxiety, fear and pain adversely influence the let-down reflex and may even prevent you from letting down your milk at all. During the first few weeks or months a woman's let-down is more vulnerable than later when her milk supply is established and she is more confident. This goes part of the way to explaining why women breastfeeding second babies are more successful at the beginning than they were with their first babies.

When people talk of 'the establishment of the milk supply', they really mean that the let-down reflex has become so well-conditioned through practice that it virtually never fails. They also mean that a woman's breasts have adapted themselves to match their milk supply to the baby's demands, with no surplus or shortage.

A poor milk supply caused by an unreliable let-down reflex is one of the commonest problems of breastfeeding but once you understand what's happening, you'll have every chance of putting it right. Successful breastfeeding depends as much on good emptying of the milk (which of course depends on a well conditioned let-down reflex) as on the actual amount produced.

—In one interesting set of experiments women who said they hadn't enough milk were given an injection of oxytocin (the hormone that lets milk down) after a feed. The researchers then measured the amount of milk let down after the injection. Most of the women let down about as much milk again as their babies had already taken! In other words, 50 per cent of their milk was still in their breasts after the initial feed. But because they hadn't let it down adequately with their own oxytocin, it wasn't all available to their baby.

If your let-down usually takes two to three minutes to work and you normally restrict suckling time to, say, ten minutes, your baby will lose two to three minutes of what you thought was drinking time. While seven to eight minutes' drinking time is enough for some babies, it leaves others very hungry.

Remember that you may let your milk down several times at each breast, especially if your baby stays at the breast for a long time. Stopping him before he's ready may mean he'll miss out on one of these let-downs.

How do you know you're letting your milk down? You may notice some or all of these signs:

- 'After-pains' in your womb early in a feed in the early days (see page 21).
- Tingling in your breasts immediately before the milk comes.
- Milk spraying or leaking from your breasts.
- Your breasts feeling warmer than usual.
- Initial nipple pain disappearing as the milk comes down (equalizing the negative pressure created by the baby sucking).
- Your baby sucking with rhythmical, one-per-second sucks. This is 'nutritive' sucking – the sort which mean he's swallowing milk as it's let down. You may hear him swallowing too.

Some women don't have any of these sensations yet let their

milk down perfectly well. The only way they know they're doing it is by:

- The baby settling at the breast and swallowing in a steady rhythm.
- The baby thriving and growing.

How to make your let-down more reliable. You can do several things to help:

a) Condition your let-down reflex

- Try to get into a routine before a feed – a regular chain of events will condition your let-down into working reliably.
- Don't be tempted to skip night feeds: you'll need them to stimulate your milk supply.
- When your breasts feel tense and full, wake the baby for a feed.
- Try not to let him sleep for long periods, because your breasts need regular emptying.
- If your milk lets down unexpectedly, wake him and feed him.

b) Be calm, unhurried, and enjoy the feeds

- Have everything you might need during a feed – for you, the baby and any other children – to hand.
- Decide in advance what to do about the phone (a cordless phone is ideal), the front-door bell and other people who may be with you in the room (see page 228).
- Cut down on activities which you find stressful but which are inessential, such as unnecessary entertaining, letter-writing, phoning and cooking.
- Cut down on other activities so that you always have time for feeds and are never in a hurry to do something else. This might mean not promising to be anywhere at any set time. Simply explain that you'll come when you're ready. You may have to make some exceptions, such as visits to the doctor.
- Relax both before and during a feed and try to clear your mind of any worries. While this may sound difficult, it comes with practice.

Enjoy the feeds. Instead of thinking of them as times to get as much milk into your baby as quickly as possible, calm down, stop pressuring yourself, and try to consider them as unique and special times together. Babies grow up quickly and the time will come soon enough when your child will want to be independent, so it's worth enjoying this time while you can.

c) Try switch-nursing – ('Nursing' is the American term for breastfeeding.) Switch-nursing is a well-tried technique to encourage a baby to suck more strongly so as to stimulate both the let-down and the milk supply. It's useful for coaxing tired, jaundiced, pethidine-doped, ill, pre-term or other weak feeders into sucking more strongly and milking the breast more efficiently.

Switch-nursing means swapping your baby from one breast to the other as soon as his sucking slows down and you can hear or see him swallowing less often. So instead of simply giving first one breast, then the other, you carry on by switching back to the first and then perhaps switch ing to the second again. Try giving him ten minutes each time you switch. If you're feeding two-hourly to stimulate your milk supply, this will mean you'll be feeding for about forty minutes every two hours. Alternatively, you could switch from side to side just twice – going, for example, from your left to your right to your left breast again. The time this takes is a small price to pay for increasing your milk supply.

Switch-nursing is effective because each time you switch from side to side, there's immediately some milk in the reservoirs of the 'new' breast for him to drink. This means that he's likely to suck and milk you more enthusiastically as he drinks, and this in turn will stimulate another let-down. If you end up having more let-downs in a feed than usual, it's good both for your milk supply and for conditioning your let-down reflex.

However, if you usually need several minutes of breast-stimulation before you let your milk down, leave your baby at the first breast and then at the second until he comes off each of his own accord, otherwise he may not have long enough after you let your milk down to get any hind-milk but will fill up with fore-milk instead. He'll then be too tired and full to go on sucking. However, the low-calorie fore-milk won't satisfy him for long, and your let-down won't get the stimulation it needs.

d) Keep fit – Take the time and make the effort to find forms of exercise which you enjoy and can do at least three times a week and preferably five. Exercise boosts the levels of endorphins (natural feel-good chemicals in the blood) and having a fit body helps you relax, which in turn makes it easier to let down your milk. It also increases the blood-flow through the breasts and thus stimulates milk production.

e) Look after yourself – Avoid getting over-tired: try to have at least one nap during the day; put your feet up whenever you sit down; don't do unnecessary housework or other chores; organize shopping to make it as easy as possible; and cut down on outside commitments. If you allow yourself to get exhausted, you'll be less likely to let your milk down reliably.

f) And:
- Make sure you're comfortable when feeding because things such as aching shoulders or a draught round your feet won't help.
- If you have sore nipples, try to get your let-down to work before the baby feeds. Remember the pain will eventually go and is anyway unlikely to last throughout a feed (see page 307).

- Have a small alcoholic drink just before a feed. This will relax you and help your let-down (but see page 242).
- Some women find that a hot shower helps their let-down, though obviously this isn't practical before every feed. Sometimes you might like to feed in the bath, where the warmth will help you relax and encourage your let-down. Your baby will like it too!

6. Encourage your baby to keep alert and awake
(see page 335)

You can help your baby stay awake enough to feed well by talking to him, stroking him and switch-nursing (see no. 5 (c) above). Staying wide-awake allows him to suck and milk your breasts more strongly and also to avoid getting into the habit of snoozing for long periods at the breast.

7. Help your baby suck and milk more effectively
(see nos. 1, 5 (c) and 6 above and also page 365)

8. Get help

Get help from your midwife (in the UK, your health visitor), doctor, lactation consultant or breastfeeding counsellor if your baby isn't gaining weight well, or is losing weight. They can help you improve your breastfeeding technique and this, in turn, is very likely to increase your milk supply. The doctor can also check that your baby's health is good.

9. Avoid formula if at all possible

Giving your baby formula will probably diminish your milk supply. This is because once he no longer has to rely on your milk, he's unlikely to want to feed often or for long enough to stimulate your breasts well. In this case it's best gradually to cut back on the amount of formula he has and to take steps to increase your milk supply. Check that he wets and soils his nappies as he should (see page 265) and stay in touch with your doctor (or, in the UK, your health visitor).

Even if your baby had unnecessary complements of formula in hospital, you're highly likely to be able to breastfeed fully once you get home.

Reduce the amount of formula by 15ml (½oz) at each feed, so that he receives more breast milk each time. Give the formula by cup or spoon (or, if necessary, via a supplementer, see page 449) rather than from a bottle, otherwise he may get so used to a bottle that he may be loath to breastfeed.

Feed him more often and let him stay at the breast as much as he wants – even just for comfort at an empty breast. Your milk supply will begin to increase after two or three days. Be prepared for long and frequent feeds – perhaps as much as forty minutes every two hours. Sometimes he may want to suck and nap on and off for several hours. Look after yourself by doing as few other things as possible – just rest and cuddle the baby. You *can* build up your milk supply. All you need is information, confidence and patience.

— In 1980, the Department of Health recommended that women should give nothing but breast milk at least for the first three months. However, by 1985 their figures showed that one in three six-week-old breastfed babies was receiving formula as well.

10. Avoid a dummy (pacifier)

It's also better not to give your baby a dummy if you think you may not have enough milk. A dummy will satisfy some of his need to suck and may stop him asking for as many breastfeeds as you need to stimulate your milk supply.

11. Eat an enjoyable and healthy diet

Provided you eat and drink well, your diet should make no difference to your milk supply, bearing in mind that you may need to eat slightly more than normal and drink according to your thirst. Severely malnourished women produce less milk but the quality of their milk is little affected. (See page 236).

12. Exercise to increase the circulation in your breasts

Over any given period of time the blood-flow through the breasts is 400–500 times the volume of milk produced. The greater the blood-flow, the more milk there is. Regular exercise may not only encourage your let-down (see no. 5(d) above) but also increase the circulation in your breasts and the amount of milk you make.

13. Wear a comfortable bra

A breastfeeding woman who wears too tight a bra may find that her milk supply decreases. Constricting the breasts reduces or even stops the milk supply and is a well-known method of drying up the milk. If you have small or medium-sized breasts, leave your bra off altogether while you get your milk supply going again, then wear a more comfortable bra.

14. Keep positive

Women who really want to breastfeed produce more milk. One study of women's attitudes to breastfeeding found that those who'd said at first that they preferred bottle-feeding were three times more likely to find that their baby refused the breast, and twice as likely to say that their baby was a bad feeder, compared with women who intended from the beginning to breastfeed. This indicates that positive attitudes are very helpful. Interestingly, in the same survey, women who wanted to breastfeed reported that their babies refused the bottle.

But the fact remains that many women who really want to breastfeed fail because they believe they haven't enough milk. Indeed, many a woman's greatest single concern before she embarks on breastfeeding is that she won't have enough milk.

A concern about not having enough milk seems to be engrained in modern women. It's tempting to wonder whether this is symbolic of a deep-seated, albeit unconscious, feeling of not being good enough, or not having enough to give.

15. Get plenty of rest and relaxation

Looking after yourself in this way is a very good idea while you are putting so much concentration and energy into building up your milk supply.

16. Come off the combined Pill

The contraceptive pill, unless of the progestogen-only type, usually reduces the milk supply. (See page 123 for alternative methods of family planning.)

17. Stop smoking – or at least cut right down

Smoking can decrease the milk supply by lowering the prolactin level. It can also hinder the let-down.

18. Drink more fluid?

Lots of people will tell you to drink plenty but be careful only to drink what you want because drinking more than you feel like usually isn't helpful. Having said that, some women find that drinking more than they have been doing seems to help.

19. Consider traditional milk-boosters?

Throughout the centuries women around the world have used amulets, potions, herbal skin rubs and other remedies, special foods and drinks, chants and prayers to ensure they produce enough milk. These purported milk-boosters are collectively known in medical jargon as galactogogues.

There's no harm in trying any of them *provided you also carry out the proven methods (above) for increasing your milk supply.*

Let's look at some of these 'milk-boosters':

- Alcohol, especially heavy beers and stouts. Alcohol increases the prolactin level but babies tend not to drink much milk when it tastes of alcohol, so they don't stimulate the breasts as well as usual. Having small amounts of alcoholic drinks may help but only by making you relaxed and therefore encouraging your let-down reflex. Drinking too much may interfere with your let-down.
- Vitamin B. If your diet isn't very good, the benefit of this vitamin could be to improve your sense of well-being. This may help if you've been feeling tense and haven't been letting your milk down well. But it's better to eat well.
- Vitamin E. There's no scientific proof that this helps at all.
- Cows' milk. It used to be said that this helped breastfeeding women make milk, but if you're eating a healthy diet there's no need to have any cows' milk unless you like it.

- Carrots are reputed by some to increase milk production but, confusingly, carrot juice is said by others to decrease it!
- Corn, peas, beans, lentils, chickpeas, oats and barley are traditionally said to boost a woman's milk supply. However, there are no research data to back up these claims.
- Walnuts and almonds are said to be good for milk production, as are sunflower, sesame, celery and fenugreek seeds. You can add any of these to your meals. Animal studies show that fenugreek seeds have oxytocin-like activity.
- Parsley is said by some to increase the milk supply and by others to decrease it!
- Caraway seeds, dill and fennel – made into tea or used in your diet – are said to be 'warming' and ease tense muscles, which may aid the let-down.
- Borage leaves and seeds, ginger, coriander, cumin and nettles, made into tea or added to meals, have been used for centuries to increase the milk supply.
- Chaste tree (*Vitex agnus-castus*) seeds stimulate the pituitary gland and enhance a low prolactin level. A study of 125 women found that chaste tree increased milk production in 80 per cent; after twenty days the average milk production was three times as high in the women taking chaste tree as in those not taking it. You can take it as a tea.
- Saw palmetto berries are reputed to help the breasts function properly and can be made into a tea.
- Herbal teas made from raspberry leaves, cinnamon or blessed thistle can help if you're feeling stressed, which may in turn help you let your milk down better. But beware of drinking too much of any herbal tea: in one report, mothers who drank 2 litres (3½ pints) a day of a herbal tea (containing liquorice, fennel, anise and *Galega officinalis*) said to stimulate milk production found that their babies reacted badly, with restlessness, vomiting, floppiness, tiredness and a weak cry, as well as poor growth. Their symptoms disappeared when their mothers stopped drinking the tea!

- Essential oils of geranium and fennel added to a base oil (such as sweet almond oil) and used for a whole-body massage are said to boost your supply. Add about 10 drops of essential oil to one tablespoonful of base oil.
- The homeopathic remedy *Agnus castus* is said to help.

20. Consider taking prescribed drugs?

Chlorpromazine, other phenothiazine drugs and the rauwolfia group of drugs can increase the milk supply but have side-effects.

Metoclopramide is a drug which is normally used to reduce nausea and vomiting. It also stimulates prolactin and can increase the milk supply. Small trials with mothers of pre-term babies (using 10mg of metoclopramide by mouth three or four times a day for a week, then tapering it off over the next week) show that it usually increases the milk supply within two to four days. However, it can have unpleasant, possibly even serious side-effects and isn't licensed for boosting the milk supply.

Does your age matter?

Older women having their first baby tend to produce less milk than do younger ones. However, this is only at first so it's well worth persevering.

Does the number of children you've had matter?

Women breastfeeding their first baby tend to produce less milk at first than those who've already breastfed one or more. However, this is only at first. They can readily make more milk if they know how.

WHAT IF YOU CAN'T BREASTFEED?

With the best will in the world and with the very best help there is, a tiny percentage of women are unable to breastfeed. If you are one, there are several things you can do:

- Don't despair. It isn't the end of the world.
- Be grateful you have an alternative.
- Focus on the positive aspects of your experience and recognize them as successes. An example might be the enjoyment you and your baby have had during some of the feeds you've done together. Remember that such breastfeeding as you've done is better than none. Your baby is lucky to have a mother who has tried her best – no one can expect 'straight As' for everything in life.
- Be forgiving of yourself. And if you later discover that you might have been able to breastfeed, had you known more, received more support and done it differently, don't blame yourself or other people but work out what to do next time.
- Consider giving the occasional feed – perhaps in the early morning – if you still have some milk. With the relief of your anxiety over not having enough milk, you might even start letting your milk down better and, as a result, produce more than you thought you could.
- Allow yourself time to recognize, name and come to terms with your feelings about being unable to breastfeed. You may experience a whole mass of conflicting emotions about what's happened. Sadness and disappointment may mingle uneasily with anger, frustration and helplessness.
- It may help to talk to someone who's prepared and able to listen, or you might find you want to write – either about what's happened, or about your feelings, or paint or do something else creative. In this way you'll be able to move on and enjoy your baby as he grows without dwelling unproductively on what might have been.
- Don't transfer any of your disappointment, anger or guilt to your baby. It isn't his fault and it isn't yours either. Your love for your child is more important than your milk, so don't allow difficult feelings to make you lose sight of your unique relationship.

- When you bottle-feed your baby, hold him as you did when breastfeeding, not like a doll held at arm's length.
- Consider giving just as much breast milk as you can at the same time as your baby drinks formula. Increasing numbers of women who, for whatever reason, aren't producing enough milk, use a nursing supplementer (see page 449). This gadget enables their babies to be at the breast, get what milk there is, and at the same time receive formula through a fine tube (which enters the baby's mouth along with the nipple). It also allows his sucking and milking to stimulate the milk supply, and gives both woman and baby the pleasure of breastfeeding while assuring adequate nutrition.

If at first you don't succeed

If you go on to have another baby, try breastfeeding again. Many women breastfeed second or later babies successfully even though they failed before. You'll be more confident and experienced as a mother next time, which should help. Remember that failing to breastfeed for as long as you wanted the first time may mean you'll need more encouragement, practical back-up and skilled support next time. It's up to you to make sure you get it.

WHAT IF YOU DON'T WANT TO CONTINUE BREASTFEEDING?

It's usually easy to make milk dry up – it isn't advisable to use dry-up pills. Simply reduce the length of time your baby spends at the breast by gradually cutting down the number and length of feeds over a period of several weeks, if possible. Too rapid weaning may cause problems such as painful engorgement (see page 302), blocked ducts and even breast infection. As your baby receives less breast milk, give more formula and other drinks by bottle.

Some women find that in order to produce enough milk they have to spend more time with their babies at the breast than they are prepared to devote. Giving complementary bottles eases the pressure for such mothers. Breastfeeding a baby shouldn't be seen as a gruelling or annoying chore. If it is, a woman is well advised to reconsider what she's doing. It's better for a baby to have a happy mother who happens to be bottle-feeding than an unhappy breastfeeding one who may get to the stage of being depressed or bearing a grudge. Sometimes practical help is all that's needed to sustain a woman who finds her baby too time-consuming and tiring, so don't be too proud to ask.

Drying up your milk after giving birth (see also page 433)

If you are intent on bottle-feeding, your milk will still come in and your breasts may feel very full, especially between the third and fifth days. Whenever they start to feel tense and full, express (or pump) only just enough milk to make them comfy. The engorgement will dry up your milk. Neither restriction of drinks nor diuretics (drugs to remove water from the body) works, and Epsom salts are best avoided because they can cause diarrhoea. Neither heat, ice, nor a tight bra seems useful, but some women find that putting cold cabbage leaves over their breasts inside their bra makes them feel better. Herbalists suggest eating plenty of garden mint, sorrel and sage to help dry up milk and French women sometimes eat a parsley omelette when they want to stop breast-feeding. (See also suggestions for herbal remedies to reduce engorgement, page 306.)

Doctors once used oestrogen (stilboestrol) to dry up milk. However, this sometimes had serious side-effects, such as blood clots in the veins, and stopping it often caused a rebound increase of milk production. A synthetic oestrogen called chlorotriansene may be safer. Another drug, bromocriptine, is effective but unnecessary, expensive and banned in many countries as a lactation suppressant because it can produce side-effects (headache, nausea, heartburn, dizziness and, rarely, high blood pressure, a temporary stroke-like illness, and even a heart attack).

In southern India women traditionally put strings of jasmine flowers on their breasts to dry up their milk. Research has shown that these are just as effective as bromocriptine.

An advantage of not using drugs to dry up your milk is that if, like many women, you change your mind and decide after all to breastfeed, you'll find it easier to build up your milk supply (see page 271) if you haven't suppressed it artificially.

IS YOUR BABY HAVING TOO MUCH?

In the early days, before your milk supply matches your baby's demands, you may have too much milk. Over a few days your supply will gradually adjust but the abundance can cause problems, especially towards the end of the first week. A newborn baby can be bewildered and almost choked by an over-exuberant flow of milk. He'll turn his head away, cough, splutter and be reluctant to go on feeding. He may also swallow too much air as he tries to drink from this 'fire hydrant' and then suffer from colic (see page 199).

You can cope with an over-abundant milk supply by expressing some milk before a feed, either by hand or by allowing the milk to leak away if you let your milk down before your baby goes to the breast.

A similar problem can arise if you allow your breasts to become over-full by letting your baby sleep too long between feeds. Instead, either wake him when they feel full and tense, or express enough milk to soften them between feeds.

Many women overcome the problem of too much milk by feeding from one breast only at each feed (see page 214). The presence of stagnant milk in the unemptied breast, together with its pressure as it builds up, stops the milk-producing cells making so much. If you feed from only one breast in any one feed, though, do ensure that you don't allow the unemptied breast to become overfull at any time before you offer it to your baby at the next feed. Express just enough milk to remove any lumpiness or tension.

And if necessary express a little milk just before a feed so your baby can easily take the breast into his mouth.

It may also be a good idea to stop your baby comfort-sucking and snoozing at the breast and allow only 'nutritive' sucking (when he is actually swallowing milk). You can recognize this sort of sucking by its rhythm of one suck per second.

You may find that your baby prefers to feed in an 'uphill' position if your milk flows fast and furiously, as this position prevents a strong spray of milk from catching him in the back of his throat. Hold him facing you on your lap and guide his head on to your breast, holding your nipple if necessary.

As your baby grows, he'll be better able to cope with an efficient, fast let-down reflex without choking.

If you still have too much milk, think about donating the extra to a milk bank, where it would be used for pre-term or sick babies whose mothers don't want to or can't breastfeed. Ask your doctor or midwife how to go about this in your area.

Knowing what affects your milk supply will stand you in very good stead if, like many women, you're challenged by some sort of breastfeeding problem (Chapter 12). And, as we'll see in the next chapter, it also helps you to persist with breastfeeding if you decide to go out to work.

ELEVEN

The working mother

When women talk about why they don't want to breastfeed it often isn't long before the subject of going back to work crops up. This is hardly surprising as women are now such an important part of the work-force in many industrialized countries. It's difficult to know exactly how many mothers with young children work, because many do so part-time or at home and much of this activity is unrecorded by government agencies. What is clear, though, is that only a small minority of mothers with young babies go out to work. The majority choose to stay home to look after their babies.

> — A UK government survey (1996) found that only 16 per cent of mothers of families in which the youngest child was under five worked full-time; 30 per cent worked part-time and 48 per cent were full-time mothers.
> — A large survey of over 5000 women in Great Britain (1990) found that only 8 per cent of mothers with babies between six and ten weeks old had returned to work. One in five had paid work when their babies were four months old; and one in three when their babies were nine months.
> — A large US survey (1987) found that at six months, about one in four mothers who had chosen to breastfeed and who were not employed were still breastfeeding. This compared with only one in ten mothers who had chosen to breastfeed and who were employed.

We saw in Chapter 1 how young Western women are often brought up to think of themselves as important economic units, and how this militates against breastfeeding. Nowadays a job comes first to some young women and raising children has to fit in with maintaining their standard of living. Having said this, such statistics as are available show that only a few women give up breastfeeding to go back to work when their babies are very young. However, over the last ten years increasingly more women have stopped breastfeeding older babies to go back to work.

— In the British study mentioned above, 14 per cent of breastfeeding mothers of babies between two and three months old, 23 per cent with babies between three and four months, and 15 per cent with babies between four and nine months stopped breastfeeding so that they could work. The corresponding figures ten years ago were 6, 2 and 6 per cent respectively!

Those who want to breastfeed either carry on as long as they want and go back to work later at a time to suit themselves, or find ways of continuing to breastfeed when they return to work. But let's be clear: full breastfeeding and work don't mix in this society – at least, not without a lot of effort.

The International Labour Organization recommends that nursing mothers should have a break of at least half an hour twice during the working day. Many countries recognize these breaks and in some they are shorter but more frequent. Two breaks during the day that mean a breastfeeding woman can feed before work, once during the morning, once at lunch-time, once in the afternoon and then as much as necessary at home in the evening and night.

In many countries employers must, by law, provide a room for breastfeeding mothers. For example, in France establishments employing more than 100 women over the age of fifteen must provide nurseries. And if an employer in Denmark has twenty-five or more women on the payroll, he or she must provide a breast-feeding room. Breastfeeding at work is almost impossible in the UK as so few organizations have nurseries. In contrast, in parts of Africa relatives bring the baby to the working mother so that she can feed him, or mothers take their babies to work and have them by their sides. Only a very few breastfeeding women take their babies to work with them in the UK.

But although it's difficult to combine breastfeeding and working, it can be done. Before we see how, we'll discuss why some women want to or have to combine the two.

PROS AND CONS OF WORKING AND STAYING AT HOME

Women's expectations have changed a great deal over the last two generations and both they and society as a whole have had relatively little time to adjust. Their reasons for deciding whether to return to work or stay at home may be many and complex:

Money

Many women say the cost of living is so high that their partner's income (if he has a job) simply isn't enough to run a home. However, it may be worth challenging this assumption. Think what you'd actually have to go without if you didn't work, then weigh up the advantages of being able to be with your baby and to breastfeed more easily. Some women, on reflection, prefer to cut back financially for a while and enjoy staying home with their child.

Don't forget to take the real financial cost of working into consideration when making your decision, including such things as clothes, travel, meals away from home and so on. Equally, make sure you're clear about your long-term financial plans if you put work on hold for a while. For example, make sure that you understand the position over your pension.

Quite a few women say they need to work for the money when in fact they also have other – and to them more important – reasons. In effect they shroud these reasons for working in economic excuses which may seem more acceptable.

Career

Some women don't want to lose their place on the career ladder. While it's true that this can be important, it's equally true that many women have returned to a rewarding and even illustrious career after a long break to mother their children. There are no absolutes.

You could consider having a break while you breastfeed for as long as you want to and then, if you return to work, starting again in a completely different way, perhaps even working from home. If you work for a large organization it may be worth discussing with your employer whether there's any way you could take a career break and return to work when your child is older. Job-sharing is another option that can work well for breastfeeding mothers of young children.

Self-image

Some women are disturbed by the thought of becoming a full-time mother. They want to maintain the status quo by returning to work and thereby retaining the image they have of themselves as an independent working woman. Indeed, increasing numbers of women measure their self-worth by their ability to earn money.

However, having some time away from work doesn't necessarily extinguish the part of them which thrives in the world of work, it simply puts it on hold until such time as they choose to return. Many women see motherhood, being with their baby and breastfeeding as ways of *adding* to their self-image, their understanding of who they are, and their maturity – not detracting from them.

Company and stimulation for the mother

Some mothers of young children are lonely and crave adult company. Others are bored and miss the buzz of their jobs. Many of us today get most of our need for company and stimulation met at work. However, many women who stay at home find ways of meeting people and making friends in their local community, and it's very important to do so.

Some women admit to taking a job to have a break from the baby or to 'keep sane'. This last is an understandable, if sad, result of the isolation experienced by increasing numbers of mothers of young children. With today's small family units some women are alone much of the time with their young children and it isn't surprising that some of them don't enjoy the experience and try to find a way out.

Things are different in many parts of the world. For example, in rural Africa a mother and her baby aren't parted at all for the first fifteen months. Researchers studied a sample of such mothers to see if they became irritated by being with their children so closely for so long. They found no ill-effects in either the mothers or their babies. However, these women are generally surrounded by other people and never lack for company or practical and emotional support, as well as having access to wide open spaces.

Company and stimulation for the baby

It's a popular myth that babies benefit from attending a nursery while their mothers work because they need exposure to different people – adults and children – if they are to develop socially. There's no evidence that this is so. Young babies benefit most from sensitive and responsive one-to-one attention. If you spend time playing with, talking to and listening to your baby, and if you get out and about together and meet people so as to get *your* needs met, there's no reason why he should miss out at all and every reason why he should gain a great deal. This said, your baby will probably benefit from having other people around while he is with you.

To work or not to work?

When you're making your decision about whether or not to work, remember that the opportunity to do so will always be there but the chance to be with your baby won't. Babies don't last – working does!

Overall, though, some women consider paid work essential for financial survival and many more find the extra money helpful, especially as a baby can prove an expense in itself. Yet others feel strongly about working for personal reasons. However, many wish, just as strongly, to carry on breastfeeding. Is it possible to do both?

COMBINING WORK AND BREASTFEEDING

If you intend to work, the easiest solution is to work at home if you possibly can. All kinds of home-based jobs, from making things and word-processing, to telephone-selling, could enable you to breastfeed and fit in your work to suit you and your baby.

The next easiest option is to work part-time and locally. Working locally cuts down on commuting time and means you can pop home easily and quickly in an emergency. With local part-time work your baby may need feeding only once while you're away. If you leave him with a minder, you can put expressed breast milk in the fridge to be given by cup or spoon.

Working part-time a long way from home, or full-time anywhere, means being away from your baby for a lot longer. You can express enough milk to leave for him while you're away, but it requires considerable effort, time and determination. While it's good because he will have breast milk while you're at work, and you'll keep your milk supply going, it also means that both you and he will miss out on the pleasure of breastfeeding. And, of course, he'll have no chance to be at the breast when he wants to be close to you for reassurance or comfort.

Some women manage to leave enough milk for their baby while they're out just by expressing after the early morning feed, when their breasts are usually fuller than at any other time of day. However, most need to express milk after each feed at home. And many find they can't leave enough milk for their baby unless they also express at work and take this milk home for their baby to have the next day. This can become very time-consuming.

Expressing your milk (see page 189)

You'll probably get only a very small volume of milk when you express after a feed, but you can add small volumes together and they soon mount up. You'll soon learn what works best for you.

Make sure your minder knows how to shake and warm your milk and, unless you're sure you've left enough, tell her what to give your baby if he's still hungry after your milk. Boiled, cooled water will fill his tummy until you get home. If he does need water while you're out, take steps to increase your milk supply (see page 271) so that you'll be able to leave more in future. Keep formula as a very last resort.

Reasons for expressing at work:
1 So that you can add it to the milk you express at home and leave enough for your baby the next day.
2 So that your breasts don't become too full. If they do, you risk not only discomfort but also a blocked duct or breast infection, and a gradual reduction in your milk supply. You can always throw away the milk if your baby doesn't need it.
3 So that you can make more milk. Expressing boosts your prolactin level, which encourages the breasts to produce more. However, expressing doesn't stimulate the breasts quite as well as your baby does, so to make up for this you may have to express more often or use a pump as well.

Expressing is rather tedious, takes longer than feeding a baby and calls for privacy and somewhere comfortable to sit. However, one very good reason for doing it is the satisfaction of knowing that your baby can have your milk.

If you do this at work, express your milk into a previously sterilized plastic container, cover it and keep it cold (until it's warmed for a feed). If you can't put your milk into a fridge at work, put the container into a wide-necked vacuum flask containing some ice. Such a flask will also be useful for taking the milk home.

If you don't want to express at work, this doesn't necessarily mean you can't breastfeed. You can feed your baby before you go to work in the morning and as soon as you get back, as well as in the evenings and during the night. However, when deciding whether or not to go back to work bear in mind that getting up at night and working full-time can be very tiring. Also, some babies so like to be with their mothers that they get into the habit of waking very frequently at night, as if to make up for lost time during the day.

When you're at home in the evenings or at weekends (or at other times if you're on shift-work), feed your baby on an un-restricted basis. This, combined with continued regular expression at work, should keep your milk supply going so that you can carry on breastfeeding for as many months (or longer), as you and your baby want.

— The large British study (1990) mentioned earlier in this chapter found that by the time breastfed babies of working mothers were nine months old, 6 per cent went to work with their mothers (and could be breastfed there), 4 per cent received expressed breast milk when their mothers were at work, 39 per cent had other milk (such as formula), and the rest got by without milk while their mothers were at work. Presumably these last babies received solids and other drinks, such as water or fruit juice.

Should you get him used to the bottle?

Many women wonder whether they should accustom their baby to a bottle before they return to work. In the first few months, before breastfeeding is properly established, it's better not to. Simply carry on breastfeeding until the day you go back to work. When your baby is hungry he'll almost certainly take your expressed breast milk from a feeding cup given by the minder (though he may understandably refuse a cup if *you* offer it). In the early months a cup is better than a bottle because some babies given a bottle soon learn to prefer it to the breast (see page 185) and then make a fuss when it comes to having a breastfeed. Giving expressed breast milk from a spoon is another option. However, if you want your baby to have your milk from a bottle when he's older than four months or so, this should be no problem.

Looking after yourself

If you're a working breastfeeding mother, the odds are that you'll feel tired, especially if you have other children as well as a breastfeeding baby. This makes it even more important to look after yourself (see page 252).

Enjoying your baby

Some working mothers encourage their babies to stay awake in the evenings so that they can spend more time with them. Others say that night feeds become precious times when they and their baby can take a delight in each other's company. Whatever you decide to do, remember that you'll probably have only one or two babies in a lifetime and that they'll only be really tiny and dependent on you for a short time. Make the most of that time together and you'll both benefit hugely.

Do everything you can to stay home with your baby for at least the first three to six months. If you go back to work you can still carry on breastfeeding – but don't forget to take care of yourself as well as your baby.

TWELVE

Some common problems

To say that every breastfeeding mother and every breastfed baby is different seems obvious. However, when it comes to a problem with breastfeeding, it's important to remember that each mother–baby pair needs individual advice. What works for one woman may work for another with a similar problem but it may not, and sometimes women get round the same problem in very different ways. If you can't work out what to do by yourself, seek help from a breastfeeding counsellor or a health professional experienced in helping large numbers of mothers and babies. Not only do the baby's age and birth history influence any particular situation, so do the personalities of the mother and her baby, the home environment, any other advice given, and the parents' expectations.

PAINFUL BREASTS OR NIPPLES

Pain in the breast can be due to engorgement (see page 302), mastitis resulting from a blocked duct (see page 319), mastitis from breast infection (see page 325) and thrush (see page 315). Sometimes there's a painful, burning or shooting pain in the breast or breasts, possibly after a feed and lasting for up to an hour. Possible triggers include a badly fitting bra, tense muscles from an uncomfortable feeding position, and old scars or problems in the breast. It's been suggested, though not proved, that a particularly forceful let-down could lead to the ducts temporarily collapsing or becoming unduly sensitive; or that the pain may result from rapid refilling with milk.

The causes of painful nipples include soreness (see page 307), a cracked nipple (see page 318) and a 'blanched' nipple that has temporarily lost its blood supply (see page 317).

ENGORGEMENT

There are two types of engorgement, 'physiological' or 'vascular' and pathological.

Physiological engorgement

In the first few days, as your colostrum alters to become mature milk, your breasts naturally swell and become heavier. This swelling is caused by the increasing volume of milk together with an increase in the blood supply. This is known as physiological engorgement and is normal. Some people say it means the milk is 'coming in', though of course there was valuable milk in the form of small amounts of colostrum there before. All that is happening is that your milk supply is increasing.

With unrestricted feeding, you should soon adjust your milk production to meet your baby's needs and this swelling will lessen.

However, it's very important for your baby and, perhaps, you as well, to empty your breasts frequently enough (though not necessarily completely) to prevent them from becoming overfilled and pathologically engorged.

Pathological engorgement

If your baby and/or you don't empty your breasts well enough, milk will build up until they become swollen, lumpy, hard, tense, painful and hot. This is 'pathological' engorgement. It results from poorly emptied milk together with congestion of the blood and lymph vessels and, possibly, some leakage of fluid into the connective tissues in the breasts so that they can become extremely swollen, painful and inflamed. Unless you do something about this, your milk production will decrease and may eventually stop altogether. It's occasionally difficult to distinguish engorgement from other causes of breast inflammation or mastitis (see page 328).

Engorged breasts look red and shiny and their skin is pitted like orange peel. They may also bruise if handled roughly. Swollen ducts and reservoirs may stand out as lumps and 'cords' under the skin to such an extent that some people call engorged breasts 'stringy'. This breast swelling tends to flatten the nipples, which makes it difficult for a baby to get a good enough mouthful of areola and nipple to feed well.

If you have engorged breasts you'll probably feel hot and shivery and may sweat profusely. You'll also be more thirsty than usual and should drink as much as you want, *not* limit fluids as some people used to suggest. Some women feel weepy, either because of the discomfort or because engorgement often coincides with the low feelings many women experience towards the end of the first week after delivery (see page 205).

However, these symptoms are only a part of the problem. The high pressure in the breasts also affects the milk-producing cells. They become squashed and flattened and therefore unable to produce much milk. While this may be a good thing in the short term, in that the reduction of milk production lessens the further build-up of pressure in the breasts, it's very bad in the long term because the cells' ability to produce milk can be damaged so much that their milk production shuts down completely.

In fact, allowing engorgement to occur is the commonest method of drying up milk (see page 289). A woman who doesn't breastfeed becomes engorged towards the end of the first week when her milk naturally comes in. The build-up of pressure in her breasts so damages the milk-producing cells that her milk dries up.

But all is not lost if your breasts become engorged. You can restore your milk-producing cells to their former healthy state (see below). However, if you were to carry on breastfeeding half-heartedly, limiting the number of feeds, you might relieve your engorgement but your milk production might never again regain its former potential and would eventually dry up.

Poor management of engorgement is one of the commonest reasons for failure of the milk supply in the early days, yet this failure is entirely preventable. Women who say that their milk vanished after a week could, in almost every case, have breastfed successfully if only they had known what to do.

Preventing pathological engorgement

If you follow the advice in Chapter 7 about breastfeeding in the first few days, *you're unlikely to become engorged at all*.

However, if you've had poor advice (and one leading American doctor says that in his opinion engorgement is a disorder caused by doctors!) you can take steps to deal with the resulting engorgement and lay the foundations for successful breastfeeding in the months ahead.

Dealing with engorgement

If you are painfully engorged, you – and your helpers – need to check that your baby is taking milk well. Ask yourselves three questions: Is he swallowing regularly and purposefully? Is he satisfied by feeds? And are your breasts softer after a feed?

TEN STEPS FOR TREATING PAINFUL ENGORGEMENT

1. **Feed your baby frequently.**

2. **Encourage your milk to let down before you feed (or express or pump).** Do whatever helps you relax. Swing your arms round vigorously, going first in one direction twenty times, then in the other twenty times. Although heat encourages the let-down, it's better not to have a hot bath or put hot flannels on the breasts because heat also encourages congestion.

---

3. **Feed your baby whenever your breasts feel full**, even if he hasn't asked for a feed or is asleep.

4. **Express or pump before a feed if you need to soften your areola** to make it easier for your baby to feed. A baby allowed to suck on a tense areola is unlikely to take the breast into his mouth properly. Instead he'll chew on the nipple and make it sore. He'll also obtain very little milk. This is because he can't take a big enough mouthful to drain the milk reservoirs, and also because the pain he causes by chewing on the nipples prevents you from letting your milk down. If you're badly engorged, an electric pump will be more comfortable than a hand pump or hand expression.

5. **Make sure your baby is well-positioned** at the breast (see pages 166 and 310) so that he can suck and milk effectively.

6. **Feed your baby at least for long enough to remove fullness and lumpiness.**

7. **Express or pump after a feed to remove any lumpiness.** This lumpiness is most likely to occur if your baby is too tired, apathetic or poorly to suck and milk the breasts effectively for long (see page 335). You can empty your breasts either by hand expression or by pumping, though there's no need to empty them fully.

8. **Express or pump between feeds** if your breasts feel at all full, tight or tender and you don't want to wake your baby.

9. **Relieve tenderness and pain** (see next page). This is *as well as*, not *instead of*, nos. 1–8 above.

10. **Give yourself a pat on the back.** You're doing a grand job by breastfeeding and taking steps to overcome this temporary problem. Keep going.

Relieving tenderness and pain

There are many ways of relieving tenderness and pain while you take steps to cure your engorgement.

- Cool your breasts with, for example: 1) Ice packs. These can be packs of frozen vegetables (such as peas), plastic bags filled with ice (crushed is more comfortable than cubes), gel-filled cool-packs from the fridge or freezer, or washed cooled cabbage leaves. It's sensible to put a protective layer of cloth between your skin and the pack. 2) Cold flannels. First put them in ice-cold water then wring them out. 3) Cold water splashes for your breasts. Coldness decreases congestion and makes the breasts feel more comfortable. Cool your breasts after a feed for about thirty minutes on and off, and repeat as necessary, though not in the half-hour before you're likely to feed, because it might hinder your let-down. Don't get too cold, though!
- Aromatherapists suggest *very* gently massaging or smoothing in a little oil or cream containing rose or peppermint essential oil (two to three drops to a tablespoonful of carrier oil or cream). But don't get this on your areolae or nipples as its taste might put your baby off feeding. You could also put a few drops, in total, of one or more of the essential oils of rose, lavender, geranium or fennel into a bowl of hot water. Lay a large hanky with a round hole cut in the middle on the surface of the water to pick up the film of oil. Then apply the hanky to your breast with the hole over your areola and nipple. Cover with a towel and leave for five minutes. Repeat every few hours. Avoid putting any oil on your areolae and nipples as your baby might not like its taste.
- Medical herbalists suggest: 1) Making a herb tea by pouring 570ml (1 pint) of boiling water over 28g (1oz) of dried cleavers (*Galium aparine*) leaves, stems and flowers; cover and steep for ten minutes, then strain. Put two flannels into a bowl of this tea, wring out a little and apply to the breasts. Repeat frequently. Cleavers is traditionally used for engorgement as it has a cooling action and is said to relieve congestion. 2) Making a decoction of poke root by grinding 28g (1oz) of the root using a pestle and mortar, covering with a little over 570ml (1 pint) of water in a pan, simmering for ten minutes, then straining and using in the same way as cleavers tea.

Like cleavers, poke root is a traditional remedy for engorgement. You can buy these herbs from a medical herbalist or a herbal supplier.

• If you happen to be engorged in summertime, and if you're lucky enough to have jasmine flowers in your garden – or know someone who has – you might like to copy the women in southern India and cover your breasts with jasmine flowers!

You'll notice that we haven't mentioned pain-killers for this condition. This is because they do not seem to be very much help and because it is best, if at all possible, to avoid taking any drugs while you are breastfeeding. Treating the causes, as above, is by far the best approach, but if you need to take something, paracetamol is safest.

SORE NIPPLES

Most women say that their nipples hurt at some time while breastfeeding, especially in the early weeks and particularly the very first week after delivery. Surveys estimate that up to 80 per cent of mothers have sore nipples at some time. It isn't always possible to prevent soreness, but several things can help and nearly everyone finds that pain and soreness lessen in time.

Why do nipples hurt? There are several reasons. Sometimes they are completely undamaged. More often, they are roughened; there's usually reddening and swelling of the small projections (papillae) on top; and there may be a crescent-shaped stripe of tiny blood-spots (petechiae) across each nipple. There may also be some crusting.

The pain of a sore nipple begins as soon as the baby starts feeding and generally lasts only a minute or two, not throughout the feed. In women breastfeeding on demand, the peak of nipple soreness occurs on the third day and starts decreasing by the fourth day, whereas in women breastfeeding on a four-hourly schedule, the soreness continues to get worse until the fourth day. Babies fed on a schedule may damage the nipple skin more as they tend to suck more strongly because they are so hungry. Large babies tend to cause more soreness than do small ones for the same reason.

The pain of sore nipples is very characteristic. It's usually described as feeling as if the baby were biting the nipple. It usually goes as soon as the milk lets down, and perhaps for this reason it's nearly always less or even non-existent in the second breast.

The most reasonable explanation for the pain, with or without actual skin damage, would seem to be the very strong suction exerted by the baby before the milk lets down or while he sleeps at the breast. The crescentic stripe represents the area of nipple exposed to maximum suction, with the baby's palate resting above the stripe and his tongue below. Women with no visible damage may have tougher skin which resists the suction better. The pain stops (provided that the nipple skin is not too damaged) when the milk lets down because the baby no longer needs to suck so strongly.

Towards the end of the first week after delivery, when milk is being produced freely, there's always some fore-milk available when the baby starts to feed (and before the hind-milk lets down), so strong suction from trying to get milk from empty reservoirs shouldn't be a problem.

The occasional woman with soreness in later weeks may have no fore-milk available for her baby at the beginning of a feed. The reason for this may be because her ducts are constricted and not allowing milk through because she's cold, in which case she should have a warm shower or bath before feeding, put some more clothes on or turn the house-heating up, or bathe her breasts with warm water.

A baby who has the nipple and areola positioned poorly in his mouth (because of being held awkwardly or because his mother has poorly protractile nipples or engorged breasts) is more likely to cause soreness by damaging the nipples.

As any experienced breastfeeder knows, nipple soreness can be extremely painful! Don't be surprised if you wince at the beginning of a feed or even cry out: this doesn't mean you have a low pain threshold or you're a coward. Just remember that nipple soreness can be cured. As the days go by, your nipples will grow tougher and more pain-resistant. Then when you stop breastfeeding, you'll notice that they gradually return to their former state.

TWENTY STEPS FOR TREATING SORE NIPPLES

The cardinal rule is to carry on feeding: DON'T STOP.

1. Change your feeding position several times a day. This ensures that no single part of the nipple takes the force of the baby's suction every time. For example:

In the morning: At each morning feed after you get up, hold your baby in the 'normal' position on your lap, with you sitting up.

During the afternoon and evening: Hold him in the 'football hold' (his legs pointing backwards under the arm of the side you're feeding him from, with his body supported by a cushion if necessary) and you sitting up.

During the night: Lay your baby at your side.

With a little ingenuity you can work out other variations. Some mothers learn the knack of lying by their baby and feeding him from the breast opposite to the side he's lying on by leaning over him carefully and half lying on their tummy.

2. Treat any painful engorgement (see page 302). A baby finds it difficult to feed effectively from an engorged breast and is very likely to chew the nipple as the areola may be too tense to be taken into his mouth.

3. Encourage your let-down to work before you put your baby to the breast by going through a routine of preparing for a feed. Then your baby won't have to suck and milk your breasts so strongly and for so long to stimulate the let-down. This is good because fear of pain as your baby sucks on sore nipples, as well as actual pain, delays the let-down reflex.

4. Make sure your baby is positioned well. If your nipples look sore, with stripes across them or blood blisters, it's highly likely that your baby is having to suck too strongly simply to hold the breast in his mouth. He's unlikely to have enough of the breast in his mouth, so the nipple won't go far enough back in the mouth. This means that when he sucks, the nipple will be drawn in and out of his mouth and easily made sore. Also, and most importantly, a poorly positioned baby doesn't milk the breasts well, so milk production and flow are poor. This means that milk doesn't flow into the reservoirs and from there into the baby's mouth quickly enough to fill the vacuum and reduce the high suction pressure.

Some experts suggest that nearly all nipple soreness results from poor positioning! Check that you're holding your baby correctly as follows.

Sit upright, or lean slightly forward, with your baby's head supported by your arm. Use this arm to turn him towards you so that his face, chest, tummy and knees are all facing your body, and so he doesn't have to turn his head to get to the breast. Make sure his chin is against your breast because you want him to have a good mouthful of that part of the areola under your nipple.

Hold your breast with your thumb and first finger spread out, your thumb on the upper part of your breast (above the areola) and the other fingers below it. Tickle your baby's upper lip very gently so he opens his mouth very wide. He should have part or all of the areola (depending on its size) in his mouth, and certainly not just the nipple itself. Pull your baby's bottom in towards you so that it's no further away from you than his chest is. He should now be feeding in a good position. However, if you think he may not be able to breathe well, simply lift your breast up slightly .

5. Feed your baby frequently. This encourages your mature milk to come in sooner and helps establish your let-down reflex. You may develop sore nipples sooner than your schedule-feeding neighbour in the next bed but your soreness will disappear before hers, your breastfeeding will almost certainly be more successful and you'll be less likely to develop mastitis from a blocked duct and/or infection.

6. Don't limit drinking time but limit total suckling time. Suckling to comfort your baby while he goes to sleep after he's finished drinking is good practice when your nipples are not sore. But if you have sore nipples you may find it helps them heal if you take him off the breast when he's finished drinking. By doing this and by encouraging your let-down to work before he feeds (see no. 3 above) you'll limit his total sucking time but not his actual drinking time. It isn't always easy to know when babies have finished drinking, because they often have breaks between bouts of sucking, and sometimes even short naps too. However, if your baby spends long at the breast without swallowing regularly and showing signs of 'nutritive' sucking (one suck per minute), although you try to keep him alert and interested by encouraging your let-down, it's time to stop. When a baby is doing 'non-nutritive sucking', while snoozing or sleeping, he'll tend to suck faster, at a rate of two sucks per second, with pauses between short bursts of this 'flutter' sucking.

When nipple soreness eases after a day or two, go back to letting him suck for as long as he wants or else your milk supply may start to diminish.

7. Always offer the less sore nipple first. By the time you offer the sore one, your milk should be flowing well and you should have little or no pain.

8. Distract yourself by reading or watchng TV, and try breathing exercises and other relaxation techniques to help in the first part of a feed when your nipples feel most sore. Anything that takes your mind off the pain may help because the power of positive thinking can be very effective.

9. If your nipples are poorly protractile, try using breast shells for half an hour or so before a feed. These may temporarily make the nipples stand out enough for your baby to take a good mouthful of breast and avoid sucking on the nipple alone. Keep the shells clean to avoid introducing infection into the damaged skin. A word of warning here. The still, warm air inside breast shells can make the nipple skin swollen and moist. This may cause more soreness and can also make a cracked nipple worse. Shells may or may not help but they could be worth a try once or twice to see.

10. Care for your nipple skin as described on page 187. If you are washing your bras, nighties and any other clothing in contact with your skin with a biological washing powder, there's a very small chance that your nipple soreness may be caused by a sensitivity, so try using a non-biological powder instead.

11. Think twice before using any cream, ointment or hydrogel. Nature provides her own lubrication in the form of natural oils produced by nipple skin. Also, trials have shown that the routine use of proprietary skin preparations is largely ineffective at preventing sore nipples. If you do use one, gently wipe off any excess before a feed so your baby doesn't end up swallowing it! And do a patch test for skin sensitivity first by applying a small amount of the cream to your skin and waiting a few hours to see whether you react adversely. Many women are sensitive to lanolin (or substances such as pesticide residues in lanolin); there is some lanolin in both Masse cream and the chamomile-containing cream called Kamillosan. Lanolin comes from sheep's wool and because sheep are dipped in pesticide solutions (sometimes containing organochlorines), may contain pesticide residues. However, lanolin free from pesticide residues is available. See also page 188.

12. **Avoid antiseptic spray.** In the UK some women use an antiseptic (chlorhexidine) spray on their nipples in the mistaken belief that it prevents soreness, cracks and mastitis. However, there is no evidence either that this spray prevents soreness or cracks – or that it's effective against them once they have developed. Provided that your breastfeeding technique is good and you take adequate precautions against infection in hospital, there is no reason to use such a spray.

13. **Express some milk after each feed, rub it on to your nipples and let it dry.** This is a successful, simple and traditional tip for helping sore nipples heal. Breast milk contains growth factors (see page 51) which encourage cells to grow as well as soothing and anti-infective factors.

14. **If you have to stop your baby feeding, break the suction by putting a fingertip into the corner of his mouth and pushing the nipple to one side.** Pulling him off may increase any soreness.

15. **Take an aspirin or small alcoholic drink** twenty minutes before a feed if you feel the pain is hindering your let-down.

16. **Carefully expose your nipples to ultra-violet (UV) light**

from a sun-lamp (or a UV bulb in a lamp socket) to speed up the healing of damaged nipple skin. Sit three or four feet away from the lamp and protect your eyes with goggles or a thick towel. Expose your nipples for half a minute on the first day, one minute on days two and three, two minutes on days four and five and three minutes on day six. If there is any reddening of the skin, reduce the exposure time. If you can sunbathe with your nipples exposed, the sunlight will help a lot, but don't get sunburnt! If you have no garden, sunbathe indoors with the window open as very little UV light comes through glass. If you have access to neither a sun-lamp nor sunlight, try exposing your nipples to the light from a 60-watt electric light bulb for 20 minutes two or three times a day. This is better than nothing.

17. Don't remove any crusts appearing on the nipples – they are part of the healing process.

18. Try using a very thin rubber nipple shield over the sore nipple *only* if all the other measures fail. Such a shield has a teat for the baby to suck through and may or may not help. One danger is that it can introduce infection into the damaged skin if it isn't properly cleaned after each use. Another drawback is that a shield reduces skin stimulation, reduces the milk supply and prevents a baby from getting all the milk in the breast. Even the thinnest shield keeps back 22 per cent of the milk, while ordinary ones can keep back 65 per cent! If you're determined to use a shield, don't do so for long because both your milk production and the establishment of the let-down depend on actual skin stimulation by the baby.

19. Cool your nipples immediately before you put your baby to the breast. Try putting some ice cubes into a small polythene bag, covering it with a flannel or cloth and holding it against your nipple. A gel-filled cool-pack or a splash of cold water would do as well. However, because anything cold can hinder the let-down, it's probably best to encourage your let-down to start working before you cool your nipples.

20. Keep your nipples dry. Dry your nipples before covering them, and if you use anything inside your bra to mop up leaks, be sure to change it frequently to prevent your nipples from being enclosed in soggy material for long. Some women use a piece of one-way nappy liner or absorbent paper inside their bra to help keep their nipples dry. Waterproof-backed bra pads aren't ideal as they retain moisture next to the skin and encourage nipple soreness.

Rarely, a sore nipple bleeds and the baby swallows tiny amounts of blood. This can look horrifying if it's regurgitated in a mouthful of milk but there's no need to worry because your blood won't do your baby any harm. Treat the soreness and carry on feeding.

If your nipples stay sore during a whole feed, consider whether it may be caused by dermatitis from detergents used to wash clothing or from substances in creams or other remedies you may have put on your nipples. Once you have tracked down the cause, remove it and treat your nipples if necessary with hydrocortisone cream from your doctor.

THRUSH

This infection with the fungus or yeast *Candida albicans* (also known as Monilia) can make the skin of the nipple and areola sore. There may be particularly severe burning pain in the nipple and areola beginning after the first week following delivery and becoming worse after a feed. Indeed, this pain may continue for the entire time between feeds. There may also be deep shooting pains going deep into the breast during and between feeds.

You may also have itchy nipples with flaky pink, red or purple areas and possibly a bright red ring on your areola. Sometimes the areola is shiny and slightly swollen, and there may be fine cracks around the nipple, perhaps with white matter inside. Very occasionally thrush on the nipples shows as adherent white spots.

Candida is a normal inhabitant of our skin and bowels but in certain circumstances it can multiply and cause an infection. And if mother or baby has a Candida infection (for example, in the baby's mouth or nappy area, or the mother's vagina or bowel), they can easily pass it to each other. Thrush thrives in warm, moist situations and likes milk, so a baby's mouth and a mother's nipples and areolae (particularly if encased in a bra pad and bra) make very suitable breeding grounds. A woman is more likely to get thrush if she's recently taken antibiotics, has sore or cracked nipples, or is on the Pill.

As it's very easy for a breastfeeding woman and her baby to pass thrush backwards and forwards to each other, it's important to make sure that both are treated simultaneously, promptly and vigorously. If a mother has vaginal thrush, this should be treated at the same time. Treatment of both mother and baby is best carried out for two weeks even if both seem better beforehand. There is no need to stop breastfeeding.

Anti-fungal medication

Your doctor can prescribe anti-fungal preparations such as nystatin, miconazole or clotrimazole for you and your baby. Miconazole appears to be better absorbed and more effective on the nipples. Rinse your baby's mouth carefully with water after each feed and put a little (1 ml) nystatin suspension into his mouth. You should wash your nipples and areolae after each feed, dry them well, then put some anti-fungal cream or ointment on your skin. If you use breast pads, make sure you change them after each treatment.

If your thrush still doesn't clear up, your doctor can prescribe some 1 per cent aqueous gentian violet solution for you to use on your nipples and in your baby's mouth. Apply it just once a day but for no longer than three days. The stain will make your nipples and your baby's mouth look dramatically purple.

Other measures

A baby can become reinfected from anything that has previously been in his mouth, so boil daily for twenty minutes any dummy (pacifier) you may have given him. If you have repeated vaginal thrush, cut down on the amount of added sugar and other refined carbohydrates in your diet, as well as yeast-containing foods and drinks, including alcohol.

Home remedy?

Research shows that treating thrush on the nipples by applying a vinegar solution (made by mixing a teaspoon of vinegar with one cup of water) after each feed, and treating thrush in a baby's mouth with bicarbonate of soda solution (made by mixing a teaspoon of bicarbonate of soda in a cup of water) may help stop itching. They don't *cure* thrush, though.

Sunshine or ultra-violet (UV) light from a sun-lamp or UV bulb (used carefully, according to instructions) may also help get rid of thrush on your nipples.

Blanched nipple and areola

A few women find that nipple pain is sometimes followed by their nipples and areolae turning white and going numb, presumably because the blood supply has suddenly been reduced. The pain is like a cramp; it begins during a feed and continues afterwards, and the blanching and numbness begin either during the feed or very shortly after the baby comes off the breast. It may persist for half an hour or longer until the blood supply and colour return. If this happens to you, keep as warm and relaxed as you can and adjust your baby's feeding position (see pages 166 and 310).

NIPPLE CRACK

A few women develop a crack or fissure in the nipple. The crack may follow poor treatment of nipple soreness. It may develop at the base of the nipple, usually along a line representing the baby's maximum suction pressure while feeding. Indeed, if you have sore nipples and can also see a white 'compression' streak across your nipple after feeding, adjust your baby's position (page 310) because otherwise the skin may crack along the line of the streak.

A crack is acutely painful and needs careful and prompt treatment if the pain isn't going to put you off breastfeeding. Thrush sometimes infects a fissure (see above).

What to do

The best prevention and treatment is to take steps to treat sore nipples (see above). In particular, changing your feeding positions, avoiding non-nutritive sucking, and letting some expressed milk dry on your nipples after each feed speed up healing markedly.

However, it may be better not to let your cracked nipple dry by letting air get to it. Although research is lacking and this is an about-turn on previous advice, dermatologists point out that cracked skin elsewhere heals better if kept moist. They see no reason why this shouldn't apply to cracked nipples too. The outer layer of the nipple skin, the *stratum corneum*, cracks if it's dehydrated because it contains insufficient internal moisture. Applying cream, ointment, oil, hydrogel or a non-adherent burns dressing on cracked skin might possibly increase its moisture content, allow slower, more gentle drying, and give the distorted contours of the *stratum corneum* time to return to normal without rapid drying and scabbing creating tension on the skin either side of the crack. If you use any type of skin preparation, gently wipe away any excess before your baby feeds.

Dermatologists say it is a good idea, though, to remove any surface moisture remaining on the nipples after a feed or after leaking. Surface moisture is different from internal skin moisture.

One Australian hospital suggests putting washed geranium leaves over cracked nipples. The leaves contain tannin which apparently helps prevent cracks from getting worse.

If a crack doesn't heal within a few days you may need temporarily to take your baby off the breast because of the pain, and either express your milk or use an electric pump for a while – sometimes for as long as four or five days, though usually only for one or two. Give the expressed or pumped milk to your baby by spoon. Avoid using a bottle as some babies find it difficult to breastfeed afterwards.

Using a nipple shield so that you can carry on breastfeeding with a cracked nipple is not wise. The problem with nipple shields is that they reduce breast stimulation, which eventually adversely affects the milk supply. One Australian study showed that women preferred to treat their cracks by other methods (changing their breastfeeding technique as above, or temporarily stopping breast-feeding and expressing).

When a crack has healed, gradually resume breastfeeding, starting twice a day and continuing to express or pump regularly between feeds. Prevent it reopening by regularly changing your baby's feeding position (see pages 166 and 310).

BLOCKED DUCT (see also page 330)

This causes a red, tender lump or an area of inflammation (local mastitis) in the breast. And a woman with a blocked duct may also feel flu-like and achey.

A duct becomes blocked either because of pressure from a badly fitting bra, or from engorgement with inadequate emptying of one particular duct. Milk builds up in the duct behind the blockage and causes a lump. When the baby feeds, the let-down works even in the area of the breast supplying the blocked duct, so the pressure in the duct builds up more, often making the lump very painful as the milk lets down.

If you treat a blocked duct at this early stage, the lumpy area should subside with no further problem. But if you do nothing, the affected part of the breast will probably become inflamed. This inflammation results from fluid and certain constituents of dammed-up milk escaping from the blocked duct into the surrounding breast tissue. This makes the overlying skin red and causes the body temperature to rise as inflammatory products get into the bloodstream. The fever can be as high as 40°C (104° F) after a feed.

Treatment of a blocked duct is an urgent matter because stagnant milk in the milk gland and duct behind the block, and in the surrounding breast tissue, can so easily become infected. Simple measures, started at the first suspicion that anything is wrong, should do the trick in every case.

TEN STEPS FOR TREATING A BLOCKED DUCT

1. **Make sure your whole breast is emptied thoroughly each time your baby feeds.** Complete emptying is not usually necessary but, in the case of the blocked duct, the lower the tension of milk in the breast, the better chance you'll have of clearing the blockage. Check that your baby is well positioned at the breast (see page 166 and 310); let him feed as long as he wants; then express the remaining milk.

2. **Feed your baby more often** if your breasts – or even a part of a breast – still feel lumpy after a feed. This ensures

frequent drainage of the ducts. Fit in as many extra feeds as you can, even if you're already feeding on demand.

3. **Offer the affected breast first** to ensure the best possible emptying and return to it later in the feed.

4. *Gently* **but firmly massage the lump towards the nipple** during a feed (and after if it's still there) in an attempt to release the dammed-up milk.

5. **Check that your bra isn't pressing anywhere** and causing the block, especially if you wear an old-fashioned nursing bra with a band across the top of the breast when the flap is open, or if you pull the cup of an ordinary bra down to feed.

6. **Vary your feeding position** at each feed (see page 309). This simple tip is one of the most helpful.

7. **Relieve the pain** with hot, wet compresses applied every hour, or put a covered hot-water bottle over the area. Splashing the breast with hot water while leaning over a basin before a feed may help. Even better, immerse your breast in comfortably hot water for five to ten minutes, perhaps in a bath of deep water.

8. **Take a course of antibiotics suitable for a breastfeeding woman, if the lump is still there after twenty-four hours in spite of all these measures**. This will prevent infection. Your doctor can prescribe these for you. *Don't stop feeding when you're on antibiotics.*

9. **Get plenty of rest and relaxation.** Actually go to bed; even if this is for only one day it will make you feel better and may boost your resistance. This will help prevent any local inflammation (local mastitis) from your blocked duct from progressing to mastitis of the whole breast. It's been

suggested that blocked ducts may sometimes result from stress. The reasoning on this is that stress produces more adrenaline; adrenaline leads to the release of fat into the blood; and with more fat entering the milk, the milk is more likely to thicken and to coat the duct lining – much as fatty blood can lead to fatty deposits on artery linings. This theory is, however, unproved.

10. **Take more exercise** – especially of the shoulders, arms and upper half of the body – as this may help disperse a painful swelling caused by a blocked duct. Do both general body exercise to boost your circulation and chest area-stretching exercises to give a blocked duct every chance to unblock.

One extremely unusual – and unproven – therapy for lumpy breasts and mastitis comes from the field of kinesiology and is said to reduce congestion by increasing lymph drainage. There seems to be no known medical explanation. However, as it can do no harm and some women have found it helps, we've included it here. You can either do it yourself or – and this is said to be more effective – ask someone else to do it for you.

Touch the lumpy area of your breast very lightly with one hand. With three fingers of your other hand, you then massage a particular part of your leg on the same side of your body. The area to massage is from just below the knee up the outside of the leg to the hip – along a line similar to that of the side-seam of a pair of trousers. Use a firm circular motion for about ten seconds in one place, then move your fingers up the line and repeat the process. When you reach the hip, repeat if necessary with your first hand on another lumpy area of the breast.

Expressing a 'plug'

Some women notice that if they persevere with gently trying to express milk from a blocked duct, they eventually express a very small firm 'plug' of white or yellow, cheesy or granular matter from the opening of that duct at the nipple. This plug is probably made of dried-out milk that has been dammed up behind the blockage. The milk that they then express from that duct is usually thicker than normal and may flow slowly of its own accord for a while. When the milk that was dammed up in the blocked duct and gland has all been expressed, the newly-produced milk looks normal. The thickening of the milk is simply due to stasis and water absorption.

If a plug is right at the nipple, you may be able to see the swollen milk reservoir bulging in the areola – rather like a varicose vein, though not coloured.

Repeated blocked ducts

Some women are plagued with repeated blocks. If this happens to you in spite of taking the ten steps above, it may be worth considering a dietary change.

Something may be making your milk too 'sticky' and encouraging certain constituents of the milk (such as the fat globules) to adhere to the lining of your ducts, thus reducing their diameter and making a blockage more likely. There are several things you can easily try which will hurt neither you nor your baby and might just help.

Look at your diet – Eating too much fat, particularly saturated fats, can make blood more sticky, so it's possible, though unproven, that the same might happen to breast milk.

Check that your diet is healthy, with plenty of vegetables and fruit and not too much meat, dairy food and other sources of saturated fats. If you eat a lot of fat, consider adjusting your diet so that you eat less, and change the balance of fats so that you eat more polyunsaturated fats and fewer saturated ones. However, make sure you have enough fat in your diet. Now is not the time for a low-fat diet!

Eat some oily fish two or three times a week, as these contain certain omega-three essential fatty acids (DHA or docosahexaenoic acid, and EPA or eicosapentaenoic acid) which not every woman can make in large enough amounts from other foods to meet her body's needs.

Also include in your diet some of the following: onions; garlic (about three cloves a day); pineapple; ginger; avocados; and foods rich in vitamins B_1 (thiamine, such as whole-grains, peas, beans, lentils, brown rice and meat), B_6 (in whole-grains, bananas, avocados, nuts, seeds, green leafy vegetables, meat, fish and egg yolk), C (most fruits, green vegetables, potatoes) and, possibly, E (nuts, seeds, soya, lettuce, vegetable oils); flavonoids (bright pigments found in many vegetables and fruits); and salicylates (naturally-occurring chemicals found in many vegetables and fruits). These, together with oily fish, emulsify blood fats (that is, disperse them into smaller globules). It's reasonable to suggest they might do the same with milk fats.

Take a GLA supplement – Take starflower (borage) or evening primrose oil. These contain another essential fatty acid (GLA, gamma-linolenic acid) which, again, not every woman makes from other foods in the amounts her body needs.

Look to your stress levels – Your reaction to stress could hinder the production of essential fatty acids. You can't avoid stress – indeed, it's a normal part of life – but you can learn more effective stress-management techniques.

Smoking – If milk behaves in any way like blood, then smoking (and even passive smoking) might make it stickier. Smoking is known to make one particular type of breast inflammation (periductal mastitis) more likely.

Check your sleeping position – Some women find that sleeping on their fronts can result in a blocked duct.

Homeopathy – The homeopathic remedy Phytolacca is said to help. The dose of Phytolacca (either 30C or 12C) is one tablet two or three times a day. It should not be taken within half an hour of food or drink.

Herbal remedies – Medical herbalists recommend drinking dandelion root tea (not more than a cupful three times a day), and smoothing some linseed oil combined with a few drops of essential oil of rose or geranium on to inflamed breasts.

MASTITIS

The term 'mastitis' isn't very helpful because all it means medically is that the breast is inflamed. Many people assume that every inflamed breast is infected. However, several things other than infection can make a breast inflamed. Studies show that out of every two women with mastitis, one has engorgement (see page 302) or a blocked duct (see page 319), while the other has an infection.

It's important to distinguish non-infected mastitis from infected mastitis. This is because breast infection is potentially serious and needs antibiotic treatment. On the other hand, it isn't a good idea to have unnecessary antibiotics. Fortunately, lab tests usually solve the problem (see below).

Mastitis is most likely to begin in the upper part of the breast and in the side nearest the arm. If left untreated, the inflammation can spread and the tissues can become infected.

BREAST INFECTION (mastitis with infection)

Breast inflammation due to infection can be called mastitis with infection, infected mastitis or, simply, breast infection.

Infection may affect only one area of the breast or the whole breast. If infection is present, the breast is red, swollen, hot, painful and tender, with shiny skin, and the woman feels shivery, ill and achey, as if she has 'flu, with a fever of 38° C/100.4° F or more. She may feel nauseated and might actually vomit. It's sometimes possible to squeeze pus from the nipple.

If just a part of the breast is involved, the symptoms are like those of a blocked duct but worse. And usually only one breast is affected.

If the infection involves the whole breast, it may look as if it's badly engorged (see page 302), but unlike severe engorgement, which nearly always affects both breasts, mastitis due to breast infection usually affects only one.

Unless it's obvious, how can you and your medical advisers tell that your breast is actually infected?

Distinguishing inflammation due to breast infection from inflammation due to severe engorgement or a blocked duct

It can be difficult to be sure of the underlying cause of mastitis, though usually a woman's story helps.

Ideally it's best to send a sample of your milk to the path lab before you start taking an antibiotic. Immediate examination of the milk enables the lab to tell your doctor whether you need antibiotics at all. If you do, you can start on one then more time-consuming culture and sensitivity tests can identify the organism causing the infection and determine whether an antibiotic other than the one you are taking would be more appropriate.

Some information for doctors

- *There's probably engorgement* if there's a normal leucocyte (white blood cell) count (less than ten to the 6th/ml of milk), and a normal bacteria colony count (less than ten to the 3rd/ml of milk), indicating that the milk is sterile or contains normal amounts of skin bacteria.
- *There's probably a blocked duct* if there's an increased leucocyte count (more than ten to the 6th/ml of milk) and a normal bacteria count

(less than ten to the $\frac{1}{3}$/ml of milk) indicating that the milk is sterile or contains normal amounts of skin bacteria.

- *There's a breast infection which needs antibiotics* if there's an increased leucocyte count (more than ten to the 6th/ml of milk) and an increased bacteria count (more than ten to the 3rd/ml of milk). It's important for the lab to do culture and sensitivity tests of the milk to show which bacteria are responsible for the infection and which antibiotic is the most appropriate. However, these tests take several days, so if a woman's leucocyte and colony counts are high and she has obvious signs of infection, her doctor will start her on the antibiotic which is most likely to help. When the test results come through she may need to change to a different antibiotic, because taking the wrong one makes recurrent infection more likely.

Test for thrush – Ideally the laboratory should test your milk for fungal infection with thrush (*Candida albicans*) as well. One survey showed that one in two women with mastitis had *Candida*, though of course that doesn't necessarily mean that it was causing the inflammation, because *Candida* is a normal inhabitant of most people's skin. However, if *Candida* does seem to be the culprit, you'll need anti-fungal treatment, not antibiotics.

What to do if you have an infection

- Take antibiotics early. The best one to start with – as long as you aren't allergic to penicillin – is flucloxacillin (in a dose of 500mg four times a day). If you are allergic to penicillin, you can take erythromycin (500mg twice a day). (Antibiotics which are *unsuitable* because they enter milk and can harm a baby are tetracycline, ciprofloxacin and chloramphenicol.)
- Check your feeding technique and in particular keep your breasts well and frequently emptied by your baby (see below) and/or by expression or pumping. This maintains your milk supply and helps healing. If you let your breasts remain too full – or if you try to let your milk dry up – you run a serious risk of an abscess developing.
- If you've had a blocked duct, turn to page 319.
- If you've been engorged, turn to page 302.
- If you've had a cracked nipple, turn to page 318.

- Rest more. One study showed that women with mastitis due to a breast infection had had fewer hours of sleep at night than other women, and were less likely to be taking daytime naps. Take special care of yourself when life is busy, for example, around Christmas or other holidays.
- Treat the pain with aspirin and hot flannels.
- If you smoke, cut down or give up. If you can't, take a supplement of vitamin C (at least 100 mg a day), as smoking reduces the levels of this vitamin.
- If you're in hospital, ask for a disinfectant hand-wash solution. German researchers reported that if breastfeeding mothers – and the staff who touch them – carefully and regularly wash their hands with such a solution, there's very much less chance of getting mastitis.
- Find effective ways of managing the pressures in your life, as high stress levels can lower your resistance to infection. Various relaxation methods can reduce both physical and emotional tension.
- Check that you are eating a healthy diet with plenty of fresh fruit and vegetables, and consider taking supplements of vitamins C (at least 100mg a day) and E (10mg of tocopherol acetate daily).
- Several remedies can be helpful. These include: gently smoothing in some vitamin E cream, or cream scented with the essential oil of geranium (three drops to one tablespoon of a simple cream)

Causes of breast infection

Breast infection can occur at any time. The underlying triggers for any individual woman becoming vulnerable to infection with bacteria which are usually normal residents of their skin often aren't clear.

In some women who have been breastfeeding successfully for several weeks or months, certain breast infections follow poor or delayed treatment of engorgement, a blocked duct or a cracked nipple. Others are thought to enter the breast via the nipple from the baby, who is likely to have picked them up in hospital, carrying them in his nose, without symptoms. When several mothers and babies have a breast infection at once in hospital or soon after they leave, their mastitis is called 'epidemic' mastitis. This sort of infection may begin in the milk ducts themselves.

The organism which causes breast infection is nearly always *Staphylococcus aureus*. Occasionally *Staph epidermidis* or *streptococci* are responsible.

Interestingly, a doctor we know who worked in a totally breastfeeding hospital unit in Africa saw no breast infections in four years of looking after several thousand mothers.

Can your baby have your milk from an infected breast ?

Generally, the answer is yes. It's almost always better to go on breastfeeding: better for the baby and better for you.

However, if – and only if – your milk contains particularly large counts of bacteria (dead or alive) there's a very small possibility of gastroenteritis or even septicaemia and your baby shouldn't drink it even it's sterilized. You can breastfeed if your baby is well, but if you want to avoid any risk, then temporarily either feed only from your unaffected breast, or give donated breast milk or formula. Pump or express your infected breast and discard the milk. When the bacteria count drops you can breastfeed again.

What if the infection doesn't get better?

If, despite excellent treatment as outlined above, your breast is still inflamed and infected, yet there is no abscess (see below), your doctor may change the antibiotic to co-amoxiclav (taking care to monitor your baby carefully for signs of jaundice).

If this, in turn, does not help, then to be on the safe side he should check that you don't have a cancer.

BREAST ABSCESS

This usually follows poor or delayed treatment of mastitis (breast inflammation). One survey showed that *abscesses occurred only in women who stopped feeding when they got mastitis*. A lump caused by an abscess isn't tender.

Treatment is as for breast infection but if the abscess doesn't resolve, either repeated aspiration (drawing off the pus through a needle) or, as a last resort, surgical incision and drainage, will be necessary. Only very occasionally does a woman with an abscess need a general anaesthetic.

You can feed your baby from the affected breast if you and your doctor are reasonably sure that the infection is contained within the abscess (which is usually the case). Otherwise, carry on feeding from the other side and temporarily discard the expressed milk from the breast with the abscess.

LUMP IN THE BREAST

Women of all ages and at all stages of their lives can develop a lump in their breast. The important thing to remember is that breastfeeding is no sure protection against cancer so continue to be 'breast aware' – look at them carefully each month and feel for lumps. It's more difficult to feel lumps if your breasts are larger and firmer, but if you do, take it seriously. Having said this, the lactating breast is often lumpy. Such lumps are usually 'here today and gone tomorrow', whereas a significant breast lump stays.

The causes of lumps during breastfeeding are much as at any other time with the addition of those related to milk production.

A blocked duct causes a lump which should become much smaller within 72 hours with suitable treatment (see page 319). If it doesn't see your doctor.

Lumps such as fibro-adenomas that are commonly found in the breast, lactating or not, may appear for the first time during lactation. Four times out of five, such lumps are not cancers and if necessary can simply be removed (preferably under local anaesthetic) and breastfeeding continued.

A woman who develops breast cancer will probably be advised

to wean because the drugs used for chemotherapy will enter her milk and harm her baby.

A galactocele (milk retention cyst) is a non-tender, smooth, rounded, cystic swelling filled with milk. It's thought to be caused by a blocked duct which never opened again. If a cyst becomes infected, it forms an abscess. Sometimes gentle expression can empty milk from a cyst via the nipple. It's wise to try both this and other ways of dealing with a blocked duct (see page 320). If you ignore it, the milk in the cyst will gradually become thick and creamy, cheesy or oily. If the cyst is aspirated (emptied via a hollow needle), it refills with milk. A cyst like this can be surgically removed under a local anaesthetic. You can safely carry on breastfeeding.

CHALLENGING FEEDERS

Some babies take to the breast within a few minutes of being born and never give their mothers any trouble. Others, however, seem completely disinterested, feed briefly, then let go and cry, or even seem to have a battle with the breast. There's nearly always a reason for such behaviour; the challenge is deciding how to manage.

Whatever the cause of the difficulty with feeding, keep your milk supply going. Although a few babies never feed enthusiastically, they virtually all feed eventually given the chance. An unenthusiastic baby may not stimulate your milk supply well enough, so you'll need to express or pump after each feed. You may need to keep this up for some weeks, so be prepared.

Before you even think of labelling your baby as a 'difficult feeder', get rid of any engorgement (see page 302) and check that you have him well-positioned (see page 166 and 310). Some women have to take special care at first because they have poorly protractile nipples.

Poorly protractile nipples (see page 158)

A few women still have poorly protractile nipples at the end of their pregnancy, though they tend to improve after several weeks of breastfeeding.

If your nipples don't stand out well, you may find it helps to wear breast shells for a few minutes before a feed: this brings the nipples out just long enough for the baby to get a hold. Using a breast pump for a short while before a feed has a similar effect. Once your baby latches on, your nipple should stay out for the duration of the feed. When he stops feeding, it'll probably go back in.

You can also help your baby latch on by taking your nipple and areola between your finger and thumb and gently making a flat 'biscuit' for him to take hold of. This biscuit should be held so that it is parallel with the line of the baby's lips and not at right angles to it. However, release your grip as soon as he's feeding well because otherwise you may obstruct the reservoirs and ducts and stop the milk flowing.

Baby kept from you after birth

The best time to start suckling is in the first half-hour after birth. After this the baby's urge to feed gradually lessens (see page 164), although of course you can still teach him, with patience. Learning to feed is best done in the first few hours; after that you'll have a slower pupil on your hands.

Baby affected by your pain-killers in labour

In the UK pethidine is a common offender, while in the US many babies are also affected by barbiturates. Such babies may be drowsy and apathetic about feeding for up to five days, though the effects usually wear off more quickly.

You might not be able to get your sedated baby to feed well but you can avoid giving a bottle and you can keep your milk supply going by expressing or pumping after each feed. You can also give him expressed milk from a cup or spoon when he's finished at the breast, and make sure he has a chance to go back to the breast if he wishes. Wake him often – every two or three hours at least – for a feed, as the sooner he learns how to breastfeed, the better. While you or a nurse may be able to get him to bottle-feed even if he won't feed from you, this isn't a good idea as he'll then be far less likely to take to the breast once the sedation wears off.

The key to managing this problem is perseverance. You can cope if you know what to do.

Jaundiced baby (see page 359)

A jaundiced baby is often sleepy and difficult to interest in feeding. Frequent small feeds are best. As the jaundice clears, he'll become more interested, so be patient and keep your milk supply going by expressing after each feed (see page 189).

Baby has been given a bottle

A baby who learns to bottle-suck will try to breastfeed using the same technique. Unfortunately, this often doesn't work and the baby has to relearn how to breastfeed. You'll be able to get him to feed from you, with patience, but it's far better to avoid giving a bottle in the first place. Once a baby has fed from the breast for many weeks, the occasional experience of bottle-feeding shouldn't matter, although some older babies quickly learn that milk comes from a bottle more easily and are then reluctant to take the breast if there's the slightest chance of a bottle!

The technique a baby uses for bottle-feeding is easier than the one he uses for breastfeeding. When bottle-feeding, a baby applies a little suction, lets the milk pour into his mouth and then swallows. There isn't much movement of his tongue and there's little jaw movement.

If a baby bottle-sucks the breast, he gets very little milk. There's much more work involved in breastfeeding so it's hardly surprising to find that the muscular effort expended is good for the development of the baby's jaws.

If you're teaching a baby to breastfeed once he's been given a bottle, it's no help if you constantly muddle him by giving both breast and bottle. If you want to breastfeed, don't give your baby a bottle at all. If for some reason he isn't getting all his nourishment direct from the breast, give him complements of expressed breast milk (or formula if you must) by cup or spoon or from a supplementer (see page 449).

You can tell whether your baby is trying to bottle-suck during a breastfeed because you'll occasionally see him sucking his cheeks in (caused by him sucking his tongue). He may stick his tongue out (known as 'tongue-thrusting') and do a lot of 'non-nutritive' sucking (a fast, fluttering sort of suck at a rate of two or three sucks per second) rather than slower, 'nutritive' sucking. Your baby won't swallow very often (check this by listening and by watching for the ear movement which accompanies a swallow) and there are long intervals between bouts of sucking. Feeds take a long time because your baby's poor milking action doesn't encourage you to let your milk down.

Even one bottle can make subsequent feeding behaviour difficult. In the rare event of a mother being so ill that she can't feed her baby, her baby should have his milk from a cup or spoon (or from another mother), not from a bottle.

Full baby

If, however unwisely, you are feeding on a hospital schedule, and your baby has had a bottle of formula since you've fed him, he's unlikely to be hungry for the next scheduled breastfeed. This is because formula stays in the stomach much longer than breast milk. Complements of formula are rarely necessary, so tell the nurse you would rather feed your baby more often and for longer and that you don't want him to have anything other than breast milk to drink, day or night. Remember that you need your baby to feed often so that your milk comes in quickly and you produce plenty of milk. A baby full of formula is no help to your breasts as he simply won't feed.

Exhausted baby

If you feed your baby according to a schedule in hospital, he may cry from hunger for some time – perhaps as long as an hour – before it's time for the next scheduled feed. This is especially likely to happen at visiting times and at night. By the time you get him he's exhausted and goes to sleep after feeding for a very short time, even sometimes before your milk even lets down.

This is obviously ridiculous. You must insist on feeding your baby as soon as he cries. Remember that the smaller the baby, the more often he'll need feeding, and the earlier crying will exhaust him.

Sleepy baby

A sleepy baby may be suffering from you having had a long labour or from the effects of the pain-killers you had in labour (see page 332); he may be jaundiced or unwell; he may be tired out from crying between feeds; or he may simply be a baby who likes a lot of sleep.

You'll find it helps if he is alert (but not crying) when you start to feed him. You may be able to wake him up more by taking his clothes off (though don't let him get chilled), rocking him gently, or stroking his back firmly. Watch for any of the little signs that show he may be ready to feed even though he isn't asking for a feed. These include eyes darting around beneath closed eyelids, sucking movements, putting his hand to his mouth, moving in general, and making small sounds.

Encourage him to continue sucking by gently expressing a little milk into his mouth while he's actually at the breast. If he is too sleepy to get enough milk, however much you try to keep him awake and interested in feeding, you can help by making sure he gets your hind-milk. Do this by expressing your breasts *after* you've finished each feed. Collect the milk – which will be fat-rich hind-milk – and give it to your baby by cup or, even better, by a supplementer (see page 449) halfway through the next feed.

Baby overwhelmed by milk supply

If your let-down is so powerful that the milk gushes into your baby's mouth and nearly chokes him, you'll find it helps to collect this early milk in a sterilized container and allow him to feed only when the milk stops flowing so exuberantly. You can give him the collected milk by cup or spoon afterwards.

Babies who try to swallow quickly enough to cope with an exuberant milk supply often swallow too much air and develop colic or regurgitate more than usual after a feed. Some babies bring up almost a whole feed because of this. Expressing or simply collecting the initial milk you let down, as described above, should get over the problem. If you simply allow the baby to bring up a whole feed and then feed him again, he'll certainly keep the milk down because the flow will be much slower and he won't swallow as much air, but your milk supply will increase because of the law of demand and supply and your let-down will subsequently work even better, making the problem worse at the next feed.

One way to overcome the problem of too much milk is to give one breast per feed, letting your baby suck on the empty breast for comfort. Give the other breast at the next feed. This allows him to suck for comfort without getting two breasts full of milk at each feed. Express some milk from the unused breast if necessary to keep you comfortable. See also page 290.

Crying baby (see pages 196 and 224)

Baby wants feeding very often

How often a baby wants to feed depends on his personality, how hungry and thirsty he is, how tired he is and on whether or not he is well and happy. In other words, there may be some specific reason why your baby sometimes or always wants frequent feeds, or he may just be asking for what is perfectly normal and desirable for him.

The first thing to do is to check whether you're making enough milk. If not, take steps to increase your milk supply (see page 271). Second, if he feeds very frequently just at a particular time of the day (which is most likely to be in the evening), and cries if you don't feed him, see page 198. However, if your baby is healthy, thriving and gaining weight, he may simply have got into the habit of feeding frequently. If you are not happy to go along with this, you may be able gradually to lengthen the gaps between feeds by distracting him with various activities. A good tip is to get him used to larger feeds. Try expressing some milk in the morning (a time when most women have most milk). Keep this milk in the fridge. When your baby starts wanting frequent feeds – perhaps in the evening – give this milk to him from a cup after one of the feeds. This may fill him up and allow you to have a longer break.

Excited baby

A baby who is so excited by the idea of feeding that he 'bounces' at the breast as he searches and lunges for the nipple, and at the same time waves his arms around, may be too active to settle down to a feed. He disturbs himself so much that he becomes overwrought and ends up frustrated and crying. If your baby fits this picture, you could try wrapping him (firmly but not too tightly) in a shawl or cloth to keep his arms by his sides. Encourage your milk to let down before he goes to the breast, so there's milk there for him as soon as he starts to feed. Rub a little milk over your areola to see if the smell of it helps him focus and concentrate. If his behaviour puts you off so that you find it difficult to let your milk down, you could try using a supplementer (page 449). This will provide a stream of your expressed milk from a tube which he takes into his mouth along with your nipple.

Baby fights at the breast

A baby who fights at the breast may have had the experience of being smothered by the full breast while feeding and learnt that, for him, getting milk means not being able to breathe through his nose. Make sure your breast isn't obstructing his nose. You may find it helps to lift your breast gently with your fingers from underneath. With patience on your part he'll forget his early unpleasant experiences.

Alternatively, a baby may be frustrated because you don't have enough milk. Three months is a common time for the supply to dwindle, usually because of insufficient stimulation of the breasts by too few feeds. He may also be going through a growth spurt and be dissatisfied by the amount of milk you have. Try increasing your milk supply by feeding him much more often and for as long as be wants to suck. He should be happier within two or three days. See also page 271.

If he sleeps through the night, this may jeopardize your supply as your breasts will remain unemptied for a long time. Wake him to feed him, or express some milk when you go to bed and if you wake during the night with tense breasts. However, best of all, wake him for a feed as this is a much more efficient and quicker way of boosting your milk supply than expressing. See also page 215.

Don't confuse fighting at the breast with the common fussing or playing and butting some babies do while they're waiting for milk to let down. These babies are happy once the milk is flowing, whereas true fighters carry on thrashing around and never seem to feed properly.

If your baby is still reluctant to take the breast, try the trick of popping a bottle teat, perhaps filled with expressed milk, into his mouth. Once he latches on, withdraw it and substitute your nipple.

Baby refuses one breast

Occasionally a baby takes a liking to one breast and refuses to feed from the other. He may be more comfortable one side or the milk may just come more easily from that breast. Unusual causes include blindness in one eye, and deafness or an ear infection in one ear.

To overcome the problem of refusing one breast, try starting a feed from the side he prefers, so that the milk starts flowing from the other side. Then transfer him to the other breast without turning him round, letting him feed in the 'football hold' or 'twin' position (see page 309). This may do the trick.

If not, express milk from the unused breast to maintain its milk supply and keep trying at each feed time. He'll almost certainly come round to the idea of feeding from both sides again. Many babies (and, come to that, many mothers) prefer one side to the other. It's quite possible to end up rather lopsided if you feed your baby more from one side than the other. The side which isn't stimulated as much will, in time, respond by producing less milk. Most women have breasts which are unequal in size before they become pregnant. This doesn't matter at all, though they may find they always have more milk on one side.

Baby throws his head back

This behaviour is most often seen in pre-term babies and generally disappears by eight weeks. Try gently bending your baby forward, so that his back curls up, to see if this more relaxed position helps him settle at the breast. Wrapping him firmly in a small blanket can help keep him in a curled position. You may find that he relaxes as soon as he sucks.

If your baby arches his back at the same time, feeding him as you hold him firmly in the 'football hold' (see page 309) may help. Try to arrange yourselves so that his bottom is right against the back of your chair and his legs bent upward, so that his body is bent forward at the hips.

Floppy baby

If your baby is floppy, he probably has a very relaxed muscle tone and may not feed very effectively. Breastfeeding such a baby can be extremely time-consuming. You may find that expressing your milk after and between feeds and using it in a supplementer (see page 449) helps you continue breastfeeding.

Baby has a cold

Let your baby stay at the breast as much as he wants so that he gets the nutrients, fluid and comfort he needs to see him through his infection. He'll probably have to keep stopping a feed so as to take a breath through his mouth, and he'll need longer to get as much milk as he needs. Feed with him as upright as possible so as to help the mucus drain from his nose down the back of his throat. Gently wipe away any obvious stuff in his nose with a soft tissue before a feed. Smear a little petroleum jelly or silicone cream just inside his nostrils so that mucas is less likely to obstruct his nose.

If your baby is so distressed by being unable to breathe through his nose that he can't feed, put a few decongestant nose drops into each nostril ten minutes before a feed. However, it isn't a good idea to use these more than you have to because long-term use can damage the lining of the nose. You might like to put some decongestant vapour rub on his neck and chest before a feed too.

If necessary, you'll have to express your milk and give it to him by feeding cup or spoon, as this may be easier for him. And don't forget to express milk after a feed (or between feeds) if he hasn't been able to feed well and your breasts are still full and tense.

Finally, make sure that you are eating a healthy diet with plenty of fruit and vegetables and consider taking a supplement of vitamin C (at least 100 mg a day). This may help his cold go quicker.

LOW BIRTH-WEIGHT

About 7 per cent of newborn babies are of low birth-weight – officially defined as less than 2.5kg (5–6lb). Two-thirds of these are born early, after less than thirty-seven weeks of pregnancy, and are called 'pre-term' babies. The others have a weight appropriate for their gestational age and are known as 'small-for-dates' babies. Worldwide, 22 million low-birth-weight babies are born each year.

Breast is best

Both pre-term and small-for-dates babies do best on breast milk if they are able to have milk at all (see below). While pre-term formula is better than ordinary formula, breast milk is superior to both, though it may need enriching – or fortifying – with certain nutrients (see below).

As we explained in Chapter 3, breast milk has many known advantages for all babies. But it has additional specific advantages for pre-term babies. The composition of a pre-term baby's own mother's milk is specifically tailored to his level of maturity (see next page). Also, pre-term babies digest breast milk better than pre-term formula and are less likely to bring it up, which is good news as they need the nourishment.

Breast milk is valuable not only because of its nutritional composition but also because of its immunological advantages. A pre-term baby, even more than a full-term one, needs the protection against infection and allergy that only breast milk provides.

What's more, a mother who breastfeeds her pre-term baby may find it easier to feel close to him. This is important because enjoying your baby can be difficult amidst all the technical paraphernalia of a special care baby unit.

Last but not least, a baby whose mother cuddles him close (when he is able to leave the incubator for short periods) is greatly advantaged by the pleasure and stimulation of being so near her: hearing her voice, heartbeat, breathing and tummy rumbles, sensing her delight and interest in him, smelling her unique natural body scent, and – when he's able – tasting the sweetness of her milk.

Pre-term milk

A woman who has a pre-term baby produces milk of a different composition to that of full-term milk. Her milk is naturally and specifically designed to meet the needs of her baby; as her baby grows, her milk will gradually alter .

Pre-term milk contains relatively more protein, ionized calcium, chloride and immunoglobulin A, and less lactose. It also has more lactoferrin and lysozyme.

Very low-birth-weight babies 1.5kg (2–3lb) or less

The very smallest babies can be fed only via a drip of nutrients into a vein. But breast milk is best for a very low-birth-weight baby when he is mature and well enough to have milk via a tube into his tummy. Indeed, many experts strongly recommend breast milk for these vulnerable babies. Some mothers of very low-birth-weight babies find it difficult to produce enough milk – possibly, some experts think, because their shortened pregnancy didn't give the glandular tissue in their breasts enough time to mature. Other mothers choose not to breastfeed. In such cases breast-milk banks can provide donated milk (see page 353). As this is mature milk, not pre-term milk, it may not provide enough protein, calories or minerals and will almost certainly need to be enriched, or combined with pre-term formula.

Try to be with your baby as much as you can and when he can leave the incubator for short periods, cuddle him a lot. You'll find you'll let your milk down better when you're near him and he'll benefit from being near you.

— A UK study (1988) found that very low-birth-weight babies who had plenty of cuddling next to their mother's naked skin cried less when they were six months old. Their mothers also breastfed them for longer than mothers who hadn't had this skin-to-skin contact.

Sucking reflex

The more premature a baby, the less likely he is to have a sucking reflex (see page 22). A baby who weighs less than 1.5kg (2–3lb) doesn't yet have a sucking reflex and must be tube-fed. As he matures and reaches the age when, had he stayed in your womb, he would have been thirty-two to thirty-four weeks old, his sucking reflex gradually appears. Once low-birth-weight babies (and even those weighing 2.5kg (5–6lb) start breastfeeding, it tends to be some time before they feed effectively, so they need to continue being tube-fed or cup-fed with your expressed or pumped milk.

By the equivalent of thirty-four weeks, your baby will have developed not only his sucking reflex but also his swallowing reflex, his rooting reflex, and his 'gag reflex' (a protective reflex allowing him to choke on milk that goes the wrong way).

Providing breast milk for your pre-term baby

With patience, perseverance and support, you can provide breast milk for your baby and at the same time build up your milk supply until he's mature enough to suck.

If your pre-term baby isn't mature, heavy or well enough to suck yet, he can still benefit from your breast milk via a fine tube (gavage or nasogastric tube). This passes down his nose and the back of his throat into the gullet and stomach. It stays in position between feeds. You or a nurse can give tiny and frequent – perhaps hourly – feeds of your milk down the tube.

Collecting your milk – For the first few days it's best to collect your milk by expressing it (see page 189). When it comes in, you can pump (see page 443) instead or as well. Expressing takes longer at first but some women prefer it. It's wise to learn to express as soon after delivery as possible, because it's easier to learn the technique before your breasts fill up on the third or fourth day.

Start collecting milk as soon after delivery as you can. It won't take long in the first two or three days because you'll only have small amounts of colostrum. However, this is particularly valuable for a pre-term baby, so treat it like liquid gold.

To collect your milk, you'll need to empty your breasts as well as possible at short, regular intervals – every two to three hours during the day. Aim for at least eight sessions in twenty-four hours, although there's no need to stick to a rigid schedule. Whatever you do, don't collect your milk fewer than six times a day.

Although some women find that they can go six or seven hours at night without being woken by full breasts, and manage to fit in enough times to express during the day, it's best at first not to let more than four or five hours pass during the night without expressing, and always to express at any time if your breasts feel full.

Collecting your milk frequently in this way builds up your milk supply, even though your baby won't need large volumes for some time. It's also just as important to start expressing or pumping your milk soon after birth as it would be to breastfeed very soon after birth had you had a baby of normal size. And it's important to prevent engorgement (see page 302).

Remember to wash your hands before expressing or pumping, using a disinfectant solution in hospital. Encourage your milk to let down by making sure you're warm and by very gently massaging or stroking each breast towards the nipple. Pump for ten minutes on each side and switch from side to side every two or three minutes if necessary to encourage the milk-flow.

Any milk that your baby doesn't need straight away can be stored as a reserve supply (see page 349).

Ready for breastfeeding?

Your baby may be able to coordinate sucking and swallowing as early as an age equivalent to when he'd have been thirty-two weeks had he stayed in the womb. He'll probably weigh 1.3–1.5kg (2½–3lb) at this time. Research shows that babies can coordinate sucking and swallowing earlier at the breast than they can at the bottle.

However, well before this you can hold him at your breast several times a day to get him used to the warmth, smell and feel of being there. Every so often put a few drops of expressed milk on to his lips and tongue to give him a taste of things to come. A tube-fed baby misses out on the sweet taste of milk in his mouth. Ideally it's best if you can do all this with your baby somewhere quiet and comfortable.

When he seems to be at all interested in sucking, offer your breast several times a day. The tube can stay in place for the time being. There's absolutely no need to give a rubber teat to test for his readiness to suck. Be guided by your intuition and keep trying.

At first he probably won't suck at all. This is to be expected and doesn't matter. You'll need to persevere for days or even weeks, keeping your milk supply going by expressing or pumping frequently in the meantime.

Don't be surprised if your pre-term baby just licks your breast during the first few sessions, or seems to go to sleep for up to twenty minutes between bouts of one, two or three proper sucks. He's just regaining his strength and as long as he's warmly wrapped up next to your warm body he'll be all right. It's difficult to coordinate sucking and swallowing at first but every day makes a difference, and practice makes perfect.

Eventually your baby will take three, four or five sucks, then, if you listen well enough, you'll hear him swallow.

Encourage your milk to let down (see page 275) before he starts sucking and don't be afraid to adjust your position until it seems right (see pages 166 and 310). The nursing staff will offer you skilled advice on positioning your baby at the breast in such a way that he càn feed most effectively. Change him from side to side every so often during a feed and let him go on feeding as long as he wants, remembering that he'll need frequent breaks because it's all so tiring.

As your baby gets used to the breast, try to fit in *at least* eight to ten breastfeeds a day. A full-term baby would have this sort of number of feeds and a pre-term baby, who has smaller feeds, needs at least the same number and ideally more in order to take enough milk.

When your baby seems to have finished, express or pump the rest of your milk. You or the nurses can then give this to him by tube until he is breastfeeding efficiently enough to get all he needs directly from you.

It's very important that you and your baby between you empty your breasts frequently, as it's the breast stimulation from frequent feeding/expression/pumping that'll build up your milk supply. You are no different from the mother of a full-term baby in this respect.

During the transition from full tube-feeding to full breast-feeding, you'll find it much easier if you can live in the hospital and be as near your baby as possible.

Have confidence that you'll be able to provide enough milk. Experience in the US shows that pre-term infants who received sugar water and formula complements lost more weight than those who are breastfed frequently at the breast and given nothing else. If you want to increase your milk supply, plan an intensive campaign of more frequent feeds for two or three days at least, and read Chapter 10.

With enough support from the nursing staff and paediatrician, and with the knowledge that you couldn't do better for your pre-term baby than give him your milk, you'll probably succeed. Try to relax and enjoy this time as you mother your baby in such a special way. If you can, talk to other mothers breastfeeding pre-term babies. Some hospitals have regular group support meetings.

If you go home without your baby, borrow an electric pump to use at home so that you can take your milk to the hospital each time you visit.

You'll probably find you'll express or pump milk in very small quantities but they are well worth collecting. Liaise with the nurses to find out how much your baby takes down the tube at each feed. Amounts as small as 10–15ml (a dessertspoonful to a tablespoon) are normal for a baby weighing just over 1kg (2lb). When you put your milk into a bag or other container, close it securely and label it with your name and the date.

Ideally your baby should have your milk as fresh as possible so that he gets full benefit from all its anti-infective properties. This means staying in hospital with him. But if you can't stay with your baby you can store your milk and take or send it in for him to have when you aren't there (see page 349).

THE FIVE STAGES OF TUBE-, CUP- AND BREAST-FEEDING

With your help and with skilled support for you, your baby can progress from being fully tube-fed to fully breastfed as follows:

1. *Full tube-feeding with breast milk* (if he is sufficiently mature and well enough to digest milk at all).

2. *Part tube-feeding and part cup-feeding* with expressed or pumped breast milk. Usually start when he reaches an age equivalent to about thirty to thirty-two weeks had he stayed in the womb. He'll probably take only 5–10ml (one or two teaspoonfuls) at first. Hold your baby on your lap, sitting half upright, and gently tilt the cup so that he has to work to get the milk. You may see him lapping with his tongue like a kitten when he gets used to cup-feeding. Whatever you do, don't pour milk into his mouth.

3. *Part tube-feeding, part cup-feeding and part breastfeeding.*
He'll probably be able to suck and swallow your milk directly
from your breast when he reaches an age equivalent to when
he'd have been about thirty-two to thirty-four weeks had he
stayed in the womb (he'll probably weigh more than 1.5kg
(3lb). Continue until he can take all he needs from a feeding
cup and breast, then the tube can be removed. This will be a
red-letter day.

4. *Part cup-feeding and part breastfeeding* (and gradually
more breastfeeding and less cup-feeding). If you prefer, you
can give expressed milk via a nursing supplementer (see
page 449). This device enables your baby to have expressed
milk while he is breastfeeding. An advantage of using a
supplementer is that your baby can get more milk more
quickly, which is useful if feeding tires him out. A disadvantage might be that he gets it so much more quickly that he
doesn't give your breasts the stimulation they need to make
plenty of milk. You can get over this by allowing your baby
to comfort as much as he wants, and by making sure that
you empty your breasts well after each feed (and storing this
expressed milk to put in the supplementer for your baby's
next feed).

5. *Full breastfeeding.* Most low-birth-weight babies are the
equivalent of between thirty-two and thirty-six weeks before
they can suck well enough to take adequate nourishment
from the breast alone.

Your pre-term baby never actually needs a bottle. If he were to
get used to bottle-feeding, he might later have problems learning
to breastfeed effectively (see page 323).

Studies in Chicago have shown that pre-term babies don't
breathe as well while bottle-feeding as when breastfeeding, which

means they get measurably less oxygen. Some pre-term babies are already short of oxygen (from the respiratory distress syndrome or from a heart defect) so this is especially bad for them. Pre-term bottle-fed babies also have a slower heart rate than breast-fed ones.

What if you go home ahead of your baby?

If your baby stays in hospital and you go home, you can take or send your milk in for him, as you obviously won't be there every time he needs a feed. Ask the nurses to give your milk from a cup, rather than by bottle. Ideally, it's preferable for you to stay in hospital alongside your pre-term baby until he can come home too. But this isn't always possible.

Store your expressed or pumped milk in the fridge for up to twenty-four hours. Your baby should have it within forty-eight hours of you expressing or pumping it.

Mothering your pre-term baby

Pre-term babies are nursed in incubators in special care baby units (SCBUs) to keep them warm and to protect them from infection. Unfortunately, not many SCBUs have beds for mothers to stay. This means you'll have to go to your baby when you want to see him, although someone else can take your milk to him if necessary.

Physical contact is very important both for your baby and for the development of the mothering instinct. If possible, hold him as often as you can. If he has to stay in his incubator, stroke him gently through the armholes.

You may like to consider sleeping with your baby too. In Pithiviers in France, pre-term babies who slept in their mother's beds gained weight faster than the others. However, bed-sharing isn't a good idea if you are a smoker.

It's all too easy to take your cue from the nursing staff as to how to handle your baby. However, the nurses are expert at nursing care and may not have time to give their small charges the physical contact (cuddling, stroking and holding), attention and talking to that they need. Try to mother your baby as warmly and intimately as possible, even though you will almost certainly feel awkward at first.

Perhaps a lack of mothering is partly why babies who are born pre-term tend to cry twice as much as full-term ones. No one will laugh at you if you talk to your pre-term baby, if you spend time looking at him, or if you ask to do as many routine nursing jobs, such as nappy-changing, as possible. And when you take him home, take all the time in the world to get to know each other and to enjoy one another's company.

Kangaroo care

Researchers have found that pre-term babies can go home sooner if their mothers have spent a lot of time with them next to their bodies, safely tucked into their clothing between her breasts, rather like a young joey kangaroo in his mother's pouch. According to South American researchers, most babies weighing 1.2kg (2½lb) or more can be cared for like this. And researchers at the Hammer-smith Hospital in London also found that babies of over 1.5kg (3lb) do better if cared for like young kangaroos! Your husband or partner can carry the baby next to his naked chest in the same way if he wishes.

Looking after yourself

You'll have a lot to deal with if you have a pre-term baby and it's very important to look after yourself (see Chapter 9) and to ask for all the help and support you need, from family, friends and hospital staff. This is especially important if you are a single parent and if you have other children.

The more people you have backing you up, the better – and the longer you're likely to breastfeed. It's even more vital for you because you'll be spending so much time in the busy, high-tech atmosphere of the special care baby unit, away from your family and friends, and sleeping in a busy hospital.

Take every opportunity to relax and enjoy yourself. For example, make sure you are as comfortable as possible in hospital. You might like to take a tape-cassette player and headphones in so that you can listen to your favourite music; and you can ask relatives and friends to bring in favourite foods and drinks or take you out for a meal. Your partner could give you a shoulder or back massage as you feed your baby and all three of you could have a cuddle together.

You and your baby are priorities now and need high maintenance. In your role as breastfeeding mother of a pre-term baby, you are a very special person and are doing the very best you can for your baby's future.

Confidence, support and encouragement

Although pre-term babies do so well on breast milk, many hospital staff strangely seem reluctant to encourage mothers to breastfeed. This may be partly because they perceive it as difficult and time-consuming – for the mothers and themselves. It's also because they don't want to make women who don't breastfeed feel guilty (but see page 457). *However, if you know what to do and have enough skilled advice, encouragement and support, you are very likely to be able to breastfeed your pre-term baby.*

— Research in the US (1995) found that most mothers who continued breastfeeding when they took their pre-term babies home reported a turning-point after two weeks of being there. Their babies stayed awake at the breast for longer (which is much more rewarding for a mother) and breastfed more effectively. Many pre-term babies start to suck really strongly at the breast only at about the time they were originally expected to be born.

— A study in North Staffordshire (1994) found that encouraging mothers of pre-term babies to breastfeed raised the proportion who left hospital exclusively breastfeeding from 1 per cent to 58 per cent!

— Researchers in a special care unit in Bombay (1985) found that encouraging mothers to breastfeed their pre-term babies resulted in 95 per cent doing so successfully. A big bonus was that the babies were very much less likely to develop infections and to die from them. The cost of running the unit also decreased as more babies received breast milk.

Small-for-dates babies

Occasionally a baby is smaller than expected from the duration of the pregnancy: that is, 'small for gestational age' or 'small-for-dates'. This is almost certainly because he has been poorly nourished in the womb. At first some small-for-dates babies suck poorly and have a poorly coordinated swallowing reflex. They also tend to produce a lot of mucus, which can make them gag and regurgitate.

Your small-for-dates baby may have a sucking reflex in spite of weighing very little, so it's worth giving him a chance to suck every so often, whatever his weight, unless he's also very premature. He'll need frequent feeding and this will help keep his blood-sugar level within normal limits. He'll also need to be kept warm.

Fortifying/enriching breast milk

Breast milk for tube-fed pre-term babies is thought to be even better for some of them if it's fortified or enriched. Although most pre-term babies do well on breast milk alone, very small ones tend to grow only slowly and have a higher risk of developing rickets.

So if your baby is mature enough to manage milk feeds, your paediatrician may recommend fortifying or enriching your own milk with protein and certain vitamins and minerals (calcium, phosphorus, zinc and copper). After about two weeks your baby may benefit from an iron supplement too. If your baby is being given donated breast milk, he'll certainly need extra protein and calories. This is because donated milk is mature milk and differs in composition from pre-term breast milk; it's also likely to contain a high proportion of low-fat fore-milk collected while dripping from the breast.

A tube-fed baby may need extra calories to replace those lost when breast-milk fat sticks to the lining of the feeding tube and is therefore lost. If you have plenty of milk, it's possible to discard the fore-milk and just give your baby the higher-calorie hind-milk.

Commercial human milk fortifiers are added to expressed breast milk. Once a baby weighs 2kg (just 4lb), or when he is discharged from hospital, fortification is usually stopped.

BREAST-MILK BANKS

Breastfeeding women with milk to spare can supply it to a breast-milk bank. Donated milk can be transported from milk banks by road or rail if necessary to pre-term or sick babies in other hospitals.

Babies whose own mothers are not feeding them and who may particularly benefit from donated milk include very low-birth-weight pre-term babies in the first week of life (as they tolerate donated milk better than pre-term formula at this time), those who aren't growing and thriving, those who have had bowel surgery, and those who have a poorly functioning immune system. Sometimes older babies with diarrhoea and other bowel symptoms from severe food intolerance benefit from donated milk too.

Donor mothers are carefully screened before their milk is accepted. Their medical history, blood tests and drug intake are important. If a woman is taking any drugs, including nicotine (from smoking), alcohol, aspirin and the Pill, her milk is not accepted.

An accepted donor mother receives detailed instructions about how to collect and store her milk. It is cultured to make sure the bacteria colony count is low enough, and then pasteurized and frozen for up to six months.

Pasteurization is best done by the 'flash' method to protect the milk's natural antibodies and enzymes as much as possible. Ideally, donated breast milk shouldn't be sterilized at all. Pasteurization destroys live cells. It also destroys lipase, and babies fed on pasteurized breast milk put on less weight than do those given 'raw' milk, as they need lipase in order to absorb fat. Another problem is that donated milk is often collected as 'drip' milk – milk that drips from one breast while the donor's baby feeds from the other. And drip milk is in itself low in fat, containing only two-thirds of the calories of expressed milk.

Donated breast milk has helped save the lives of many sick or tiny babies whose own mothers could not or would not feed them themselves. If you have milk to spare and want to donate it, mention this to your doctor, midwife, health visitor, or the staff at your local hospital's special care baby unit. They will advise you what to do.

Addresses for health professionals and others who would like to know about milk banks can be found on page 450.

COLOURED MILK

Milk naturally varies in colour. For example, colostrum is yellower than mature milk and fore-milk is more translucent than the whiter hind-milk. However, very occasionally other colours are seen.

Yellow milk – Taking a supplement of beta-carotene (made by the body into vitamin A) can colour milk yellow. Probably eating a large number of satsumas on a daily basis could do so too, as they can temporarily colour the skin yellowish-orange. Eating a lot of carrots or pumpkin can also turn milk, like skin, orange-yellow.

Red, pink, brown or orange milk – Eating beetroot stains some women's milk pink. Seeing blood in your milk can be quite a shock but it's rarely anything to worry about. Having said this, it's wise to check your breasts and if you are concerned about anything, to consult your doctor.

The most likely cause of blood in the milk is a cracked or sore nipple (see pages 318 and 307).

However, some women have blood-staining in the first week after delivery with no sign of anything else wrong. This is rare, generally disappears within two to five days, and doesn't harm the baby. You can continue breastfeeding. The most likely cause, according to one researcher, is a tendency for an affected woman's blood vessels to leak red blood cells. There are normally a few red blood cells in milk, but quite a lot are needed to colour it.

Blood in the milk occasionally comes from a tumour. This is almost always non-cancerous and the discoloration stops once breastfeeding is well under way. However, you should discuss with your doctor whether investigations are necessary.

Green milk – Milk can go green if a woman eats dark green leafy vegetables or asparagas or if she takes an iron-containing drug called ferritin.

Milk of assorted hues – As milk stagnates in a blocked duct, a milk-retention cyst (a cyst that develops behind a block in an untreated blocked duct), or the swollen ducts of a condition called duct estasia, it can turn one of many colours. These include deep yellow, brown, green and even blue-black. The colours occur as a result of various substances being present, including cholesterol, cholesterol 5, 6-epoxides, oestrogens and fluorescent compounds, including lipofucsin complexes, formed from oxidized fats. They are visible only when milk is expressed or drawn off.

Smokers who express milk from such a collection of long-stagnant milk may see even darker-coloured milk.

THE BABY WITH TEETH

Some babies are actually born with one or two teeth, though most don't get their first tooth until six months. There's no reason why teeth should interfere with breastfeeding as the baby's gums aren't used for feeding: the pressure comes from the tongue below and the palate above.

Your baby may, however, try the odd bite when he's older and will be very interested if you make a big fuss. It's best to say 'No' firmly and gently take him off the breast. If you smile, he may think you like it and do it again! A few such babies actually think it's a good game.

Some babies bite only towards the end of a feed. You can easily handle this. You'll soon get to know when he's about to bite, so simply take him off the breast before he starts.

Some babies bite from frustration if the breast is too full or if there isn't enough milk. You can cope by dealing with the underlying problem.

Managing problems with breastfeeding – like managing any problems – can be both challenging and rewarding. The same applies in various special situations and these are the subject of the next chapter.

THIRTEEN

Some special situations

TWINS OR MORE

Because two babies stimulate the breasts twice as much as one, you'll automatically be able to make enough milk for them. Many mothers have breastfed twins successfully for as long as they wanted to, so don't let anyone try to persuade you that you'll have to give either one or both of them formula feeds as well or instead.

It's easiest at first to feed each twin separately. However, to save time later it's worth learning the knack of feeding them both at once, although there'll always be times when you'll enjoy the luxury of feeding them, enjoying them and getting to know them individually.

You can feed twins together in one of several positions. The easiest is probably to hold each one in the 'football hold' with his legs under your arm and sticking out behind you; cushions or pillows under their heads will take the weight off your arms. Or you could hold one baby in the conventional position, while the other lies facing the same way at the other breast, parallel to him, while you support his head with his hand. Yet another idea is to have both babies in the conventional position, with one lying across the other.

Make sure you position each baby properly as your nipples may become sore if either of them drags on the breast. Once you get into the swing of feeding them both, you'll find it works well.

Should you wake the second baby for a feed every time the first one wakes? The answer is 'Yes' if you want to save time and 'No' if you would like the occasional chance to suckle one at a time. If you're at all unhappy about your milk supply then you should always wake the second baby and feed them both.

How about alternating the breast that each twin feeds from? The usual advice is that this is to be recommended, so that the twin that sucks more strongly stimulates each breast alternately. However, each newborn animal in a litter usually chooses a nipple and keeps to it, so it's possible that human babies might prefer to do the same. Certainly in the first few weeks, if you always feed one baby from one breast and the other from the other, and if one sucks more strongly and so drinks more each time, you'll find that your breasts become rather lopsided. Most women say that once their milk supply is established, their breasts almost always become more equal in size.

Many mothers of triplets have successfully breastfed them, though sometimes formula is necessary as well, especially early on. However many babies you have, it's good for them if you can provide at least some milk for each one.

Mothers of 'multiples' say that the more support and encouragement they get while breastfeeding, the better. So don't be shy to ask for as much as you need, and to be really clear about exactly what you'd like done to help.

The Twins and Multiple Births Association (TAMBA) in the UK (PO Box 30, Little Sutton, L66 1TH) can provide information about breastfeeding, details of support groups, and telephone support for mothers of twins or more.

Last but by no means least, take as much care of yourself as you can (see Chapter 9). For example, you'll need plenty of good food to eat, and plenty of rest.

— Research in the Gambia (1986) found that all the women studied were able to feed their twins successfully.

BABY ILL OR IN HOSPITAL

Unless your baby is so ill or immature that he can't have milk, he'll do better with your milk than with any other. He'll also recover more quickly after illnesses such as gastroenteritis if he doesn't have to cope with the stress of digesting formula.

If he has to go into hospital, it's best if you go too so that you can comfort and support him emotionally and feed him. If you can spend the day with him but not the night, leave expressed or pumped milk for the nurses to give from a cup.

If you can visit only infrequently, you may need to bring enough milk to last for several days. It calls for real patience to express or pump your breasts frequently (more often than your baby usually feeds) day after day. However, it can be done and is easiest if you hire or buy an electric breast pump (see page 443).

BABY JAUNDICED

In the first few weeks of life there are many causes of jaundice (yellow skin colour caused by high blood levels of the yellow pigment bilirubin). These range from the normal 'physiological' jaundice found in many babies, both breast- and bottle-fed, to abnormal jaundice from one of a variety of conditions (including bowel obstruction, infection, a congenital defect, drugs, an underactive thyroid gland, diabetes in the mother, and ABO or rhesus blood group incompatibility). Abnormal jaundice can be serious if not treated properly. The diagnosis depends on the time of onset of the jaundice and on blood tests.

Only a few full-term jaundiced babies need medical treatment. This will depend on the type of jaundice and the bilirubin level. Repeated blood tests indicate whether the bilirubin is rising or falling.

Babies with moderately raised bilirubin levels for whatever

reason are often given phototherapy (light therapy). In this they are placed naked and uncovered for short periods of time in a cot 16 inches beneath a strong blue light with their eyes covered with a mask or coloured Perspex shade. Some hospitals lay babies on special blankets that emit blue light. The light changes the shape of the molecules of bilirubin in the blood, which allows them to be removed from the body. Light therapy may hinder frequent and unrestricted breastfeeding. However, if the nurses agree you can take your baby from under the light and feed him two-hourly (or more often if he wants).

If your baby is otherwise well, your paediatrician may agree to your taking him home and giving him daylight phototherapy. Do this by placing him, uncovered, in a cot or somewhere safe by a window in strong daylight. Beware of sunburn and don't let him get too cold or hot. You'll have to take him to the hospital for blood tests to monitor the bilirubin level. The advantage of being at home is that you can breastfeed much more easily there.

Pre-term babies are affected adversely by lower raised levels of bilirubin than are full-term ones, so any treatment must be started sooner. Breastfeeding is very important for these babies and skilled help and support from the nursery staff make all the difference to its success.

Physiological jaundice

This follows the normal breakdown of red blood cells in a newborn baby, appears on the second to fourth day of life and usually disappears by about a week. It's more common in breastfed babies but there's no evidence that it causes any long-term problems.

This early-onset jaundice is less likely in babies breastfed soon after birth and on a frequent and unrestricted basis. The fewer feeds a baby has, the more likely he is to have jaundice. All many jaundiced babies need is more breast milk. You can arrange this by increasing your milk supply by feeding more often and for longer.

One expert suggests that the minimum number of breastfeeds a day for reducing the risk of jaundice is ten to twelve.

Colostrum helps a baby's bowel get rid of meconium, the first bowel motions which contain a lot of bilirubin. If meconium isn't excreted quickly it can be reabsorbed into the bloodstream. Frequent breastfeeds help a baby get rid of meconium more quickly.

Studies show that giving an infant water isn't helpful and may interfere with his mother's milk supply. This is because he will want fewer breastfeeds if his tummy is filled with water. If your jaundiced baby is inadvertently given water in hospital, stimulate your milk supply by expressing after and between feeds.

Breast-milk jaundice

Some healthy breastfed babies become jaundiced a little later, towards the end of the first week of life. This is known as 'breast milk jaundice'. It is worst during the second to third week and lasts from four to sixteen weeks. One or two in every hundred breastfed babies develop this sort of jaundice.

Most paediatricians aren't too concerned about bilirubin levels below 20mg/dl. And although higher levels than this from other sorts of jaundice can damage a baby's brain, such brain damage has never yet been attributed to breast-milk jaundice. In fact, there's considerable evidence that breast-milk jaundice has no serious long-term effects.

However if, as happens in a few babies, the bilirubin level rises to 20mg/dl and above, many paediatricans prefer to be cautious and suggest that a woman do one of two things:

1 Stop breastfeeding for a while (the time recommended varies between twelve and forty-eight hours but you may like to start off with twelve hours and extend it if necessary). If this happens to you and your baby, keep your milk supply going by expressing or pumping more frequently than you would have fed, and discard the milk until you can breastfeed again. Your baby can have donated breast milk or formula in the interval. His

bilirubin level willl fall significantly and you can then resume breastfeeding. The bilirubin level usually then rises slightly before falling slowly and steadily. If it were to rise significantly again, interrupt breastfeeding once more. If the bilirubin doesn't fall significantly after a short break, extend the break by six to twelve hours; the hospital stafff will measure the bilirubin level every four to six hours. Clearly if the level rises during the breaks from breastfeeding, the jaundice isn't due to breast milk.

2 Carry on breastfeeding but at the same time dilute her milk by giving donated milk (from a milk bank) or formula via a supplementer (see page 449). If you do this, be sure to empty your breasts after each feed by expressing, because your baby may feed for a shorter time as he'll also be getting milk from the supplementer. The bilirubin level will fall more slowly than had you interrupted breastfeeding, but it'll be more comfortable for you and will allow your baby to go on getting some of your milk.

The cause of breast-milk jaundice isn't clear. One theory is that it's due to a chemical in milk which interferes with bilirubin metabolism. Another is that it is caused by high levels of fat-splitting enzymes (lipases) in milk which break down fat and release fatty acids which then inhibit the breakdown of bilirubin.

Abnormal jaundice

Babies with abnormal jaundice look yellow actually at birth or within twenty-four hours and need medical attention. Whatever treatment is necessary, they need early, frequent and unrestricted breastfeeds for the reasons outlined above.

DIARRHOEA

Breastfed babies are very much less likely to suffer from diarrhoea than are bottle-fed ones (see page 64). However, if a baby does get diarrhoea from a bowel infection, studies show that it's better and safer to carry on with breastfeeding. Babies who stop breastfeeding are five times as likely to become dehydrated as those who continue. If your baby is severely ill, he may need to drink a solution of oral rehydration salts from a cup as well as breast-feeding. Even if a baby becomes so dehydrated that he needs intra-venous fluids, he can continue to breastfeed. Only extremely rarely does a baby with a bowel infection need to stop breastfeeding.

HYPOGLYCAEMIA (LOW BLOOD-SUGAR)

Breastfeed your baby as soon after birth as possible, and then on an unrestricted basis with frequent feeds to help keep his blood-sugar (glucose) level within normal limits. Your first milk, colos-trum, is the best food for your newborn baby. Breast milk is a good source both of sugar and of the other nutrients from which a full-term baby makes glucose – the sugar needed by each body cell.

Quite a few pre-term, newborn babies develop a low blood-sugar level as they adapt to having intermittent feeds instead of a continuous supply of nutrients, including sugar, via the umbilical cord. Very immature pre-term babies may have difficulty in digesting any type of milk, but especially formula. This makes it stay in the stomach a long time, delays the release of its glucose and allows the blood-sugar level to fall.

Signs of low blood-sugar include sweating; weakness/limp-ness/floppiness; disinterest in feeding; tiredness; a high-pitched or weak cry; blueness; a rapid pulse; irritability; 'jitteriness' – frequent juddering or shaking movements – particularly when disturbed; and, at worst, fits, collapse of the circulation and a coma. If the blood-sugar level repeatedly dips or if it stays low for a long time (for days rather than hours), a baby's brain can be damaged. This is why doctors are careful to monitor the blood-sugar level in any baby who shows signs of a low blood-sugar or who is likely to have a low level.

A low blood-sugar level is unusual in a healthy full-term baby of normal weight who is fed frequently. Many experts consider that such a baby needs blood-sugar tests only if he has symptoms suggestive of a low blood-sugar. If so, he may need other tests to find out whether an underlying condition (such as an infection) is responsible.

Certain babies are more likely to have a low blood-sugar level. They include those who are pre-term or small-for-dates, have an infection, were short of oxygen during labour, or have become chilled; and those whose mothers had pre-eclampsia, have diabetes, or have taken certain drugs. Such babies need routine blood-sugar monitoring in hospital.

All these babies, including those pre-term babies who are mature and well enough to have milk, should ideally have undiluted breast milk (their mother's own milk is best), by tube, breast or cup, as soon as possible after birth. They need this milk frequently and on an unrestricted basis. If a mother can't increase her milk supply, her milk can be topped up by formula (special pre-term formula for pre-term babies), with or without donated breast milk. If she doesn't want to breastfeed, her baby can have formula. If necessary, sugar solution can be dripped into a baby's vein.

RHESUS ANTIBODIES

Some mothers who know they have rhesus antibodies in their blood worry that if they breastfeed, these may pass to the baby in their milk. It is certainly true that if a woman has rhesus antibodies in her blood she'll have them in her milk too. However, they have no effect on her baby because they're inactivated by his gut. It's therefore perfectly safe to breastfeed your rhesus-positive baby if you are rhesus-negative and have rhesus antibodies. Indeed, it is the best way to feed such babies, according to several studies. It's also safe to breastfeed after having an injection of anti-D immunoglobulin.

SUCKING AND MILKING PROBLEMS

Medical reasons for poor sucking and milking include the effects of drugs given to the mother in labour (see page 332), the after-effects of a poor oxygen supply in labour, and a pre-term birth.

Less common reasons include certain neurological and neuro-muscular problems (see page 373) and hypothyroidism. These conditions are uncommon and you can be sure that your paediatrician will diagnose them.

Mechanical factors which can affect a baby's sucking and milking action include a large tongue, cleft lip, certain congenital abnormalities of the gums and jaws, and severe tongue tie (see page 369).

A baby may have difficulty in swallowing for a variety of reasons including cleft palate, inflammation following intubation for breathing difficulties at birth, and a small lower jaw. If swallowing is difficult, a baby milks the breast poorly too.

Some of these conditions are relatively easy to treat and the baby's sucking and milking action improves after treatment. Others improve spontaneously. A baby with an untreatable or less easily treatable condition will need a lot of help to breastfeed.

Apart from medical reasons for sucking and milking poorly, a baby may be tired, jaundiced, or full (see pages 335, 359 and 334). There may be practical problems such as poor positioning at the breast (see pages 166 and 310), poorly protractile nipples (see page 312) or engorgement (see page 302).

Many breastfeeding babies have had one or more bottles of formula. This can play havoc with breastfeeding simply because it's so easy for a baby to learn to bottle-suck and sometimes so difficult for him to breastfeed when he's used to bottles (see page 185).

The usual story of a baby with a poor sucking, milking or swallowing action who fails to gain enough weight in spite of unrestricted breastfeeding is that he wants the breast very frequently, sometimes hourly or even more or less non-stop day and night. Some aren't interested in feeding; they are 'happy to starve' (see page 269) and may sleep a great deal. The mother may be tired out and desperate for help.

Such a baby probably gets only fore-milk because poor sucking and milking hasn't been stimulating the breast well enough to let down the hind-milk. Fore-milk, while high in volume, is low in calories and fat. This means that although the baby has frequent feeds, he doesn't put on much weight. A poor let-down eventually decreases milk production, so continuing like this is doomed to failure.

A baby who sucks and milks well encourages the milk to let down by:

- sucking with a rapid fluttering movement
- then sucking slowly and swallowing after each group of several sucks ('nutritive sucking')
- then waiting for a while before starting the whole process again, up to eight times in one session.

However, a baby who doesn't suck and milk well may swallow very little because he sucks with rapid 'fluttering' movements ('non-nutritive sucking'). He often swallows only for the first few minutes, when getting fore-milk, and then stops.

A good way of telling whether your baby is swallowing is to watch for little movements just in front of his ears, and to listen. He may sleep for twenty minutes or so between bouts of only two or three sucks, and may keep his eyes closed much of the time. You may also notice that his cheeks are occasionally hollowed by being sucked in. This is caused by tongue-sucking: if you pull his lower lip down you'll see that his tongue is above the nipple instead of below it. Sometimes he sticks it out (tongue 'thrusting') which makes him come off the breast.

The best thing to do is to find out why your baby is having trouble in sucking, milking or swallowing and, if possible, to put it right.

If there's no apparent reason, if the cause is untreatable, or even if it has been treated successfully, you can try ten steps to help your baby get your milk.

TEN STEPS TO HELP A BABY WHO BREASTFEEDS INEFFECTIVELY

1. Check your feeding position (see pages 166 and 310)

2. Offer your nipple and areola attractively – Soften your breast first, if it's very full of milk, by expressing a little; encourage your nipple to erect; put some of your milk on to it so your baby can smell and taste it straight away; encourage your milk to let down before he feeds; consider using a supplementer so milk flows immediately; either hold your breast as if on a shelf, with your opposite hand supporting it from below, or use a cigarette hold to make a 'biscuit' of the nipple and areola in such a way that the 'biscuit' is in parallel with the baby's mouth (but release this hold as soon as possible as it may obstruct your milk ducts). Some experienced counsellors say the 'shelf support' works best for a baby with sucking and milking difficulties; try gently touching your baby's lower lip with the nipple and when he opens his mouth, draw him closer to the breast.

3. Change sides as soon as he stops swallowing – every five minutes or so). You can do this during a feed. This so-called switch nursing (or 'burp and switch technique'), encourages the baby to suck better and also stimulates the let-down. As you are changing him over, encourage him to wake up, if he's sleepy, by burping him (bending him at the waist is a good way). See also page 278.

4. **Feed somewhere quiet** – or try talking or singing to rouse him. Praise him after a good sucking session: even a very young baby may respond by doing it again.

5. **Experiment with his clothes** – See if he feeds better when firmly wrapped and warm or unwrapped and not too warm.

6. **Try feeding with you and him both naked** – See if the skin contact stimulates him to suck better.

7. **Rock or jiggle** – Do this to arouse him, if necessary.

8. **Feed more frequently** – As your baby's sucking and milking are improved by nos. 1–4 above, don't forget to wake him for feeds if he's been in the habit of sleeping for long periods. Your milk supply needs stimulating now and it's no good getting him to suck properly if there's little milk for him because you haven't been feeding (or expressing or pumping) often enough. While his improved sucking will in itself increase your milk supply, it needs to be combined with reasonably frequent, unrestricted feeds, with no long gaps between them. Aim at first for no more than two hours (from the start of one to the start of the next) between feeds during the day, and three hours at night, though if your baby wants more, of course put him to the breast (see page 175).

9. **Aim for realistic goals** – If your baby has been putting on no weight, then a gain of two ounces (60g) in the next week is very good. If he's been losing, then staying the same is excellent.

10. **Try a supplementer** (see page 449) – This is recommended if you can't improve your baby's sucking and milking actions. Fill the container with milk you expressed or pumped after each feed. Your baby will get your milk both directly from your breast and from the supplementer.

However, he'll get more of it more quickly and easily. A supplementer is also useful if he needs extra milk immediately. If you can't produce enough to put in it, use formula or donated breast milk. At the same time you can increase your milk within a few days by expressing or pumping regularly and frequently. As a last resort, bottle-feed your baby with your expressed or pumped milk.

TONGUE TIE

A few babies are born with a frenulum – the midline membrane between the tongue and the floor of the mouth – which is shorter (from top to bottom, with the baby upright), longer (from back to front), thicker or tougher than usual. This can tether the tongue so badly that it is said to be 'tied'. You or your advisers may be able to see that the tongue is unusually tethered to the floor of the mouth so that its tip can reach neither the upper nor the lower gums. However, the back of the tongue may 'roll' forward over the gums because its tip is held back by the frenulum. This can make the front edge appear notched, puckered or heart-shaped.

A baby with tongue tie may not be able to push his tongue far enough forward over his lower gums to feed effectively. This means he holds the breast in his mouth between his upper and lower gums, instead of between the upper gums and the tongue. This can cause a problem with breastfeeding. He may make a 'clucking' noise as he tries to milk the breast. He may not be able to hold the breast in his mouth very well and milk may dribble from the side of his mouth. His mother is also more likely than other women to have sore or cracked nipples. And the ineffective sucking can lead to a poor milk supply and blocked ducts.

The best way of dealing with minor degrees of tongue tie is to be particularly careful over your breastfeeding technique. The odds are that your baby will manage and the more practised he becomes at feeding, and the older he gets, the easier breastfeeding should be.

However, tongue tie which causes continuing breastfeeding problems responds very well to minor surgery to cut the frenulum, and shouldn't be delayed unnecessarily.

BABY WITH A CLEFT LIP AND/OR PALATE

The initial shock and disappointment of discovering that your baby has a cleft lip, with or without a cleft palate, may make you reluctant to breastfeed. Once you get over this initial feeling, you'll remember that you never see older children walking around with a noticeable deformity of their lips. The plastic surgery available today is so good that the defect can be almost perfectly repaired.

A cleft lip in itself needn't interfere with breastfeeding. Some milk may leak around the cleft but you'll soon learn how to press the lip around your breast to form a seal (something you couldn't do with the rubber of a bottle teat if you were to bottle-feed). Your baby will still be able to suck (unless the cleft is exceptionally severe) and milk your breast. Prevent engorgement and try not to let your breasts become too full as both these conditions make it more difficult to form a seal around his lip. If your breast is very full before a feed, soften it by expressing.

Many hospital units now repair cleft lips within two days of birth, though others still wait the traditional three months or so before operating. Early surgery is by far the best from the feeding point of view. Not only does it make feeding easier for the baby but it also makes the mother more inclined to breastfeed.

Different surgeons advise waiting for different lengths of time before letting a baby suck after a cleft lip repair. Because of the danger of the scar splitting, some suggest waiting for three to four weeks; others allow sucking at ten days; and yet others immediately after surgery. From both the mother's and the baby's points of view, the sooner the baby starts feeding, the better, but obviously the healing of the scar must be given priority.

— Sixty out of 100 babies resumed breastfeeding immediately after their operation in a survey reported in 1987. There were no complications and the breastfed babies gained weight faster than those fed from a cup.

While you wait to resume breastfeeding after surgery, keep your milk supply going by frequent and regular expression or pumping. You can give your milk to your baby in a feeding cup.

If the operation is postponed for several months, you'll need a lot of patience while breastfeeding, as babies with a cleft lip tend to take a long time over their feeds.

If your baby has a severely cleft lip and you find it impossible to breastfeed, you can give him your milk from a cup, from a specially shaped spoon, or from a bottle with an adapted teat. Ask your paediatrician about these.

A baby with a cleft palate can't suck well because he draws air in from his nose when he tries. Make up for the loss of suction by holding your nipple and areola in his mouth while he feeds. He'll be able to suck and milk your breasts satisfactorily with practice. You may find a supplementer useful while he is learning to milk your breast (see page 449).

Unlike formula, breast milk doesn't irritate the mucous membranes of the nose of a baby with a cleft palate. Most mothers, though, prefer to breastfeed their baby with a cleft palate in a relatively upright position to minimize the chance of milk going into the nose.

Breastfeeding is associated with less otitis media than is bottle-feeding, which is good because babies with a cleft palate are particularly prone to ear infections.

— In 1994 researchers recommended that babies with a cleft palate should be breastfed for as much of their first year as possible.

An affected baby can use a plastic dental plate ('feeding plate') until the cleft is repaired, usually after he's a year old. The plate is made from impressions of his palate. It can be inserted as early as three days after birth (sometimes not until ten days) and not only helps him feed satisfactorily but also improves the shape of the dental arches. Some hospitals make plates routinely and others only for severe clefts.

BABY WITH A LEARNING DIFFICULTY

There's every reason why you should breastfeed your baby if he has a learning difficulty. He'll gain the same benefits from being breastfed as any other baby and it will help develop your relationship.

Many women whose babies have a learning difficulty feel that they deserve every possible help and chance in life and consider, rightly, that breastfeeding is the best starting point.

Just like your baby, you will need plenty of encouragement and support as you learn to breastfeed. Don't be afraid to ask for as much as you need from the hospital staff and from your family and friends.

Down's syndrome

One mother of a baby with Down's syndrome commented: 'I'm sure that breastfeeding and the closeness that comes with it helped me to love and accept him just as he was.'

Babies with this condition are particularly prone to infections, especially respiratory infections, so the protection provided by breast milk is really valuable.

Some feed apathetically and slowly because of muscle weakness, a poor sucking reflex or general sleepiness (see page 335). However, bottle-feeding would be just as time-consuming for you. With patience you're highly likely to succeed with breastfeeding and you'll be sure you're doing the best for your baby. Just as with any baby, avoid using a bottle because learning to bottle-suck interferes with learning to breastfeed. If he is too tired to suck for long, express some milk and give it to him via a feeding cup. You may need to encourage him to suck by giving him lots of skin contact, encouraging your milk to let down before you put him to the breast, and expressing a few drops of milk into his mouth. Feed him before he has to cry, to avoid tiring him. If he's so sleepy that he doesn't wake very often, wake him for a feed every two hours or so, if necessary.

BABY WITH A NEUROLOGICAL OR NEUROMUSCULAR CONDITION

Babies with a neurological condition benefit from being breastfed just as much as any other baby. However, they can have particular feeding problems. Such babies include those with cerebral palsy, infantile spinal muscular atrophy, congenital muscular dystrophy, neonatal myasthenia gravis and infections of the central nervous system.

For example, a baby with cerebral palsy may sometimes arch his back while feeding (see page 339). Because of their condition, other babies may be apathetic during feeds (see page 335) or have problems with sucking (a poor sucking reflex, uncoordinated sucking, or poor sucking due to muscle weakness).

It helps if you know how to recognize when your baby is doing nutritive sucking as opposed to non-nutritive sucking (see page 169), so that you can encourage the former. You also need to pay attention to his feeding position – both of his whole body and of his tongue, jaw and lips (see pages 166 and 271). See page 367 for how to encourage him to suck, milk and swallow more effectively.

It's well worth persevering because most babies affected in this way can breastfeed with enough help and most become much better at it as time goes by.

FAILURE TO THRIVE

The term 'failure to thrive' simply means that *a baby isn't growing as he should*. There are guidelines for doctors, but each baby must be assessed as an individual. For practical purposes, if a baby continues to lose weight after ten days of life, if he hasn't regained his birth weight by three weeks, if he gains at a very slow rate after the first month, if he gains at an increasingly slow rate, and particularly if he is also unhealthy, this suggests that all may not be well.

There are many reasons why a breastfed baby may not grow optimally. He may not drink enough milk (most likely because of infrequent, short feeds or poor sucking or swallowing). His mother may currently not produce enough milk (because of poor technique, an unhealthy diet, illness or exhaustion), or she may not let her milk down well (for psychosocial reasons, because she's a heavy smoker or drinker, or because of certain drugs). See also Chapter 10. Eventually a poor let-down leads to poor production.

The baby may be losing nutrients (because of malabsorption, diarrhoea or vomiting); he may have an infection (for example in his urine); or he may have high energy needs which aren't being met (for example, a baby who is small-for-dates or who has a congenital heart disease). And several of these problems may be combined, which is why a doctor needs to take a careful and complete medical, social and dietary history, examine the baby thoroughly, look at the mother's breasts, watch a feed and arrange for lab tests.

BABY NEEDS AN ANAESTHETIC

If a baby needs an anaesthetic before an operation, US research (1994) concluded that breastfeeding could safely continue until up to three hours beforehand.

RARE ILLNESSES

Galactosaemia is an inborn condition caused by an enzyme deficiency. This can sometimes be fatal if an affected baby is not put on a diet free of lactose (milk sugar). There is no alternative but to wean your baby from the breast at once and give him a special lactose-free formula.

Certain other 'inborn errors of metabolism', for example phenyl-ketonuria, can be diagnosed soon after birth. This condition causes high levels of phenylalanine in a baby's blood which can lead to brain damage and learning difficulties. Breast milk contains lower levels of this amino acid than does formula. This means a baby can breastfeed. Monitoring the phenylalanine levels means that if they were to rise dangerously high, the baby could have a combination of breast milk and a special low-phenylalanine formula or, at worst, this formula alone.

IMMUNIZATIONS

When your baby has his immunizations he may go off his milk and be more fussy than usual for about twenty-four hours. If you're over-full because he isn't sucking well, simply express a little milk every so often.

The 'triple' vaccine (diphtheria, pertussis/whooping cough, and tetanus) isn't affected by breastfeeding and a breastfed baby can have it at the normal recommended times. The same applies to polio, rubella, mumps, measles, yellow fever, cholera and typhoid vaccines.

IF YOU ARE ILL

If you are acutely ill at home and have to be in bed, you'll need someone to look after you and your baby and to bring him to you when he's ready for a feed. This assumes that you're too unwell to have him by your bed or in with you. If you have to be in hospital, you may be able to take him with you, but this will depend on what's wrong with you and on the hospital's facilities. If you can't have your baby with you in hospital, see if someone else can bring him to you for feeds. This entails a lot of work and means that you'll need to be in a hospital close to your home.

Another way of continuing to breastfeed if you're in hospital is to express or pump milk and send it home for your baby. It should be stored in a fridge and collected by a friend or relative for the baby to have from a feeding cup.

A few illnesses rule out breastfeeding. Others do so temporarily because of the drugs needed. If you have a longstanding illness such as severe asthma or kidney disease, you may feel so tired and run down that you won't be able to face breastfeeding. However, some mothers find that breastfeeding makes them rest and tires them less than bottle-feeding would.

IF YOU HAVE DIABETES

Diabetes is not uncommon, affecting about 2 per cent of the population. It's important to remember that the condition can run in families, but that breastfeeding for at least nine to twelve months reduces the risk of a baby with a family history getting diabetes himself when he's older (see page 80).

— In one US study of seventeen breastfeeding mothers with insulin-dependent diabetes mellitus, all of them breastfed successfully and fourteen fed their babies for more than nine months. Several tips came out of their experiences, particularly that high motivation and support from family, friends and health professionals are important.

A mother with diabetes whose baby goes into a special care unit after delivery needs to breastfeed, express or pump her milk frequently. After about five to seven hours she'll have an increased risk of a low blood-sugar, since the loss of placental lactogen hormone is associated with temporarily increased sensitivity to insulin. (This happens whether or not she breastfeeds). As she takes careful steps to balance her diet-insulin-exercise needs, her blood-sugar stabilizes.

Most women need less insulin in the first four to six weeks than they did before pregnancy. Some, however, need more in the first three months, probably because they eat more and exercise less.

Hypoglycaemic (insulin) reactions release adrenaline which decreases blood-flow in the breasts and can also inhibit the let-down reflex. Traces of insulin and adrenaline pass into milk but are largely inactivated by a baby's digestive enzymes in the stomach. Any minute amounts of insulin that enter the baby's bloodstream simply mean that he temporarily produces a little less insulin of his own. They are nothing to worry about.

Antibiotics chosen to treat any infections must be safe for the baby. Women who have diabetes and get sore nipples should watch out for thrush (*Candida* infection); they are prone to vaginal thrush and this can spread to their nipples (see page 315).

Any breastfed baby may suddenly want either more or less frequent feeds, perhaps because of a growth spurt. In diabetic mothers a change in the amount of milk they need to make can cause unexpectedly low or high blood-sugar levels, so they have to compensate by adjusting their diet, exercise and insulin.

Some women find that their diabetes is more stable when they are breastfeeding than it was before.

Diabetes which began in pregnancy

— Research (1993) shows that if a woman's diabetes began when she was pregnant, breastfeeding helps reduce or delay her risk of diabetes in the future.

IF YOU HAVE AN INFECTION

Several infections may temporarily produce problems if you're breastfeeding, but in no case is it necessary to dry up your milk.

If it's advisable for your baby not to breastfeed or have your expressed or pumped milk, keep your milk supply going by frequent expression or pumping, and simply discard the milk. This means you'll have no problems with engorgement at a time when you're probably not feeling too well. Once your baby is allowed breast milk again you'll have plenty of milk.

Herpes simplex (the cold-sore virus)

Women with a *Herpes simplex* virus infection causing an open sore on the breast should not breastfeed and should discard their milk until the sores have healed and no longer shed viruses.

As long as there are no herpes sores on the breast, experts recommend simply taking strict hygienic precautions, treating the infection, and continuing to breastfeed. It's *extremely* unusual for breast milk to contain herpes viruses.

A few experts, however, advise a woman with a *first* herpes attack, especially of the genital area, not to breastfeed. This is because of the danger of a newborn baby becoming infected with this potentially very dangerous virus at a time when his immune system is vulnerable and breast milk hasn't yet had a chance to develop much anti-herpes protective activity. Also, they report that there's more chance of developing an infection on the breast during a first attack.

A woman advised not to breastfeed can keep her milk supply going by frequent expression or pumping, discarding the milk. Once the infection has gone and she's no longer shedding viruses, she'll then have plenty of milk and can start to breastfeed. The anti-viral drug acyclovir has considerably brightened the outlook for treating herpes infections.

Cold sores – Neither a mother nor anyone else who has a cold sore or a sore mouth from a herpes infection – whether or not it's their first infection – should kiss a baby.

Hepatitis

Women who are carriers of hepatitis B can breastfeed as there is no evidence that this increases their baby's risk of the infection, especially if they receive hepatitis B vaccine and hepatitis B immune globulin soon after birth.

— Research (1995) reported in the *Lancet* suggested that on the evidence currently available, it is safe for women who test positive for hepatitis C to breastfeed.

Tuberculosis (TB)

If you've had lung TB and have been free from the disease for two years, you can safely feed your baby.

If you've had active lung TB in pregnancy, with a positive tuberculin test, a positive chest X-ray and positive sputum or gastric washings, and if your treatment (with 'triple' therapy: three drugs) was begun *at least a week before your baby was born*, you needn't be separated from him and can safely breastfeed *provided he is also treated with isoniazid*.

If you are bacteriologically negative, you can breastfeed even if you've only just begun treatment, provided he too is treated with isoniazid (in a smaller dose than for the baby whose mother is bacteriologically positive). It's important that your baby doesn't have too much isoniazid because he'll get some in your milk as well and an overdose can cause peripheral neuritis. Some experts suggest monitoring a baby's liver function to make sure this doesn't happen. Because one of the commonly used drugs – para-aminosalicylic acid (PAS) – in the 'triple' therapy isn't recommended for babies (though no one knows for sure how much gets into milk), a breastfeeding mother may have streptomycin or kanamycin instead. If other drugs are used, special precautions may be advisable.

If a breastfeeding mother contracts active, bacteriologically positive TB, a period of separation from her baby may be recommended for safety while drug treatment begins and until cultures of her sputum and gastric washings are negative. If her milk isn't infected, it's reasonable for the baby to have expressed or pumped milk from a feeding cup. Treatment usually makes a woman non-infectious in a very short time.

It could be argued that if a mother and baby have been together before the mother's TB was diagnosed, there's no point in separating them. However, because the complications of TB are more hazardous in newborn babies, it's worth taking every precaution to reduce a baby's risk of catching it.

There's some controversy over the management of a breastfeeding mother with TB and her baby in developed countries. In certain developing countries and among certain isolated peoples such as some American Indians, it's virtually always safer to leave a mother and her baby together, because breastfeeding is so much safer than bottle-feeding, given the lack of money for formula, the lack of water, fuel and other bottle-sterilizing necessities and the high risk of infections. In such circumstances the risk of drug toxicity is relatively unimportant. These breastfed babies should be carefully treated with isoniazid, however, and vaccinated with a special type of BCG vaccine (isoniazid-resistant). The mother's active TB needs thorough treatment at the same time.

Gonorrhoea

If this is diagnosed at delivery, your baby shouldn't have your milk or be with you until twenty-four hours after treatment has begun. Then you can breastfeed and be with your baby just like any other mother.

HIV infection

Around two million children worldwide had HIV (type 1) in 1995. Almost all contracted it from their mothers, either in the womb, during labour, or afterwards.

If a woman is HIV-positive, her decision about whether or not to breastfeed needs to be based on the particular risks and benefits of breastfeeding to her baby, and the potential dangers of bottle-feeding.

In many industrialized countries, including Great Britain, the US, Canada, France and Australia, experts currently advise HIV (type 1)-positive women not to breastfeed. However, the virus is more likely to be present in her milk if a woman becomes infected during the time she breastfeeds than if she became HIV-positive before or during pregnancy. Also, breast milk contains some anti-HIV factors and research shows that breastfeeding can slow the progression of the infection in babies who were born HIV-positive.

However, the World Health Organization recommends that HIV-1-positive women should breastfeed if they live in areas of developing countries in which many babies die because of infectious diseases and malnutrition.

Because so few babies catch HIV (type 2) from their mothers, there are as yet no specific recommendations.

Syphilis

Infection of the skin on the breasts means a baby shouldn't breastfeed but may be able to have expressed or pumped milk.

Leprosy

A mother with leprosy should breastfeed, as breastfeeding is valuable enough to outweigh any possible dangers of contact. However, she may be advised not to hold her baby at other times. Both mother and baby can have drug treatment.

IF YOU HAVE OSTEOPOROSIS

Women with osteoporosis can breastfeed if they want to and if their condition isn't too painful. They may – like other women – experience a temporary loss of minerals from their bones during pregnancy and while breastfeeding. However, bone lost while breastfeeding seems to be reversible. This means the bones harden up again some time after breastfeeding is over.

When you breastfeed, take care that you are sitting comfortably and in a well-supported position. If possible, ask someone else to pass your baby to you so as to avoid lifting whenever you can.

Two pieces of research suggest that breastfeeding helps protect against the long-term risk of osteoporosis (see page 129). It's possible, though unproven, that this may also mean it's beneficial in the long term for women who already have the conditon.

IF YOU HAVE BERI-BERI

Women with a severe deficiency of vitamin B1 (thiamine) causing beri-beri shouldn't breastfeed as there are toxic substances in their milk. This condition isn't seen in the Western world, though it is still said to exist in parts of China.

IF YOU HAVE A HIGH PROLACTIN LEVEL

Fertility problems caused by having too much of the hormone prolactin can be treated with a drug called bromocriptine. This lowers the level of prolactin and enables conception to occur.

Taking bromocriptine once a baby is born dries up breast milk, but women with a high prolactin level have traditionally been advised not to breastfeed anyway. This is, first, because breastfeeding raises their prolactin level further. Second, because there seems to be a higher risk of a breast abscess. And third, a sizeable proportion of women with this condition have a pituitary gland tumour (prolactinoma) and it's feared that raising their prolactin level further could make the tumour bigger. Because of the position of the tumour, enlargement could lead to visual disturbances, including blindness.

— However, Swedish research (1986) which followed thirty-eight women with such a tumour concluded that a woman can safely stop taking bromocriptine during pregnancy and while breastfeeding provided that: 1) she's had at least a year of treatment before pregnancy; and 2) she has regular checkups, with monthly prolactin tests and visual field measurements so she can start taking bromocriptine again at the first suspicion of any increase in tumour size. Eight out of every ten women in their survey breastfed successfully for up to two years.

CAESAREAN SECTION

Many babies today are born by Caesarean section (more than half in some US hospitals). After this operation there's no reason why you shouldn't breastfeed but you'll need to be determined in the first week or so. You'll have two main challenges. First, you're likely to have a certain amount of abdominal pain and discomfort. If you are to get your milk supply going well, it's best to feed your baby frequently day and night, just as you would had you had a normal delivery. It's just as easy to feed as it is to express or pump your milk, and you're less likely to become engorged or get sore nipples if you feed like this from the beginning.

If you've had a general anaesthetic you may not be able to feed your baby immediately after delivery but as soon as you are awake or well enough ask for him to be brought to you for a feed, even if he's asleep. More Caesarean sections are being performed today under epidural anaesthesia, which means that breastfeeding gets off to a better start.

More comfortable feeding positions

The second problem is that you'll find it uncomfortable to feed in the normal sitting position with your baby on your lap. You'll need to choose a position in which his weight isn't on your tummy and your abdominal muscles aren't strained by holding him to your breast.

Enlist the help of a nurse to position him next to you as you lie on one side in bed. When the time comes to change breasts, ring for the nurse to help you turn over and change the baby to your other side.

If you have a horizontal scar, try sitting up, with your baby on a pillow, his head facing your breast and his legs tucked under your arm on that side. Alternatively, sit up straight (to avoid straining your abdomen), lay him on a pillow at your side with his legs across your thighs, and support his head either with another pillow or with your arm (itself supported by a pillow).

If your baby is in an incubator after delivery and the nurses can't bring him to you for feeds, express or pump your colostrum (and your milk when it comes in). The nurses can then give the breast milk feeds by tube or cup, depending on the state of your baby, until you can go to him. Don't be alarmed by the small amounts of colostrum you produce – remember there isn't much in the first day or so.

A Caesarean section, especially if unplanned, can undermine a mother's self-confidence. If she's helped to breastfeed, she may think better of herself. Breastfeeding helps post-operative recovery because the production of oxytocin assists the uterus to return to its former size. A Caesarean section leaves some mothers feeling very tired for some time and it's important that they get enough rest. This doesn't mean that nights must be unbroken, with your baby given a bottle by the nursing staff, but that between feeds the day shouldn't be crammed full of activity on the ward or at home. Allow ample time to sleep or catnap. Pain-killers may be necessary, especially in the first day or two, because a Caesarean section scar can be painful while healing, especially when coughing.

By the end of the first week you should be feeling very much better and will be able to carry on just like any other breastfeeding mother.

PRE-ECLAMPSIA

Severe pre-eclampsia (previously known as pre-eclamptic toxaemia) can present initial problems with breastfeeding for several reasons. A baby may be pre-term or small-for-dates and need to be nursed in an incubator; or a mother may still be at risk of having convulsions and needing treatment, including blood-pressure-lowering drugs, sedation and bed rest in a darkened room. Most mothers recover within twenty-four to forty-eight hours after delivery. How breastfeeding is managed depends on all these factors and each mother–baby pair must be considered separately. If a woman can't put her baby to the breast, or if early feeds are unsuccessful and stressful, she may be advised to express or pump her milk. Expert nursing care helps make either as easy and stress-free as possible for her. Some doctors consider that the stress and stimulation involved in pumping or expressing is too risky for a woman who may have an eclamptic fit, and are unhappy anyway about the possible accumulation of the mother's drugs in her milk.

Points to consider, however, are that the stress factor in having engorged, unemptied breasts may be considerable in itself; that a mother may be anxious about her baby not being breastfed, unless she is heavily sedated; and that the drugs normally given have not been shown (in the relatively small numbers of women studied) to be dangerous. Having said this, care must be taken to ensure that a breastfed baby (especially if ill or pre-term) isn't 'depressed' by the accumulation of large doses of phenobarbitone.

If you are advised not to breastfeed and not to pump or express either, you can get your milk supply back later when you are well if you want to (see page 401). If your doctor is reluctant for your baby to drink your milk because of its high drug levels, you or the nurses may be able to keep your milk supply going until your medication level is reduced; the milk can simply be discarded.

BREASTFEEDING AFTER BREAST SURGERY

Plastic surgery to make breasts larger or smaller is becoming increasingly popular. Unfortunately, it's sometimes done without a woman thinking about whether or not she'll want to breastfeed one day. Some women who have a breast lump need a biopsy (sample of tissue) taken to check for cancer cells. A few have a lump removed. We'll look at each of these conditions.

Breast reduction (reduction mammoplasty)

You may be able to breastfeed after an operation to make your breasts smaller. However, whether or not you manage to do so fully will depend on the type of operation, how much glandular tissue was removed, how many milk ducts were cut, whether the cut ends of the ducts have managed to join up with open ducts so that milk can get to the nipple, and whether those milk glands with undamaged ducts can produce enough milk. In one type of operation, the nipple and areola are cut away completely before being transplanted higher up. In the other, they are left attached to some breast tissue so that after transplantation some ducts are still intact.

The longer the time between your operation and your pregnancy, the more successful breastfeeding is likely to be. Then the only way to know whether you can breastfeed successfully is to try. Even if you manage only to give your baby some milk each day, it's worth it for him and you. And if you have to give formula as well, you can give it at the same time as you breastfeed simply by using a supplementer (see page 449).

— An Australian survey (1994) of thirty women who had a baby after a breast reduction found that of the 93 per cent who wished to breastfeed, 73 per cent were doing so when they left hospital, and 27 per cent three months later (though only one woman was exclusively breastfeeding).

If you contemplate such an operation before you have children and think you might ever want to breastfeed, be sure your surgeon knows.

Breast enlargement

Many women have found they've been able to breastfeed successfully after having breast implants though these can make breastfeeding more difficult. The scare in 1994 about whether breastfed babies of mothers with silicone implants might develop a stiff gullet because of drinking silicone-containing milk from leaking implants has died down. Tests on breast milk from mothers with implants have not detected any silicone.

Biopsy or removal of a lump before breastfeeding

If you have to have a biopsy and/or a lump removed and there's any chance that you might one day want to breastfeed, have a thorough discussion with your surgeon first. As little tissue as possible should be removed, and the incision chosen should cut across as few ducts as possible. This means that if the lump isn't easy to feel, your surgeon may want to localize it first with dye or with a wire; and he may choose not to make an incision all around the areola.

If you've already had a biopsy, you won't know whether you can breastfeed until you try. However, if – even with the best advice and support – you can't feed from the side that had the biopsy, simply let the milk in that breast dry up (by not feeding from it and by expressing only the tiniest of amounts to stop it hurting). You're highly likely to be able to make all the milk your baby needs from the other breast.

Biopsy or removal of a lump during breastfeeding

Make sure your surgeon knows you are breastfeeding and wish to continue. He or she can then take great care to cut as few milk ducts as possible. Breastfeed your baby as close in time to the start of the operation as possible, and ask the nurses to bring him to you afterwards. They will also help you breastfeed from the other breast as soon as possible. Feed from the operated side as soon as you can; you may find it helps to press very gently over the dressing while you feed.

DRUG TREATMENT

Virtually every drug a mother takes passes into her milk, although some reach very much higher concentrations than others. However, many are harmless to a baby, however high their concentration in milk, while others are harmful even in tiny amounts, either because of known side-effects which affect adults as well, or because they have a different action in a young baby.

Some drugs can cause sensitivity or allergy which may be dangerous with repeated doses.

Knowledge of the effects of many drugs on a breastfed baby is far from complete because of the difficulty in doing drug trials in breastfeeding mothers. It would clearly be unethical and unacceptable to feed women drugs to see what happened to their babies. And in a social climate in which so few women breastfeed for long periods of time, the actual numbers of women on all but the commonest of drugs is very few. There's also the very real difficulty of measuring drug levels in milk.

Ideally, a breastfeeding mother should not take any drugs. However, this is obviously the counsel of perfection and there will be times when drugs are life-saving. If they happen to be dangerous for her baby, she'll have to wean, if only temporarily.

Then there are other drugs which, whilst not life-saving to the mother, may be useful in treating certain illnesses. If a particular drug is not safe for a breastfed baby, an alternative often is.

The known risks of most drugs are so low that breastfeeding is considered safe.

If you are taking any drug while breastfeeding, check with your doctor that it isn't one of the list below. It's wisest always to remind him or her that you are breastfeeding before they prescribe anything for you, as they may not know.

Rather than list the many drugs known to be safe for the breastfed infant, *we'll only look at those that are known to be either unsafe or better avoided*. If you have any doubts, ask your doctor: he can obtain more details, if necessary. The adverse effects mentioned in the following list have been noticed in breastfed babies whose mothers are on the drug in question.

Anti-infective drugs

Antibiotics – Adverse effects are usually uncommon. See individual drugs. However, they can cause diarrhoea.

Chloramphenicol – This may cause refusal of the breast, sleepiness during feeds and vomiting afterwards. Because it has been known to cause an idiosyncratic reaction which harms the bone marrow in adults and children, its use in breastfeeding mothers has been discouraged, though it can be used.

Ciprofloxacin – This is best avoided because of high concentrations in milk.

Clindamycin – Concentrations in milk may be several times those in a breastfeeding woman's blood. This drug is best avoided because of the risk of bowel inflammation.

Co-trimoxazole – This drug is now reserved only for rare conditions including AIDS. It is anyway better not taken at all in the first two weeks because of the risk of jaundice and a deficiency of folate (from folic acid, an important B vitamin).

Dapsone – This is probably best avoided.

Metronidazole – Only traces appear in breast milk but there is a theoretical risk of cancer, or of decreased appetite, vomiting and diarrhoea. High doses are not advised for breastfeeding women. One recent paper suggests that if it is necessary to treat trichomonas infection, the woman should first collect and store enough expressed or pumped milk to last for a day, then take a single 2 g dose, discard her milk for the next twenty-four hours, and give her baby her stored milk. Experts now consider that insufficient concentrations of this drug are present in breast milk to warrant advising against it.

Nalidixic acid – One case of haemolytic anaemia has been reported in a baby whose mother was also taking amylobarbitone. It has also caused raised intracranial pressure. Use with caution only if absolutely necessary and observe the baby carefully.

Nitrofurantoin – The level in breast milk is not pharmacologically significant, but this drug is not advised for mothers of pre-term or G6PD-deficient babies.

Novobiocin – Not recommended for breastfeeding mothers because of the possibility of causing neonatal jaundice.

Penicillins – Appear in trace amounts in breast milk and could, theoretically, cause allergic sensitization in a susceptible baby. Resulting levels in a baby are not high enough to treat infections in the baby. An alternative antibiotic should ideally be used, though this may not always be possible.

Sulphonamides – If a baby is jaundiced, sulphonamides in breast milk may worsen the condition. However, if there is only a trace of jaundice, the risk is negligible. Haemolytic anaemia has been reported in one G6PD deficient baby (a rare enzyme deficiency). They can cause a rash. Cautious use and careful observation have been suggested if the baby is under one month old; however, other experts recommend that it's better to avoid these drugs completely while breastfeeding.

Tetracyclines – Theoretically these can cause mottling of a baby's developing teeth, though absorption from the milk in a baby's gut is poor. Best avoided.

Anti-cancer drugs

Breastfeeding will usually have to be abandoned (although methotrexate and busulphan seem to present little hazard).

Anticoagulants

Bleeding episodes have occurred after surgery or trauma in babies. Warfarin, however, is suitable for a breastfeeding mother, as is heparin. Other drugs should be used with caution or substituted where possible with warfarin or heparin.

Antithyroid drugs

These may cause goitre in the baby. This condition can be treated by giving him thyroxine. Because some of this group of drugs have the rare side-effect of causing a potentially fatal blood disorder, a baby's blood should be monitored. So, too, should his thyroid hormone levels, though there's no evidence of altered thyroid function in a baby whose mother takes propylthiouracil. This drug is preferable because it's less concentrated in milk than is carbimazole. However, carbimazole in doses of 30 mg or less per day can be used. Iodides (found in some cough medicines and sometimes used to treat hyperthyroidism) may suppress the baby's thyroid activity and cause goitre. They can also sensitize his thyroid gland to lithium, chlorpromazine and methylxanthines.

Central nervous system drugs

Alcohol – Amounts of alcohol large enough to make you 'tipsy' reduce oxytocin levels and hinder breastfeeding. Doses higher than 1 g/kg of the mother's weight can inhibit the let-down reflex, while doses higher than 2 g/kg probably block it completely. Large amounts of alcohol can intoxicate a baby. Very large amounts on a regular basis could cause brain damage. See also page 242.

Amantadine – Contra-indicated in the breastfeeding mother, according to the manufacturer, as it may cause vomiting, urinary retention and rashes in the baby.

Anti-convulsants – All these come through into breast milk but mostly in lower concentrations than in the mother's blood. Experts recommend continuing with breastfeeding. See individual drugs.

Barbiturates – Can cause drowsiness and may also stimulate the metabolism of other drugs taken by the mother. One case of cyanosis ('blue baby') due to methaemoglobinaemia occurred in a baby whose mother was also taking phenytoin.

Bromide – Usually produces drowsiness and may cause a rash.

Cannabis – This takes a long time to be destroyed and can accumulate in a baby's body. Babies of marijuana-smoking mothers have been reported to have delayed motor development at one year. Breastfeeding women should avoid this drug.

Carbamazepine – No side-effects have been reported in babies whose mothers take the drug on its own. However, it is not advised if used in high doses or in combination with other anti-epileptics, as they are structurally similar to tricyclic anti-depressants which aren't metabolized by young babies. Significant levels can build up in a breastfed baby.

Chloral hydrate – Can cause drowsiness.

Chlorpromazine – Could cause drowsiness and may be better avoided.

Diazepam – One report of lethargy and weight-loss. Levels may build up in the baby's body and increase physiological jaundice. High doses should be used only with caution.

Dichloralphenazone – Causes slight drowsiness.

Doxepin – An alternative anti-depressant is preferable because of the risk of sedation and breathing problems in a breastfed baby.

Ethosuximide – Significant levels can build up in a breastfed baby. Poor sucking and over-excitability have been reported.

Fluoxetine – The few studies there are suggest that because this drug takes a long time to be broken down, an alternative anti-depressant is preferable for breastfeeding women.

Heroin – Can cause addiction in babies when taken by their mother during pregnancy. Breastfeeding and very gradual weaning is one way of withdrawing the drug from such a baby. However, the American Academy of Pediatrics recommends that heroin-addicted mothers should not breastfeed.

Lithium – If a mother continues with this drug she should watch her baby and report any unusual signs, such as lethargy and floppiness, to her doctor.

Morphine – Significant amounts may be excreted in the milk of addicts.

Phenobarbitone – A baby may become sleepy but the drug does not seem to be harmful. If a mother has taken big doses during pregnancy, breastfeeding followed by gradual weaning is a good way of stopping the drug slowly enough to prevent adverse withdrawal effects. One case of methaemoglobinaemia has been reported in a baby whose mother was also taking phenytoin.

Phenytoin – Many mothers have breastfed their babies safely when taking phenytoin. However, it has been associated with vomiting, tremors and rashes, as well as an idiosyncratic reaction of blueness due to methaemoglobinaemia.

Primidone – There are high levels in breast milk and these can make a baby sleepy.

Sulpiride – This can be associated with adverse affects in a breastfed baby and is not recommended.

Tricyclic anti-depressants – According to one manufacturer, these are excreted in breast milk but are not metabolized in the young baby. This could, theoretically, result in accumulation. However, no side-effects in babies have been reported and it would seem safe for the breastfeeding mother to take these drugs provided the dose is not too high and the baby continues to thrive.

Diuretics

Can decrease the milk supply. Otherwise no harmful effects have been reported.

Laxatives

May cause diarrhoea.

Hormones and synthetic substitutes

Diethylstilboestrol – If a 'dry-up' dose is given but you change your mind and later decide you want to breastfeed, you can work up your milk supply again. Drugs to dry up milk are unnecessary anyway (see page 289).

Oral contraceptives – The combined (oestrogen/progestogen) Pill can suppress quite markedly both the volume of milk produced and the duration of lactation. Two studies have shown a decrease in protein, fat and minerals in the breast milk of women on the Pill. Small amounts of steroids also appear in the milk. Isolated reports exist of breast enlargement in male babies, proliferation of the vaginal epithelium in female ones and changes in bones, though these all occurred with higher-dose oral contraceptives than are now used. One study, unconfirmed by others, showed a correlation between prior contraceptive use of these hormones and breast milk jaundice.

The progestogen-only Pill usually has no effect on the volume of breast milk. Traces of steroids do appear in the milk though. It may be preferable to use another type of contraception (see page 128), or to wait until your baby starts solids after four months of age.

It is too early as yet to be sure about the long-term safety of oral contraceptives with respect to breastfed babies developing cancers in later life.

Progestogen contraceptive implants/progesterone vaginal contraceptive ring – Studies suggest that a breastfeeding woman can use these methods with no adverse effects on breastfeeding. However, the World Health Organization suggests not starting them until six weeks after birth.

Miscellaneous drugs

Allopurinol and oxipurinol – These enter breast milk in high concentrations, which means that a breastfed baby risks the same side effects as his mother.

5-aminosalicylic acid (mesalazine) – This is considered safe but can cause diarrhoea in a breastfed baby.

Aspirin – This is best avoided because of the small risk of rashes, gastro-intestinal side-effects or, if a baby has a blood-clotting disorder, jaundice and bleeding into the brain. There is also a small risk of Reye's syndrome, which can cause fatal brain and liver damage.

Atropine – Said to diminish milk-flow and cause constipation and retention of urine in the baby but there is no good documentation of this.

Bismuth (in nipple cream) – Should not be used.

Bromocriptine – Suppresses lactation. Prolactin levels fall within a few hours.

Caffeine – See page 243.

Cocaine – Breastfeeding while taking cocaine or crack is not advised.

Digoxin – Two recent reports conclude that even if a breastfeeding mother is on a high dose of digoxin, the amounts secreted in breast milk are small and infant exposure is low.

Dihydrotachysterol – Animal studies show decalcification of the bones. Some authors recommend that mothers taking this shouldn't breastfeed.

Ecstasy and MDMA – Breastfeeding is not advised because of a lack of studies on its effects.

Ergometrine – Lowers prolactin levels. It has been suggested that multiple doses might suppress lactation. In some obstetric units ergometrine is now given after delivery only if the uterus fails to contract and expel the placenta naturally (which often takes half an hour or so) or if there is post-partum bleeding from the uterus.

Ergot alkaloids – 90 per cent of breastfed babies had signs of ergotism (diarrhoea and vomiting; weak pulse; unstable blood pressure) in one study. Many derivatives can suppress lactation.

Fluoride – Can cause mottling of teeth.

Ginseng – There has been one report of a breastfed boy of a woman taking large amounts of Siberian ginseng developing pubic hair, a hairy forehead and swollen nipples. The boy returned to normal when she stopped breastfeeding.

Gold – Can cause rashes and other 'odd' reactions. It is best avoided.

Indomethacin – There is one case report of convulsions in a breastfed baby whose mother took this drug. It is probably best avoided.

Lead – Lead toxicity (including encephalitis) has occurred after the use of both lead acetate ointment on nipples and lead breast shields!

Mercury – Mothers exposed to high levels should not breastfeed.

Nicotine – May reduce the milk supply and interfere with the let-down. Breastfeeding mothers who are smokers are more likely to give up breastfeeding early than are non-smokers (see also page 254).There is one report of restlessness and circulatory disturbance in a baby. It may also cause tummy-ache, nausea, vomiting and diarrhoea.

Phenylbutazone – Take only if there's no alternative and report any unusual signs to a doctor because of the possibility of a blood dyscrasia.

Propranolol – Only small amounts appear in the milk. However, because of the theoretical possibility of accumulation in the baby and because of the immaturity of the enzyme systems responsible for its metabolism, close observation for heart-slowing or low blood-sugar is necessary.

Reserpine – There's been one report of significant nasal stuffiness, slowing of the heart and some increase in tracheo-bronchial secretions.

Sulphasalazine – There is one case report of a breastfed baby who developed bloody diarrhoea while his mother was taking this drug. If this happens it should be reported to a doctor.

Vitamin B6 (pyridoxine) – One study showed a decrease in the milk supply with doses of over 100 mg a day. Supplements of this vitamin are often taken for the pre-menstrual syndrome or for post-natal depression, but this is inadvisable while breast-feeding.

Radioactive drugs

Experts differ in their advice to breastfeeding mothers and recommendations have changed over the years. The following is a safe summary.

[67]Gallium citrate, ^{75}Se-methionine, Sodium ^{32}P phosphate, Chromic ^{32}P phosphate – Significant amounts of all of these radioactive substances are excreted in milk. Different experts advise that breastfeeding should be interrupted and the milk discarded for between seventy-two hours and three weeks. Ask if the nuclear medicine department at your hospital will monitor radio-activity levels in your milk so you can return to breastfeeding as soon as possible.

Iodine isotopes – The latest advice is that radio-iodine studies of the thyroid gland should not be performed in breastfeeding women. Hyperthyroidism and thyroiditis can be reliably diagnosed using pertechnate (technetium [99]m) imaging in combination with clinical criteria and plasma hormone levels.

[99]Tcm-pertechnate (technetium [99]m) – Discard breast milk for twelve hours.

^{99}Tcm-MAA – Discard breast milk for twenty-four hours.

^{99}Tcm-DTPA, ^{99}Tcm-EDTA, ^{99}Tcm-MDP, ^{99}Tcm-erythrocytes, ^{51}Cr-EDTA and ^{111}In-leucocytes – No need to stop breastfeeding but some experts seek to reassure mothers alarmed by radioactivity to discard milk produced in the four hours after the test.

If you're advised to have any kind of radio-active isotope investigation or treatment, discuss with your doctor whether there's an alternative – either not using an isotope at all, or using one which comes through into milk in smaller amounts.

If the interruption is to be short, you can plan ahead and store expressed or pumped milk in the fridge or freezer to be given to the baby during that time. While breastfeeding is interrupted, keep your milk supply going by expressing or pumping frequently and discarding the milk.

Pesticides, PCBs and other environmental contaminants

Organochlorine pesticides (such as DDT, hexachlorobenzene, chlordane, dieldrin and heptachlor epoxide) are restricted in some countries and banned in others. These chemicals are fat-soluble and enter breast milk. Their concentration is higher in milk that comes from mothers living in contaminated areas or eating contaminated produce than it is in other foods. This makes breastfed babies a special risk group. However, there's a lack of information on any side-effects. And levels of organochlorines in breast milk in the UK are declining. The World Health Organization continues to monitor the situation and to recommend tight control of their use and the use of alternative, environmentally-friendly measures.

Despite the need for vigilance, experts say that the advantages of breastfeeding far outweigh any risks for all except an extremely small minority of exposed babies.

Chlordane – This insecticide and its derivatives can enter breast milk and the acceptable daily intake (ADI) is easily exceeded in contaminated areas. Its effects on breastfed babies are unknown, but chlordane and its derivatives persist in the body for at least five years. The intake for breastfed babies in the UK (1991) does not exceed the ADI.

DDT – Although DDT is present in breast milk in contaminated areas, and from mothers who smoke or have ever smoked (because DDT is used on some tobacco crops), no ill-effects have been observed.

Dieldrin – The acceptable daily intake (ADI) from breast milk is very easily exceeded in contaminated areas where some people consume up to twenty-two times the ADI! Also, Dutch research (1992) showed that the more often a woman eats meat and dairy produce, the higher are her milk levels of dieldrin.

Dioxins and furans – These are released by burning plastic made from PVC and wood treated with preservatives and are among the most toxic poisons known. They enter breast milk in industrially contaminated areas and it has been suggested that severe contamination of milk could lead to a bleeding disorder (late haemorrhagic disease of the newborn) due to vitamin K deficiency in young breastfed babies.

Heptachlor – The acceptable daily intake (ADI) from breast milk is exceeded in every exposed baby, according to one study. Some intakes are up to seven times the ADI. Long-term exposure in animals shows this chemical can damage nerves, kidneys and the immune system. The intake of breastfed babies in the UK (1991) does not exceed the ADI.

Hexachlorobenzene – Many infant deaths occurred in Turkey after mothers ate wheat treated with this grain fungicide. This is one of the most persistent organophosphates and the acceptable daily intake (ADI) from breast milk is easily exceeded in contaminated areas. Some intakes from the milk of exposed mothers contain up to 48 times the ADI.

PCBs (polychlorinated biphenyls) – The industrial use of PCBs is now banned in some countries and restricted to closed electrical systems in the European Community. The disposal of PCB-containing articles (such as transformers, capacitators and painted items) remains a problem. PCBs aren't thought to harm breastfed babies and the levels in breast milk have only rarely (after unusual exposure) exceeded safe limits.

There are literally thousands of drugs and medications available over the counter in the Western world. While most are perfectly safe in normal doses, always check the above list first. If you aren't sure what to do, talk to your doctor or pharmacist.

RE-STARTING YOUR MILK SUPPLY (relactation)

There are several reasons why you might want to do this. You may have decided initially not to breastfeed and let your milk dry up, only to change your mind after a few weeks. You may want to breastfeed an adopted baby. Or you may want to put your baby back on breast milk after an untimely weaning. In each case you can build up your milk supply, although you'll have to persevere and you'll need a cooperative baby!

If your baby has been on formula for several weeks and your milk supply has dried up, start it up again by putting him to the breast frequently. He may become frustrated at first by feeding from an empty breast, especially because the shape of the nipple isn't such a strong stimulus to suck as is the shape of a rubber teat. You can try two things. Either let him have some formula from a bottle to satisfy his initial hunger pangs, then let him feed from you, or give him formula from a cup or spoon, so avoiding the stimulus of the rubber teat, then let him feed from you. Once you start to produce some milk, try to get your let-down working before putting your baby to the breast. You may also find a supplementer helpful (see page 449).

After each feed, express or pump your breasts to encourage your milk supply to build up. Remember that the more often your baby breastfeeds, the more quickly your milk will reappear. By about two weeks you'll probably be producing enough milk to be able to do away with formula.

The keynote to success is confidence. The experience of women all over the world is that their breasts are capable of producing milk again even after several years of being dry, *as long as they have enough stimulation.*

Adopted baby

Believe it or not, many women have fully breastfed adopted babies, sometimes years after feeding their own babies. Some women have fed adopted babies *without ever having been pregnant*, though, to be fair, they had to supplement their milk with other food.

Once your breasts have been prepared for lactation by a pregnancy they always retain their ability to produce milk at a later date. If they've produced milk for any length of time, they'll be even more able to produce milk years later. This is why grandmothers in many parts of the world can breastfeed their grandchildren many years after feeding their own children.

A woman who breastfeeds her own baby has had months of pregnancy for her breasts to prepare for breastfeeding. So you must expect to take a long time to prepare your breasts too. Start building up your milk supply at least six weeks before your adopted baby arrives. Express or pump at frequent intervals. You'll probably need to give formula as well. However, some mothers have fed their adopted babies with breast milk from the baby's mother, from a breast-milk bank (see page 353) or from a breastfeeding friend until their own milk became plentiful enough.

A supplementer is a useful piece of equipment for re-lactating mothers. The original one was developed by a man for his wife who successfully built up her milk supply to feed an adopted baby (see page 449).

How long will it take to build up your milk supply? It has been done within two weeks by mothers who weaned their own baby as long as six years before. It usually takes much longer. The pleasure it gives can far outweigh the difficulty involved, though be prepared for it to take some time.

A surprising number of breastfeeding mothers and their families find themselves challanged by a special situation. However, patience, information, skilled encouragement and support and perhaps, when you're up to it, the leavening of humour, should help you find your way through to easier times.

FOURTEEN

Mainly for fathers

SOCIAL CHANGES

The role of fathers in modern society has altered over the last two decades and looks set for even more change. When we wrote the first edition of this book in the late 1970s, there was still the widespread expectation that most families would consist of a man and a woman married to one another and living together with their children. It was also generally assumed that the man would be both the main breadwinner and the father of the children.

This is still the case in most homes with very young children but things are on the move. In the US, about a third of all children are brought up in households in which there is no man and in many other Western countries similar changes are on the way. Even if a man is resident, he may not be the father of all the children. And even when the father *is* the biological parent of all the children and the family is a 'nuclear' one, living styles have greatly changed over twenty years. When it comes to fathering, many of today's families fall into one of two groups.

In the first, the man is employed and works harder than ever to keep his job and support his family. In the second, the father is out of work or employed on a temporary – perhaps contract – basis, and feels insecure much of the time. In other words, many modern fathers are either in work and, as a result, so overstretched that they have way too little time or energy for their families; or have little or no work and so feel bad about themselves much of the time.

In some ways social welfare systems have not proved beneficial to family life. Many countries are now rethinking these arrangements in the hopes of empowering fathers, mothers and their families.

These social changes have had huge implications for breastfeeding. Clearly the overstretched, overstressed man, worried about keeping his job in a precarious employment market, may not welcome a request from his partner for him to take time off work to support her after birth. In a dog-eat-dog commercial world both colleagues and employers could interpret this as a sign of weakness or lack of commitment.

The out-of-work father, on the other hand, could, in theory, because of his free time, make himself available for household support and breastfeeding back-up, but few actually do. On the contrary, many say that in a world where so many women contribute significantly to family income and where some are even the major breadwinners, they want their partner back at work as quickly as possible so that she can earn money to help keep the family finances together. In many parts of most countries it is now easier for a mother of a young child to get employment, albeit possibly poorly paid and part-time, than it is for her man. This makes bottle-feeding an attractive option for the baby's father.

But even setting aside these social changes, many men don't care much whether their partner breastfeeds. This is a pity because there are so many advantages for mother and baby and most men would be convinced if they only knew the whole story.

WHY YOU ARE SO IMPORTANT TO BREASTFEEDING

The father of a breastfed baby is a very important person because he can play several very helpful roles. Take, for a moment, an example from the animal world. While a baby gorilla is being born, the father fusses about the mother, and when she has given birth he lifts the baby up to her breast at once so that she can suckle it.

Similarly, once your partner has decided to breastfeed, you can offer help right from the start.

Even (or indeed especially) at this early stage you can take a positive hand in giving her the support and encouragement she needs for successful breastfeeding.

For example, some hospitals give breastfed babies water, glucose water or formula unnecessarily, especially at night. You can help prevent this happening. Remind the staff that you both want your baby to be totally breastfed. You'll find it's better to tell them before the birth, preferably on admission to the maternity unit. Don't be fobbed off by someone who tries to persuade you that it doesn't matter if your baby has the occasional bottle – it's up to you to hold out for what you feel is right. There's a small possibility that even one bottle of formula could trigger an allergic reaction either at the time or later in a susceptible child (most likely one with a family history of allergy).

Stay with your partner if she wants you there. She's just been through one of the most important events in her life and may want you for company and to share the experience. We'd like to see even more hospitals giving a private half-hour or more for parents to be with each other and their new baby before the pressures of everyday life impinge on them again.

It's right here in the delivery room that you can be especially supportive. She may be emotionally and physically keyed up or exhausted, and it's an interesting fact that women who have difficult or unpleasant labours are less likely to breastfeed. Anything you can do to help, support and encourage her, especially at this very early stage, could help her with breastfeeding.

In the US some women are asked immediately after the birth whether they want to breastfeed; if the answer is 'No' they have an injection to dry up their milk there and then. Of course, many women are in no fit state to decide against breastfeeding in the few minutes after giving birth and undoubtedly some later wish they'd had more time to think. In the UK dry-up drugs are only rarely given but if your partner is offered them, you can help by asking if she really needs them or whether she could instead let her milk dry up on its own. If she does have dry-up drugs, she can get her milk back if she later changes her mind, though doing so is a little more tedious.

Any breastfeeding problems are likely to feel worst in the first week because it's then that some women feel at their lowest and need most help. One experienced breastfeeding counsellor goes so far as to say that successful lactation depends on the woman's helpers and advisers, not on her ability to produce milk. Of course, one of her most valuable helpers could be you.

However useful you may be when your partner is in hospital, your real help will begin when she gets home. If you have other children you may have already been busy looking after them. Take a couple of weeks more off work if you can, so you can look after the other children and be there for your partner.

Once she's home, you'll be important as provider, protector and general helper. If breastfeeding is to succeed you'll play an even more valuable part in family life than usual for the next few weeks. Most of us have only two children in a lifetime so it's worth making an effort to give her the support and help she needs in this crucial period.

Many women expect to run the house exactly as before they had the baby – indeed many men expect them to as well! Some women feel their partners have already been coping with the other children long enough and need a rest themselves. But be under no illusions: if your partner is to breastfeed successfully, you can be a great help. Obviously you'll have to provide for her in a material sense but she'll need emotional backup too.

Breastfeeding is a deeply emotional business, so try to brush up your skills in empathic listening, putting your own concerns aside for the time being while you're with her, trying to understand how she's feeling, identifying and naming as many of her emotions as you can, and letting her know that you're aware of what's going on for her at an emotional level. It helps most of us if we feel someone understands where we're at. An additional and, usually, longer-term benefit of listening well is that this could help fend off the post-natal depression that can arise in women who feel emotionally alone – even though they may not be physically alone – in their new circumstances.

The majority of women are highly emotional after having a baby, partly because their hormones key them up to respond to their babies. But as well as responding to their baby's every whimper they may also react to the world around them in a way which is atypical for them. Even the most able professional woman who has held down a big job can collapse in tears for no apparent reason. She may even do so because she's so happy! This can be difficult to understand.

Just a word of warning. Be careful what you say. Their men play an important role in whether women carry on with breastfeeding and a casual or thoughtless remark can throw a woman completely and make her feel inadequate. So be especially sensitive.

Research the world over has shown that mammals of many species (and humans are no exception) produce less milk or even none at all if disturbed or stressed while breastfeeding. Serenity fosters successful breastfeeding and having you to listen to how she's feeling will allow her to let off steam and enjoy her baby.

Apart from tending to the home environment, you can protect your partner from well-meaning but ill-informed would-be helpers and, most of all, from herself. Children will be no less demanding now than they were before the baby came and you'll need to keep them amused – or organize others who can keep them amused – so that your partner can rest. It's a shame if a baby hardly gets to know his mother because other people's demands take precedence. However, you can act as a buffer between her and the outside world. Relatives and neighbours may be keen to see the baby, but make sure they come in small doses. Many's the time a recently delivered mother becomes so exhausted from regaling friends with her hospital sagas that she simply hasn't the energy to relate to or feed her new baby well.

Another thing you can provide is encouragement. Studies show that a woman whose partner doesn't want her to breastfeed rarely manages to do so. Even if he's merely 'neutral' the chances of successful feeding are greatly reduced. One American breastfeeding counsellor who actually guarantees success won't accept a woman as a client unless her man approves of breastfeeding. Clearly it's better if your attitude is positive right from the beginning. It can be more difficult to breastfeed than to bottle-feed in the first few days and your partner will need correspondingly more help.

See page 454 for some more ideas on how to be emotionally supportive.

SOME COMMON CONCERNS

Two things that worry men most about breastfeeding (or at least the things they most often talk about, which isn't necessarily the same) are whether their partner will (a) go off sex and (b) lose her figure. There's more about sex and breastfeeding in Chapter 15 but here let's look at the figure question.

Whether breastfeeding experts like it or not, virtually every man today thinks of breasts first and foremost as sex objects. Of course breasts are for feeding babies too, as most men reluctantly agree, but for the forty to sixty or so possible years of a couple's life together their erotic role is much more important most of the time. This makes it foolish to ignore men's fears about their partner having droopy breasts after feeding.

But let's consider what actually happens. All breasts enlarge in pregnancy, regardless of whether the woman is going to breastfeed or not. If she feeds her baby, her breasts are bigger for longer. This can be a real bonus for the man who likes large breasts! Some such men are greatly turned on by the large breasts and erectile nipples of their breastfeeding partner.

Strange as it may seem, research into breast size after breast-feeding is scanty and confused. One study reported that women who breastfed for two weeks or more thought their breasts became slightly droopier. (They also felt that their pleasure from feeding their babies far outweighed this slight change.) Many women certainly find that when they stop breastfeeding their breasts are relatively soft. This is because the milk glands and ducts can shrink in size quite abruptly. However, as the weeks and months pass and body fat redistributes itself, the contours of the breasts gradually return virtually to normal. And a point to remember is that a woman who wears a well-fitting bra by night and day (including late in pregnancy) supports her breasts which are heavy with milk and so prevents the skin over them from stretching. This in itself helps maintain their original shape.

But whatever happens, does it matter anyway? The fashion for perfect breasts is not only a little crazy but also wholly unrealistic because most men don't marry girls out of the centre-spread of *Playboy* in the first place. Breasts quite normally change with age and if breastfeeding hastens this change at all, it's only very slightly. Any man who sees his partner as a pair of walking breasts will have other problems in the relationship which are probably a lot more in need of attention.

YOU AND YOUR BABY

Many fathers like the idea of their partners breastfeeding but feel it leaves them with little they can do for their baby. In fact, some men like the idea of their baby being bottle-fed because they'll be able to give their baby the occasional feed. And at a time in history when increasing numbers of young men feel useless, helpless and even hopeless, feeding their baby is one thing they feel they can do to contribute. This is no real reason for deciding against breast-feeding though, because a father can do innumerable things with his breastfed baby, including cuddling, playing and bathing – all of which are much more fun than bottle-feeding!

Some new fathers feel shut out of the excitement of the first few days. The new mother is so closely involved with her baby that he may feel she and the baby are hogging the limelight, and this is often true to some extent. However, although a new father will have to do more than normal and won't be at centre stage, this can be a wonderful time for him. He can now practise being more self-less and learn how to support his partner in her new role as mother of their child. In many young couples this is a new experience.

Once a baby comes along things change. Now the man will spend a fair amount of time backing his partner up, servicing her, if you like, while she finds her feet as a mother and a breastfeeder. This 'mothering' role comes easily to some men but the majority find it very hard. They may have been used to being serviced by their partner, just as they were by their mother, and cannot easily change gear. Talking all this through can be helpful, and even discussing it with other men can help. Many's the man we have seen who thought all this very unmanly and 'sissy' but who, on listening to the experiences of other men with similar concerns, came to accept and enjoy their new role.

We have found that this caring for the newly breastfeeding mother can build a whole new dimension in a couple's relationship – one in which they pull together as the man grows up from being a big boy, largely supported and serviced by his partner, to a real man who gives as much, or more, than he receives. This can be a quantum leap in their life together.

BENEFITS OF BREASTFEEDING TO YOU

If your baby is breastfed there'll be many benefits to you, apart from the growth in your relationship, that you might not at first have considered.

1 To be totally realistic, you won't have to get up at night to take your turn preparing bottle-feeds – and that's no mean advantage when you're back at work.

2 The family can't run out of milk powder at awkward times and it's one thing less you'll have to buy!

3 Breastfeeding makes extra demands on the mother's body, and even allowing for the cost of extra food if she finds she has to eat more than normal, several studies agree that breastfeeding is less expensive than bottle-feeding.

4 Having a breastfeeding baby means there'll be less baby equipment to carry when you go out anywhere. This makes travelling and going out a lot easier.

5 Last is the pleasure you'll get seeing your partner enjoying the feelings of femininity, fulfilment and intimacy so many women experience with breastfeeding, and knowing you are contributing by being there to back her up. In this sense, breastfeeding is a joint effort, with you as the most important member of the fan club!

LOOKING AFTER YOURSELF

What with all the fuss, commotion and excitement over your new baby, it's all too easy to forget yourself and your needs. When a new baby arrives both the mother and the father have to get used to the physical and emotional demands of a new person and this isn't always easy. You are a very important person and you'll enjoy this time more and have more to give if your well of energy, health and well-being is full. So here's a checklist that might be helpful – of course, you'll add things to it yourself:

• Are you getting enough sleep? If you're waking a lot at night when your baby wakes and your partner breastfeeds, you may find yourself dropping off during the day. Perhaps you could learn to catnap for half an hour or so at work after lunch, or have forty winks in the early evening or when you've helped get any other children to bed.

• Are you getting enough good food? Ensure that you eat healthily so as to keep up your stamina while you are being a support to your partner and new baby.

• Are you looking after yourself outside the home? As a new father you'll benefit from being on tip-top form. Keep up your own interests and hobbies, even if you have to put a few things on ice in the very earliest weeks. There's no need for a man to give up all his interests to become a second mother to the baby. As with so many things in life, balance is everything.

- What about exercise? Time is often a problem at this stage in life but if you work those muscles and get your circulation going you'll enjoy higher levels of 'feel-good' endorphins and keep yourself in trim for your new role.

- Is there someone around for you? Your partner may be too absorbed at present while she's getting used to the new baby and, if it is her first, to motherhood, yet you too may need someone to help as you adjust to your new role. Many men, given the chance, benefit from talking about their feelings on becoming a father, with all the changes and responsibilities of their new lifestyle. Few men find it easy to 'let it all hang out', but a friendly ear, a shared joke and the sense of perspective you get from being with a friend or relative can be a godsend. Getting out with friends can help keep everything in perspective, too.

Helping your partner breastfeed is something that'll bring pleasure to you both and give your baby the best possible start. Taking a lifetime view of being a father, you'll lavish huge amounts of time, money and energy on your children. That journey starts here, so don't underestimate the importance of the time, empathy and affection you can give your partner in these first vital weeks. You can make a big difference to the way you lay the foundations for your new family.

FIFTEEN

Breastfeeding and sex

The juxtaposition of the two words ' breastfeeding' and 'sex' still raises eyebrows, even in a culture in which sex is far from a taboo subject. Indeed, it's hardly possible to open any newspaper or magazine without being confronted by some sort of sexual message. Yet for all this, many men and quite a few women still find it hard to think of the two words in the same sentence.

TWO SORTS OF SEXUALITY?

This has come about because we in the West tend to think of human sexuality as being split into two kinds of activity. The first is raunchy sex, as in 'having sex' and the second a much wider sort of sexuality that includes activities such as giving birth and breastfeeding. Many men, even today, have problems seeing their woman as both 'Madonna' (as good mother) and 'mistress' and breastfeeding is one area of life that suffers as a result.

Two millennia of Judaeo-Christian thought and dogma have created a split in the minds of many people in which a woman can be either a loving, nurturing, 'innocent' Madonna – immortalized in the figure of the Blessed Virgin Mary – or a tarty creature who enjoys sex just for itself. The majority of modern, younger women have embraced the latter concept over the last twenty or thirty years and most now see themselves as having a right to express their sexuality in ways that please them. Such women can easily separate 'fun' (for recreation) sex from 'reproductive' (for procreation) sex. Many men are delighted that this change has occurred but a well-publicized minority are fearful of it.

But a surprising number of women, and certainly their men, have problems coping with the idea that once a woman becomes a mother she somehow ought to shut off her 'sexy' side and become sexless. Several studies, and a large body of clinical experience, show that most women see motherhood as being somewhat 'unsexy'. Even today a substantial number of young women find it hard to accept that their own mothers have sex. And there is a large body of unconscious messages in our culture that tells many women that once they become mothers they somehow enter another world ... one in which sex is no longer for fun and pleasure but for procreation, duty, or whatever they think their own mother does it for.

So it is that many women enter the breastfeeding arena feeling somewhat ambivalent about it from a sexual point of view. Until this stage of their lives they had seen their breasts mainly as sexual objects from which they and their lover obtained pleasure. Now, another more 'biological' function seems to be asserting itself. Confusion reigns.

THE PLEASURES OF BREASTFEEDING

Part of this confusion is that breastfeeding can be a highly pleasurable experience and, for some women, actually arousing. Despite the guilt that such admissions can create, some women say that feeding their baby was one of the more sensual and even erotic experiences of their lives. A few even claim to have orgasms while breastfeeding.

When you think about it, breastfeeding, like intercourse, must have been somewhat pleasurable throughout human history or the race would have died out. If ever there were two things that had to be pleasant, these were they.

But for all of this, the link between sexuality and breastfeeding comes as a real shock to many women. And some don't like the link at all. One of us was broadcasting about this subject once when a woman phoned the radio station to say that she had just vomited at the mention of a woman becoming sexually aroused by feeding her baby. This extreme response reflects in a dramatic way what some women feel about the link between these two life experiences.

A few women admit to feeling more aroused while breast-feeding if their baby is a boy. And some notice that their baby boy occasionally has an erection while feeding. Such discoveries can cause real concern. How, a woman's unconscious may ask, could she possibly cause such a response in her son? Incest is a serious taboo in Western culture and this sort of incident puts some women off breastfeeding, though it's not the sort of thing that's mentioned to researchers enquiring into a woman's reasons for giving up breastfeeding! Feelings of sexual arousal are acceptable to most people – and perhaps particularly to women – only within strict boundaries. And many women consider that feeding their baby definitely comes outside them.

MEN'S AND WOMEN'S VIEWS OF SEXUALITY

But all this denies a large part of a woman's sexuality. Men, by and large, see 'sex' as being about intercourse. In fact numerous studies show that men believe that sex *is* penetrative intercourse, with one or both partners having an orgasm. However, most women say something rather different. To the average woman, sex involves mind, body and spirit. This is not to say that many, especially younger, women do not enjoy sex for its own sake, but that even these women claim that real sex goes a long way beyond this.

The reasons for this difference in perception are many and hotly debated. Clinical experience suggests that there's a fundamental difference because sex means such different things to men and women. Perhaps a helpful way of thinking about this is to say that eggs are expensive and sperm cheap. One man can impregnate many women, his semen is produced every day of his life, and he can easily lose it without biological risk.

Eggs, on the other hand, are produced only once a month and only then throughout a woman's reproductive years, and once pregnant she cannot become so again for a long time. If she breastfeeds on an unrestricted basis this could be as long as a year or more. A woman's eggs are clearly much more valuable to her and to the survival of the human race than are a man's sperm.

As a result, the commitment a woman makes to any single act of intercourse is, in biological terms, far greater than that made by a man. This has meant that over the millions of years that couples have been having intercourse, women have found it more meaningful and fateful for them. After all, it is they who carry and nurture babies, not men.

In this context, it's easy to see how breastfeeding, as part of a woman's whole sexual life, carries rather different meanings to men and women. To many men it's simply a superior way of feeding their baby, whilst to a woman, it can be an extension of her initial commitment to intercourse with a particular man, a commitment that in some mystical, let alone practical sense, lasts a lifetime, once they produce another human being together.

Women living in traditional cultures are ruled by their cycles. And in such cultures breastfeeding is still the most powerful contraceptive. Even today it is the world's most important form of contraception as a fully breastfeeding woman's cycles can be suppressed for well over a year (see page 123). Many millions of women the world over are pregnant or lactating for most of their reproductive lives, so, to them, breastfeeding is as much a part of being a woman as having periods is to a Western woman.

Today's Western woman, though, doesn't want to be ruled by her cycles, and social changes have meant that she does not seek to have babies every two or three years. On the contrary, she spends much of her reproductive life avoiding pregnancy. Modern women want to behave increasingly more like men and this involves having scanty or no periods (the Pill ensures this very effectively) and very few babies. One of us recently carried out a survey of women's attitudes to their bodies. It was illuminating that the thing that the hundreds of women who took part said they most hated about their bodies was a fat tummy, followed by big hips. Today's trend towards women looking flat-bellied, slim, and even masculine in body style goes hand in hand with their, probably largely unconscious, denial of their femaleness in an effort to become and behave more like men.

Many readers will doubtless be starting to get annoyed at all this because they may well feel that we are claiming that women should remain shackled to their hormones. But this is not the case. What is a *fact* is that men and women *are* different and that their definition of what sex means and the impact of it on their lives is understandably different as a result. And most women still feel an urge to experience the whole range of female sexuality which, of course, includes pregnancy, birth and breastfeeding. A major potential part of a woman's sexual life is incomplete if she never becomes pregnant. And some women would add, 'and never breastfeeds'.

Once we accept that a woman's whole sexual makeup revolves around her hormones we're in a much better position to understand how breastfeeding can work to her advantage and to that of her partner.

Although few people realize it, there's a considerable similarity between a woman's periods, pregnancies, orgasms and lactation. For a start, during all of these her breasts become larger. Many women say that they feel protective or 'motherly' after intercourse, after giving birth and when they are feeding their baby. And this is no accident because during all of these events the level of oxytocin, a powerful sex hormone (see page 19), increases in a woman's blood.

BREASTS AND WHAT THEY REPRESENT

Today, breasts have become *the* erotic focus for millions of Western men. This is now engrained in the fabric of our society. Advertisers and anyone else who seeks our attention cash in on this indisputable fact. It is interesting in this respect that humans are the only mammals that develop breasts in advance of their being needed to feed the young. This said, many cultures around the world do not eroticize the breasts in the way we do. It is noticeable that most such cultures breastfeed their babies for very long periods. Could it be that, as a society, we have become so deprived over the last century of the experience of being comforted and nourished at the breast – and so habituated to seeing images of the eroticised and 'unmotherly' breast – that we seek to replace those unmet infantile needs and primitive drives in other ways, albeit very much later in life? Such ways could, perhaps, include compulsive behaviours such as over-eating and promiscuous sex, and the various methods of 'oral gratification', including smoking and drinking.

With both men and women putting such emphasis on breasts as sex objects it's hardly surprising that erotic overtones can militate against breastfeeding way before a couple even get pregnant. Many studies have shown that some women won't even consider breastfeeding because they believe it will ruin their figures and so render them sexually unattractive. One of us was an agony columnist for many years, and breast size and style were among the commonest concerns that women wrote in about.

BREASTFEEDING AND YOUR SEXUAL
RELATIONSHIP

More than half of all women claim that their breasts are highly pleasurable to them, either when they masturbate or when they make love. Some experience orgasms with breast-play alone. This is hardly surprising, given that the nipples and genitals are interconnected by nervous pathways in the brain. This 'magic triangle' of nipples and clitoris can be triggered at any corner. Nipple stimulation can make a woman's clitoris enlarge and her uterus contract; and stimulation of her clitoris can arouse her nipples and breasts.

All of this means that the nipple stimulation of breastfeeding keeps many a woman in a continuously repeated state of arousal or semi-arousal. The medical literature has hotly debated whether a lactating woman feels more sexy than her bottle-feeding sister, and there is evidence both ways. The problem with all such research, though, is that there are so many variables. This means that studies trying to assess the true situation are often confounded right from the start because they are simply not comparing like with like.

The suppression of ovulation that occurs with long-term breast-feeding has been claimed to be a cause for the reduced sex drive and dry vagina reported by some breastfeeding women. But this has to be offset against the very real advantage of not having to be concerned about an unwanted pregnancy, or affected by the side-effects of contraceptives. Both these put at least some women off returning to sex in the months after a baby.

It's highly likely that it will be impossible to arrive at any meaningful conclusions about sexual desire in breastfeeding women because the scale and complexity of the study needed would be so great. At the simplest level, one woman's definition of 'breastfeeding' can be very different from another's and the effects on any given woman's body and hormones by the same type of breastfeeding so varied. Perhaps the answers to the differences between women and even within any individual woman can be explained in ways which have little or nothing to do with physiological changes.

It's inevitable that a woman's unconscious plays a large part. First, research shows that many women, breastfeeding or not, are unaware of their levels of arousal. In other words, some women can be highly aroused without knowing. Second, if at a deep, unconscious, level a woman believes that such sexual feelings are unacceptable or inappropriate in the context of feeding her baby, she will tend to 'un-know' or suppress them.

But for many women the experience of breastfeeding *is* a highly pleasurable one at not only a sensual level but also an erotic one. And, as with all facets of female sexuality, the experience can be different from occasion to occasion, according to what is going on in her life and with her hormones. So it is that some women say they feel really turned on by breastfeeding one day and completely unaffected the next.

Of course the *experience* of any given level of arousal is also very variable. Some women report that they feel simply 'nice'; others that they are aware of increased vaginal wetness; and a few that they could have a climax. Most mothers claim that they feel euphoric or contented after a feed in a way that is very parallel to their emotions after an orgasm.

Some women claim that these experiences enhance their feelings towards their man. In fact, some studies have found that breast-feeding mothers get back to sex earlier after birth than do other women. It could, of course, be that women who choose to breast-feed, especially long-term, are different in some profound sexual sense from those who do not. Clinical experience shows that this can work in both directions, with some unconsciously using their long-term commitment to their baby as a way of avoiding intimacy in their pair-bonded relationship, and others unconsciously doing exactly the opposite.

But however much pleasure and reward, be it at a mind, body or spiritual level, a woman gets from feeding her baby, her partner may not see it as entirely positive. Many men tell us how they resent their baby intruding into their sexual life. Probably many a woman fails to feed her baby, or decides not to start at all, because her partner puts her off in all kinds of subtle ways – though, to be fair, mainly unconsciously. In any human endeavour there are bound to be setbacks and bad moments. How our partner deals with these greatly affects how we proceed. And this doesn't only apply to breastfeeding – we might be discussing learning to drive, making a special meal, or whatever. A partner who encourages you when the going gets tough is likely to help make the endeavour succeed in the end. One who, for whatever reasons of his own, and many of them are entirely unconscious, cannot encourage his partner, sends unspoken messages that make it likely she'll fail.

In a culture such as ours in which a woman's breasts are seen as largely the erotic property of the couple, it's hardly surprising that millions of men are ready to jump in and declare breastfeeding a failure, a waste of time, a nuisance, or whatever, so that they can get back to the status quo.

The only way to make breastfeeding work in any one relationship is for the woman to make it clear that her man is still central and important in her life. This may not be at all easy because many men are really little boys just beneath the surface and some even give an overt 'It's the baby or me' ultimatum. A loving couple can usually sort all this out provided that they address the sexuality of the situation honestly. The real danger occurs when a woman turns herself into a cow-like figure who goes off sex and leaves her man feeling rejected and abandoned. He too has a responsibility in all this which he can show by trying to become open and aware enough to share his feelings rather than act them out in unhelpful and inappropriate ways, such as by having an affair in an effort to find the love he fears he has lost.

Some women feel less sexy during the months of breastfeeding and some more sexy. They may feel different from one baby to another, or during any one lactation. Perhaps the worst killer of sexual desire is tiredness, so if your baby wakes often at night, consider having him in or right by bed so you can easily feed him without having to wake up properly (see page 217). You can even make love with your baby alongside you if you wish. Some women say that having the two people she loves so much alongside her as she makes love adds a whole new meaning to sex.

What works best, then, is to involve your man in the fun side of breastfeeding. He can play with your breasts as he did before and even drink your milk if that's okay with you both.

Many women are shy of their breasts, some even in front of their partner. If a woman's increased bust size makes her feel more sexy, as some claim, then she may well want to show off her 'new' boobs to her man. This can turn a breast-negative woman into a breast-positive one. But the opposite can also occur, with some women saying that they feel huge, cow-like, leaky and so on, and that these sorts of things make them feel anything but sexy or attractive.

The perception of her breasts as an intrinsic part of the sensuality and sexuality of breastfeeding applies whether a woman has a lover or not. If she feels more womanly and female because of her larger breasts, or revolting and revolted by them, her whole perception of breastfeeding will be different and its chances of success correspondingly different, whatever the responses and opinions of her partner.

By and large it's fair to say that breastfeeding succeeds best if a woman is 'breast-positive'. Such a woman likes her breasts; enjoys them being played with and touched by herself and her man; and sees them as a vital part of her femaleness and femininity. A US study twenty years ago found that women who had sexual hang-ups were much less likely to breastfeed successfully. Other studies looking at women's reasons for failing to feed as they intended have discovered that a substantial minority did not do so because they found the whole thing 'distasteful' or 'immodest' in some way. Such women see their breasts as extremely private, even sometimes when with their lover, and even the thought of having to expose them other than for the purposes of washing or medical examination is unacceptable.

Then there are women who say that they are actually revolted at the thought of 'something sucking at them'. I (AS) have heard women express real horror at this. They say it all seems too animal-like, too primitive, not what they want at all. It's difficult outside the consulting room to convince such a woman that breastfeeding is for her ... the roots of such feelings are often very deep indeed and may call for depth psychotherapy if they are to be modified. Such therapy frequently unearths a deeply unconscious anger or revulsion towards breast sensations, or breasts in general, some of which may go back to the woman's own babyhood experiences of her mother's 'wicked, punishing breasts'.

But even a very breast-positive woman can have problems. Simply being a new mother, perhaps suffering from repeated sleepless nights, can make sex seem unattractive because of exhaustion.

Other women find that their swollen breasts are too tender for their man to touch, even if they both very much want him to; and yet others dislike the leaking that occurs as they become aroused or have a climax with their lover. A way around some of these problems is to encourage your man to suck your nipples before you start to make love. There's no need to worry about him stealing milk from the baby – there's plenty for both. Simply taking the pressure off your breasts before you start to make love can do the trick and will certainly help get you aroused. If your man won't do this you could express some milk yourself (see page 189).

Once you start making love again you'll probably notice quite a few changes. Some women complain that their nipples don't erect like they used to. This is, in fact, an illusion because when you're breastfeeding your nipples are always slightly more erect than usual and your breasts somewhat swollen already. Other women who like the way their breasts swell during arousal say that this doesn't happen any more. Once more, this is because their breasts are already somewhat swollen and so don't increase in size as before. Some couples change the positions in which they make love if their old favourites put pressure on swollen or tender breasts. A little thought, discussion and care can usually overcome such practical problems.

Having said all this, a couple's sexual life doesn't just revolve around *physical* sensations and pleasures. Many women say that their *emotional* response to their man changes as a result of having a baby, breastfeeding or both. For some women the experience of being a mother, of having the total responsibility for a baby and all the other pressures of, especially first-time, motherhood, is simply too much and they go off sex because they are so anxious. Other women find that the relationship with their new baby and the sensations they experience with feeding are so powerful and fulfilling that they no longer need the sorts of sensual and erotic experiences they used to have with their man. Such a woman often turns her sexuality inwards to focus almost entirely on the mother–baby relationship. Her partner, understandably, feels excluded.

To some extent this sort of intense interest in a new baby is normal, especially for a first-time mother. But by no means all of the new experiences are positive or likely to create benefits for her adult relationship. In other words, ambivalence often rears its head, with many a woman saying that the level of intimacy she feels in the relationship with her baby stands in stark contrast to the poverty of the intimacy bond with her man. It is easy to see how such a bond with her baby can be much more rewarding to such a woman. Her man has every reason to feel left out because he *is* being excluded. This sort of dilemma is the very stuff of therapy with breastfeeding couples and calls for skilful handling.

But much of this can be better dealt with, or even prevented altogether, if you do some preparatory work together as a couple to get ready for breastfeeding. Needless to say, a well-balanced relationship between mother and father gives their baby the very best chance of being successfully breastfed. Any healing of the man's over-readiness to perceive rejection where it is not intended; any preparation for the realities of sharing his partner's body with his baby; any understanding of one another's deepest sexuality, as opposed to simply genital behaviour, all help to get things off to a good start. But none of this comes about by chance. It calls for a degree of openness and frankness from both of you as you enter this new phase of your sexual life together.

The foundations for successful breastfeeding are laid in a woman's early experiences with men. If she learns to value and enjoy her breasts in her sexual relationships then they'll already be receptive to the changing experiences of breastfeeding. When a woman is pregnant her man can make breast-play an even more important part of their games together. There's no physical or mechanical reason for any breast preparation during pregnancy. However, if a woman rolls her nipples when she washes her breasts, or when she is masturbating, and if her man sucks them and rolls them in his fingers and mouth during love-making, it may help by encouraging the woman to become more breast-positive than she might otherwise be.

Once you eventually have your baby, be sure to involve your man in your enjoyment of breastfeeding, if that's what he wants. Central to this is keeping up some aspects of your 'mistress' image. Many men have good cause for believing that their partner has gone off them in favour of mothering, because these are exactly the messages that she gives. Of course, for certain women this is just what they unconsciously, or perhaps even consciously, wanted all along. After all, not every relationship is a good one and many women over the years have told us that the rewards they had from their relationship with their baby enabled them to stay with their man. The new experience of being wanted, special and needed by another human being so sharply contrasts with their experience within their pair-bonded relationship that it is indeed preferable to what their man can offer. If this seems to be an issue for you, it's probably wise to seek professional help to mend your relationship with your man rather than to 'abuse' your relationship with your baby.

As with most areas of life, honest communication is at the heart of real success. Almost every woman *can* breastfeed if she wants to. And this really is true, as our experience with thousands of couples bears out. However, it's also true that the relationship between the man and woman who created the baby is central to the success of the whole venture. Just imagine going on a major mountaineering expedition with people you didn't like, or actually had problems getting on with. The whole adventure would be unenjoyable at best and could even fail as a result. It's exactly the same with breastfeeding.

In today's world it can often take more than a well-meaning, informed and hopeful mother to make breastfeeding a success. Most women, in the absence of their mother or other older woman to help, have to look somewhere for an ally. For many this can be their partner. A large proportion of couples who make their breastfeeding experiences a source of growth together and an extension of their sexual life together succeed in nourishing not only their baby but also their one-to-one relationship.

Breastfeeding by definition involves a woman's breasts. Her feelings and those of her partner about not only this part of her body but her body in general and her sexuality as a whole inevitably affect her breastfeeding experiences. Many couples find that breastfeeding enriches their sexual insights and broadens their relationship.

SIXTEEN

Feeding the older baby

WEANING

The verb 'to wean' comes from an old English word meaning 'to accustom'. Many people think of weaning only as weaning from the breast – gradually stopping breastfeeding as they introduce other foods and drinks. However, it can also be applied to the process of getting a baby used to other foods while still breastfeeding, and that's what we'll do here. Just because you start giving your baby tastes of family food doesn't mean you have to start weaning him *from* the breast!

When, how and why you start giving other foods and drinks, and when, how and why you stop breastfeeding are mostly up to you and your baby. Here are some thoughts to help you on your way.

STARTING OTHER FOODS AND DRINKS

The day you give your baby something other than your milk for the first time is special and represents an important milestone. Some babies take to other foods and drinks enthusiastically; others are less eager, especially at first.

How do you start?

There are two ways of starting other foods and drinks:

1 Wait until your baby shows an interest in the food the family eats and let him touch it and/or pick some.
2 Give him a teaspoonful of suitably prepared food.

When do you start solids?

Official guidelines point out that breast milk *alone* is the best food for almost all babies for the first four months. They suggest offering foods other than breast milk (traditionally called 'solids') no earlier than four months.

The guidelines also recommend that if a baby has a family history of allergy or of coeliac disease (sensitivity to gluten, a protein found in wheat, oats, barley and rye), the mother should breastfeed for at least six months, avoid giving any foods before four months, and avoid giving any foods 'traditionally regarded as allergenic' before six months at the earliest.

However, some women don't know about these guidelines and others take little notice.

— In the Republic of Ireland as many as 11 per cent of one-month-old babies are already on solids.
— In Britain 3 per cent of babies are on solids by one month.
— By three months an astonishing 68 per cent of British babies are on solids; by four months, 94 per cent; and by six months, 99 per cent.

Whatever your friends do, it's better to wait until your baby is four months old before you start him on solids.

When's the latest you should start solids?

Many babies benefit from having solids in addition to breast milk by the time they are eight months old. Some, though, are satisfied and well-nourished on breast milk alone for longer.

There's no need to offer spoonfuls of food before six months, if your baby is thriving, unless you want to, as breast milk easily provides adequate amounts of nutrients for most babies until then.

Many babies who are allowed to decide for themselves when they want to start finger-feeding don't begin until around six months. This, perhaps coincidentally or perhaps not, is when many babies get their first tooth.

If left to themselves, some babies prefer to carry on with breast milk alone for longer than six months.

Surveys suggest that more women nowadays continue with exclusive breastfeeding for longer periods before starting solids. Much depends on the individual mother–baby pair and on factors such as the size of the baby and the amount of milk his mother produces. (This, in turn, depends partly on whether she knows how to increase her milk supply when her baby needs more milk.)

Studies in Africa and in Australia suggest that exclusive breastfeeding is adequate for some babies for as long as fifteen months.

Developing countries

Several surveys indicate that both fully and partially breastfed babies in developing countries are remarkably much less likely to develop infective diarrhoea than babies who have been completely or partly weaned from the breast. This may be partly because the mothers don't have access to enough suitable weaning foods, which means that babies weaned from the breast become malnourished and more likely to succumb to infection. They may also not have the facilities (fuel, water, adequate sanitation, and so on) to prepare foods hygienically. Whatever the cause, this diarrhoea is sometimes fatal and kills over a million babies each year worldwide.

Pre-term babies

A pre-term baby may not have sufficient stores of iron. The iron stores in a baby's liver increase most rapidly in the last few weeks of a full-term pregnancy, so a baby born early has smaller stores. The smaller the baby, the lower the iron stores.

Pre-term bottle-fed babies are more likely to become anaemic than pre-term breastfed ones. This is because although there's more iron in cows' milk formula than in breast milk, iron is better absorbed from the latter. However, some breastfed pre-term babies do eventually become anaemic, so your doctor will recommend iron supplements if necessary.

HOW LONG DO YOU GO ON BREASTFEEDING?

Carry on breastfeeding for as long as your baby is thriving, happy and gaining weight, and as long as you both enjoy it. Provided that he feeds fairly frequently, you'll go on producing milk for a long time. It isn't unusual for women who breastfeed into the second year to make a pint of milk a day.

Official recommendations about how long to continue breast-feeding differ. For example, both UNICEF and the World Health Organization recommend breastfeeding for two years or more. The American Academy of Pediatrics recommends one year. However, an anthropologist from Texas who has studied weaning times in different mammals suggests that it might be more appropriate if human babies were breastfed for a minimum of two and a half years and a maximum of seven.

— In the US today 5 per cent of mothers of six-month-old babies are breastfeeding.
— In Britain (1990) the comparable figure is 20 per cent. And at nine months, 11 per cent.
— However, 70 per cent of the world's mothers breastfeed for more than nine months and the average baby in a developing country is breastfed for two to three years.
— In England just three generations ago, at the turn of the century, a great many women breastfed for at least nine months and many for a year. Some continued for longer.

There are two major advantages of continuing to breastfeed after six months, even though your baby is probably having other foods and drinks by then:

- Your baby will go on receiving protection against infection. In developed countries full breastfeeding gives this advantage up to eight months.
- You and your baby probably enjoy feed times together. Breast-feeding offers emotional as well as nutritional sustenance and an older baby often turns to the breast for comfort when upset.
- You may reduce your risk of pre-menopausal cancer of the breast, cancer of the ovary, rheumatoid arthritiis and osteoporosis in later life.

Some women take a unilateral decision about when to stop breastfeeding. Many experience feelings of loss when they give the last breastfeed. Some also remember their anguish and their baby's tears and frustration when they stopped breastfeeding because they felt it was the right time.

Others take their cue from their baby and make a joint decision. And some let their baby decide.

Baby-led weaning from the breast

'Baby-led' weaning means letting your baby decide when he wants to stop feeding, whether this is at nine months or even later. Some babies lose interest in the breast relatively soon, others want to go on much longer and some don't seem to want to give it up at all.

Sudden baby-led weaning

A happily and fully breastfed baby may suddenly refuse to feed. There may be an obvious reason, such as his nose being blocked by a cold, or teething, or an unpleasant experience (such as a loud noise) while at the breast. At other times there's no apparent cause. Nourish him by giving your expressed or pumped milk in a feeding cup for the time being but offer the breast before and after each cup feed. He may be having a temporary 'nursing strike'.

HOW LONG WILL YOUR MILK LAST?

Your milk supply will last as long as you want if breast milk is the major source of your baby's fluid intake. However, as soon as you give him meaningful amounts of other drinks and only one or two breastfeeds a day, your milk will slowly dry up. Having said that, some women continue with only one feed a day for many months.

There's no hard-and-fast rule about how long a woman will produce milk. As long as your baby stimulates your breasts, they'll produce milk. Wet nurses used to feed one baby after the other for years on end and many mothers the world over feed their children for several years. The Western idea that milk automatically dries up after a few months is totally wrong.

HOW TO STOP BREASTFEEDING

If you want – or have – to stop breastfeeding, it's far easier if you do it gradually, almost without thinking. If you try to stop quickly, you may have a fractious baby and painful, engorged breasts. There's no place for drying-up pills today (see page 289).

1 Give up first the feed at which you have least milk. Most women find this is in the later afternoon or early evening. Give your baby something else to drink. If you have to wean early, remember that young babies benefit from sucking so a bottle may be better than a cup.
2 After a week or so, give up another feed. Carry on cutting out one more feed every week or so until you are feeding only once a day. You may find it's most comfortable to give up the early morning feed last, as you'll probably have most milk at this feed. Some mothers prefer to stop the final feed of the day last, as their babies enjoy this the most and sleep well afterwards.

Weaning is best unhurried and unworried. Don't wean in an emergency if you can possibly avoid it. Your baby will find it very hard to understand why he is suddenly denied the breast and might be upset for some time.

If he asks for a feed by nuzzling against your breast several days after you've stopped feeding him, and you let him suck, he'll soon realize there's little, if any, milk there – although he may want to have a go anyway.

Don't forget that if you find yourself wishing you hadn't stopped so soon you can take steps to increase your milk supply (see page 271).

WHAT SHOULD YOUR BABY EAT?

Good first foods include suitably prepared potato, apple, rice and carrot.

Finger-foods

If your baby's first foods are 'finger-foods' – foods he can pick up and suck on, chew or bite – there's a big choice. Try any raw fruit, such as a large piece of peeled apple, a rusk of baked wholemeal bread, or anything hard that won't be likely to break into pieces and choke him. He'll probably like the taste and will eat some of it by gradually dissolving it in his mouth.

Spoonfuls of food

If you begin with spoonfuls of food, remember that it must be soft enough to swallow easily because babies don't start to chew efficiently until they're around six months.

A healthy diet

At first your baby will still get nearly all his nourishment from your milk. This means you needn't worry about balancing his diet until he's eating more solids and breast milk plays a less important role.

Go easy on added sugar. Sugar can encourage tooth decay, without contributing any worthwhile or irreplaceable nutrients. The natural sugars in fruit and vegetables often taste pleasantly sweet anyway. Having said this, the occasional food sweetened with added sugar won't hurt. But it's better not to give sweetened drinks or snacks between meals or at bedtime.

Another thing best avoided is salt. Salt can be dangerous for a young baby if given in excess. Older babies enjoy food just as much without added salt and lose nothing by not having it.

Similarly, it's better to give your baby foods made from whole grains which contain unrefined carbohydrate. There's no need for him to have any refined flour, be it in rusks, bread, biscuits, puddings or cakes. Again, the occasional food made with refined flour won't hurt.

Commercial baby foods

By and large, manufacturers of commercially prepared baby foods are now very careful not to add too much sugar and salt.

Nowadays most mothers in industrialized countries – indeed, up to as many as 95 per cent – give their babies some commercially prepared foods from tins, jars or packets. But if you prefer, you can simply give your baby whatever you are going to eat, but mashed or sieved first. This is cheaper than buying commercial baby foods.

— By far the most popular first foods in the UK are rice and other cereals and rusks.

DRINKS

What drinks should your baby have to supplement the fluid from your milk as you start weaning him from the breast?

Water – Your baby will do very well if you give him only water to drink.

Fruit juice – If you want to try something other than water for a change, how about the juice of an orange diluted with water or on its own? Orange juice is best given at mealtimes, when its vitamin C encourages iron absorption from other foods. If given between meals, or at bedtime, its acid and sugar can encourage tooth decay. Apple juice is a popular drink too.

Fruit squashes or diluted syrups – Orange squash or blackcurrant syrup diluted with water are popular drinks for babies. However, syrups and most squashes contain a lot of sugar and, because they are sugary and slightly acidic, they are likely to cause tooth decay. While some contain vitamin C, not all do and many contain no natural fruit juice at all.

Herbal baby drinks – These are surprisingly popular but dentists warn that even if they contain little sugar, they encourage tooth decay if given between meals or at bedtime – especially from a bottle. This can happen even before the very first tooth shows through the gums. Dentists say that fruit-containing herbal drinks are the worst culprits for damaging teeth.

Cows' milk – Does a baby need cows' milk during weaning or after being weaned from the breast? The simple answer is, it depends.

Breast milk provides babies with an excellent balance of nutrients and you'll need to be sure that when you wean your baby he continues to have all the nutrients he needs.

In developing countries, babies have traditionally been weaned from the breast on to a diet which doesn't include cows' milk. However, they tend to get the benefit of breast milk for a far longer time than infants in developed countries.

In many developed countries in which the traditional diet includes cows' milk and other dairy foods, women are used to incorporating milk into their family's diet. Indeed, most expect to give their babies cows' milk and might find it difficult, without extra information or help, to know how to ensure that their baby gets a balanced diet, with enough fat and calcium particularly, without it. Cows' milk comes in many forms – as formula (pre-term, standard and 'follow-on' – for babies over six months) and as full-cream, semi-skimmed and skimmed milk.

Whether or not you give cows' milk depends on your baby's age and stage and on whether his drinks need to provide nutrients or just fluid. If you stop breastfeeding before four to six months (the minimum age recommended), you can replace your breast milk with cows' milk formula.

Formula provides nutrients for those young babies under four to six months who no longer have the benefits of breast milk. You can carry on giving formula until a year as a part of your older baby's diet; or you could give follow-on milk after six months and until a year. You can give your baby a little full-cream cows' milk in cooked foods after six months if you find he can easily digest it.

Cows' milk is a particularly good source of calcium and fat. Growing babies need more fat in their diet than do older children and adults, so giving your older baby some milk each day in addition to your family food readily fills this need. Semi-skimmed milk is unsuitable for children under two and skimmed milk is unsuitable for children under five.

FOOD SUPPLEMENTS

Fluoride – If you live in an area with low levels of fluoride in the drinking water, your doctor or dentist may recommend fluoride supplements in the form of tablets or drops. Ask your dentist about the local water and the amount of fluoride necess-ary, if any. Adequate levels of fluoride can cut tooth decay by half.

Children's vitamin drops – Most children don't need vitamins, but in countries such as the UK, vitamins A, C and D are recommended for all children (aged from six months up to at least two years and preferably to five years) as an insurance to protect those who do. Some breastfed babies need them because of illness, because their mothers aren't eating a healthy diet, or because neither the babies nor their mothers spend time outside in the open air each day (see below). Ask your doctor or other professional adviser for advice about your baby.

The majority of breastfeeding women neither take vitamin supplements themselves nor give supplements to their babies. These women need to be doubly sure that they protect themselves and their breastfeeding babies by eating a healthy diet and by spending some time outside each day with their babies so that both benefit from daylight directly on their skin. This is the best way of ensuring you both get enough vitamin D.

BREASTFEEDING THE OLDER CHILD

Some women breastfeed into their baby's second year or until they are two, three or even older. Breastfeeding an older child is more important for psychological comfort and pleasure than for its nutritional value as (in industrialized countries) this is by then usually supplied by other foods.

A child may feed primarily to get off to sleep, or during the night. Or there may be little pattern to feeds: he comes for a drink when he feels like cuddling and being close to his mother, perhaps when he's upset or tired.

You may notice a difficult patch between four and six months when you wonder whether you want to go on. There are several reasons why you may feel this way. First, you may be feeling much livelier in yourself and want to get going again in the outside world. Second, your baby probably wants more attention, is more aware and may cry more. Third, he may want more to eat and make you feel you haven't got enough milk. Lastly, you may have become disenchanted with breastfeeding and perhaps even feel it's going to go on for ever.

If you've had enough, give up gradually, as suggested earlier. It's better to stop breastfeeding and continue developing a loving relationship with your baby than to resent feeding him.

If you continue breastfeeding as your baby passes the one-year stage, your main problem will probably be coping with uncalled-for criticism from friends, neighbours and relatives. Many will be surprised that you want to go on long after other mothers have stopped! This can be off-putting but if you and your baby want to continue, it's up to you. To spare their amazement and even criticism – and your embarrassment – you may like to feed your older baby alone. It's scarcely surprising that a society which finds it hard to cope with the sight of a young baby being breastfed finds it even more difficult to cope with an older one. If your child tugs at your clothes or asks for a feed when you are out visiting, go into another room to feed him if you prefer. But don't make him feel there's anything shameful in what he's doing.

Just how long you go on for is a matter of personal choice. But however long you feed your baby, you'll know you've done your best for him and you'll probably have had a lot of pleasure yourself.

CAN YOU BREASTFEED DURING A PERIOD?

Breastfeeding during a period won't harm you or your baby. Some women say their babies are rather fractious around period time. This may be because they have pre-menstrual tension which their babies sense. Some babies have slight diarrhoea for a couple of days; others may seem to dislike the taste of the milk.

Changes in milk volume may occur during a period because of the alteration in the blood-flow through the breasts.

Breast milk can change in composition in the middle of the menstrual cycle (see page 156).

CAN YOU BREASTFEED IF YOU'RE PREGNANT?

You can breastfeed right through pregnancy if you want. Some pregnant women find their breasts are more tender than usual, while others simply don't like the idea of their older baby or child breastfeeding.

Others find that their breast milk decreases in pregnancy. This is probably because their pregnancy hormones affect milk production. A month before the end of pregnancy the milk supply automatically increases. The milk changes in quality during pregnancy to become richer in vitamins and fats.

BREASTFEEDING AN OLDER CHILD AND A BABY

You can carry on feeding your toddler when your new baby arrives if you want. However, let the baby have first call on your milk.

Some people in developing countries don't have enough food for the family, so weaning an older child from the breast is hazardous (see page 65).

Breastfeeding two children of different ages is known as tandem nursing.

The way to breastfeed and to wean your older baby is to be led as far as possible by him, by sensible guidelines and by common sense.

Appendix

RECOMMENDED READING LIST

When reading anything written with the aim of helping you feed, bring up or look after your child, remember that the information is there for you to sift and use if it seems right for you and your family. No author can get everything right and certainly no author can address himself to each individual reader. It's up to you to read what seems most suitable, to discuss it with friends, family, professional advisers and counsellors, and then to act on a mixture of this information plus a good helping of common sense.

The New Mothercare Guide to Pregnancy and Babycare, ed. Penny Stanway (Conran Octopus)
The Politics of Breastfeeding, by Gabrielle Palmer (Pandora)
The Complete Guide to Child Health, by Penny Stanway (Conran Octopus)
Breastfeeding: A Guide for the Medical Profession, by Ruth A. Lawrence (C.V. Mosby Company)
Breastfeeding: A Guide for Midwives, by Dora Henschel and Sally Inch (Butterworth Heinemann)

From La Leche League (*see pages 453 and 454*)

The Womanly Art of Breastfeeding (LLL)
Nursing Your Baby, by Karen Prior
The Nursing Mother's Guide to Weaning, by Kathlene Huggins and Linda Ziedrich

A Manual of Natural Family Planning, by Anna Flynn and M. Brooks
(recommended by the Family Planning Association)
The Continuum Concept, by Jean Liedloff (Futura)
Three in a Bed, by Deborah Jackson
Breastfeeding the Adopted Baby, by D. Petersen

LLL also sells a wide variety of leaflets, e.g.:
Increasing Your Milk
Positioning Your Baby
When You Breastfeed Your Baby – The First Week
Crying: Why and What to Do
Breastfeeding and Sexuality
The Breastfeeding Father
Does Breastfeeding Take Too Much Time?
Nursing with Breast Implants
Breastfeeding Your Premature Baby
Breastfeeding the Down's Syndrome Baby

From NCT Maternity Sales (*see page 453*)

Bestfeeding: Getting Breastfeeding Right for You, by Mary Renfrew,
Chloe Fisher and Suzanne Arms
Successful Breastfeeding, Royal College of Midwives (a detailed
guide for those supporting breastfeeding mothers)

NCT Maternity Sales also sells a variety of leaflets, eg:
Breastfeeding after a Caesarean Section
Breastfeeding – Too Much Milk?
Breastfeeding Twins, Triplets or More, by TAMBA (the Twins and
Multiple Births Association – see page 358)
Breastfeeding – Returning to Work

From ACE Graphics
PO Box 173, Sevenoaks, Kent TN14 7EZ

Drugs and Breastfeeding Guide 1994/95, by Jane Colvin
I've Had Enough, by Neil Matterson (a delightful book of sixty
breastfeeding cartoons)

Protecting, Promoting and Supporting Breastfeeding, The Handbook of the New Zealand College of Midwives

BREAST PUMPS

(Addresses, phone numbers and prices correct at time of going to press)

Breast pumps are necessary only in certain situations (see below) and most breastfeeding mothers never need to use one. However good a pump is, it's never as effective at milking the breast and stimulating the milk supply as is a healthy baby. And research shows that hand-expression stimulates the milk supply better than does an electric pump. If it seems likely that breastfeeding will be impossible for some weeks, for example with a very small pre-term baby, then electric pumping may help as it can be less tiring for a woman than prolonged hand-expression or hand pumping. However, it's wise to hand-express as often as possible to stimulate your milk supply.

Using a pump

Before using an electric pump, all the parts that come into contact with milk must be sterilized. This protects your baby and your nipples from infection from infected milk residues.

Position the flange (the funnel-shaped receiving end of the pump) so that your nipple rests at the inside of the upper part. During pumping, your nipple is drawn in and out. The contact with the side of the flange encourages the let-down of the milk. Spread the first few drops of milk over the skin in contact with the flange so that it can slide over the skin easily. Don't press the flange too tightly against your breast as this could obstruct the milk ducts or reservoirs. It's sensible to try to start the let-down of the milk before you begin using the pump by gently and rhythmically massaging your breast and by hand-expressing. Massaging your breast while the pump is on helps the milk flow and encourages further let-downs.

Change over to the other breast when the milk flow diminishes or stops. You can change from one breast to another several times during a pumping session, just as you would when hand expressing, or with a baby at your breast. At first you may collect only very small amounts of milk (perhaps only a quarter of an ounce or 7–8ml). It's a good idea to finish a pumping session by hand expressing the last little bit of milk as this will be the richest milk.

Because pumping is not as good as a baby at stimulating your milk supply, you'll need to use the pump at least as often as a baby would generally want a feed. Four-hourly is rarely enough – it's better to aim for a minimum of eight to ten sessions a day (two- to three-hourly). As long as your nipples don't become sore, you should be able to increase your milk supply by pumping more often and for longer each time, as the increased breast stimulation will increase your prolactin level (see page 16).

You might need a breast pump:

- When your baby is too immature or unwell to get milk from the breast directly.
- If you are taking essential medications which might pass into your milk and harm your baby. Throw away your pumped milk but keep your milk supply going by frequent, regular pumping and hand-expression until you are off the drugs and can breastfeed again.
- If you have a serious infection which temporarily precludes your baby having your milk. Throw away your pumped milk but keep your milk supply going by frequent, regular pumping and hand expression until your infection is under control and you can breast-feed again.
- If your baby has to stay in hospital without you (or vice versa). You can pump your milk for the baby to have by cup (or spoon or tube, but preferably not by bottle).
- If you are building up your milk supply before taking delivery of an adopted baby.
- If you are building up your milk supply after giving your baby bottles of formula.

- If you have already let your milk dry up after delivery – or later – but have now decided you'd like to breastfeed.
- If you want to collect milk to leave for your baby if you are going to be apart from him for a while.
- If you work away from home and want to pump and/or hand-express while you're away so you can take milk home for your baby and keep your milk supply going. Even if you don't take the milk home, it's well worth pumping and/or expressing at work as this keeps your milk supply going.
- If you have inverted nipples, when using a pump for a minute or so helps bring the nipple out before a feed.

Women often use breast pumps unnecessarily, especially in hospitals. This is because they are there, because intervention in nature's process is attractive to those who don't understand how breastfeeding works, and because many women have learnt a poor breastfeeding technique. If your baby can breastfeed, it's far better for both of you. Pump only if necessary.

Many babies who are given bottles of formula soon refuse to breastfeed because they quickly learn to bottle-suck, which is easier. Then, if their mothers are determined to breastfeed, they pump their milk and give it by bottle which makes the situation worse. If your baby can't take milk from the breast (but is mature and well enough to swallow), give it from a feeding cup.

Only rarely is it necessary to stop breastfeeding temporarily because of nipple soreness or cracking but, if you have to, it's less painful to hand-express milk than to use a pump.

Electric pumps

The prices of electric pumps reflect their sturdiness and the quality of their engineering. In general, the larger the pump, the quicker it builds up suction (or 'vacuum'). Some women find that pumping with a large pump is the fastest way of getting milk.

Electric pumps are available for hire or loan from some hospital maternity and special care baby units and from some self-help groups. They can also be bought from medical supply houses and some pharmacists.

Egnell Ameda Ltd, Unit 2, Belvedere Trading Estate, Taunton, Somerset TA1 1BH (01823 3363612) supply an electric pump, a battery-operated pump and a small electric pump which can be converted into a hand pump:

Egnell Elite Breast Pump – A Swiss electric pump distributed in the UK by Egnell Ameda Ltd, and also available from medical supply houses and on hire from many National Childbirth Trust branches (call 0181 992 8637 for your nearest one). The pump works by suction together with stimulation of the nipple and areola against the side of the flange. It is quiet, efficient, and has variable suction with a resting phase, and two sizes of funnel (for different-shaped breasts). It has two cups so that you can pump both breasts at once and the extra stimulation this provides encourages let-down and halves the pumping time compared with pumping one breast at a time. The pump weighs only 3 kg and costs £425 (plus VAT).

Ameda Lact-b Battery-operated Breast Pump is available from Egnell Ameda Ltd (see above) and also from NCT Maternity Sales (see page 453) at the special price of £25.

The *Mini Electric Breast Pump Nurture III*, made in the US and distributed by Egnell Ameda Ltd (see above), has an adjustable suction level and can easily be converted to a hand pump if you can't plug it in. It is also available from NCT Maternity Sales (see page 453) at the special price of £65. The *Breast Pump Cool Bag* is a zip bag for carrying the Mini Electric Breast Pump and comes complete with *Cool Packs* for keeping expressed milk at a safe temperature. The pump, cool bag and cool packs are also available from NCT Sales.

Colgate Medical Ltd, Shirley Avenue, Windsor, Berks SL4 5LH (01753 860378) supplies a range of four electric pumps:

The *Axicare CM12* has a variable suction strength, adjustable to three levels. The sucking rhythm can be preset or controlled by a fingertip. It comes complete with a carrying case and dust cover, weighs 2.5 kg and costs £415 plus VAT. The collection kit is an extra £11.85 plus VAT.

The *Axicare CM10* has an automatic sucking rhythm but the suction strength is adjustable. It comes complete with carrying case, weighs 5.5 kg and costs £399.75 plus VAT. The collection kit is an extra £31.60 plus VAT.

The *Axicare CM8* is a semi-automatic pump which provides constant suction. A woman can control the strength and duration of the suction with her fingertip, so as to create the sucking rhythm she finds comfortable. The pump comes complete with carrying case, weighs 2 kg and costs £280 plus VAT. The collection kit is an extra £31.60 plus VAT.

The *Axicare CM5* is a smaller version of the CM8. It weighs 0.75kg and costs £75 plus VAT. The collection kit is an extra £11.85 plus VAT.

Canon Babysafe Ltd, Glemsford, Suffolk (Freefone 0800 289064) supplies:

The Avent Naturally Battery-operated Breast Pump. This has recently been updated and costs £33 from Boots, Mothercare, major branches of Tesco, the Early Learning Centres, and branches of Children's World.

Hand pumps

Avent Naturally Single-handed Breast Pump, from Canon Babysafe Ltd (see above), is also available from Boots the Chemist for £16.99 and from the other retail outlets mentioned under their battery-operated pump (see above). This is an easy-to-use piston-action pump with a squeeze handle.

Canon Babysafe Breast Pump, also from Canon Babysafe (see above) is available in slightly different formats (colours, etc) from them direct or by order from pharmacies at £15.99.

Ameda Syringe Pump. This double-cylinder pump is available from NCT Maternity Sales (page 453) for £11.50.

Ameda One Hand Pump. This piston-action pump is available from NCT Maternity Sales (page 453) for £15.95.

You may be able to buy other hand pumps of varying efficiency from pharmacists, although they may be available by order only. The cheapest and simplest consist of a plastic or glass container with a rubber bulb to produce suction and are also known as 'breast relievers'. Milk collected by such pumps is likely to contain large amounts of bacteria because the rubber bulbs inevitably retain some milk and are difficult to clean. Bacteria thrive on the milk residue and contaminate the next collection of milk. Such pumps are also not very effective at removing milk from the breast.

FREEZER BAGS

Freezer storage bags for expressed breast milk are available from NCT Maternity Sales (see page 453) at £6.50 for a pack of twenty, or £18 for three packs of twenty.

FEEDING CUP

Suitable for pre-term and older breastfed babies. Three cups with lids cost £2.85 from NCT Maternity Sales (see page 453).

NURSING BRAS

The NCT Maternity Sales catalogue (see page 453) has an excellent range of nursing bras, both drop cup and zip cup, in a variety of sizes (up to 46HH).

Other suppliers of nursing bras include Silhouette (01295 274986 for stockists), which has three types in a variety of sizes and the Active Birth Centre (0171 561 9006).

BREAST PADS

Washable pads – Machine washable 100% cotton Ameda breast pads are available in packs of six for £6 from NCT Maternity Sales (see page 453).

Cone-shaped pads – Cone-shaped pads are available in the UK from Boots (own brand) at £2.89 for fifteen.

AVENT NIPLETTES (see page 160)

These are available from pharmacists, though you may have to ask for a special order. One costs £15.95 and two, £26.95 and are made by Canon Babysafe Ltd, Glemsford, Suffolk (0800 289064).

NURSING SUPPLEMENTERS

A supplementer, or nursing supplementer, is a device which enables a breastfeeding baby to get – at the same time – milk both from the breast and from a very thin, flexible plastic tube coming from a bag or bottle of expressed breast milk, donated milk from a milk-bank, or formula. The tube is taped to the breast with one end at the nipple, and the bag or bottle hangs round the mother's neck or is pinned to her clothing.

A supplementer is useful for:

- Teaching a baby who is used to bottle-feeding to suck properly at the breast.
- Giving a larger feed to a pre-term baby who hasn't the energy to suck for long; you express your milk between and after feeds and put this in the bottle.
- Building up your milk supply before you take delivery of an adopted baby.

- Supplementing your adopted baby's breastfeeds with formula.
- Avoiding the need for a bottle so the baby doesn't learn to 'bottle-suck'.

Some women who think they'll need to use a supplementer for only a short time make their own. If you'd like to try, you'll need some very thin, flexible plastic tubing (as used for naso-gastric tubes in special care baby units). No. 5 French size tubing is fine for full-term babies; no. 8 for babies with a cleft palate; and no. 3 for pre-term babies. Take a bottle and teat, make a hole in the teat and push the tubing through. Put some of your milk into the bottle, hang it upside down around your neck and tape the other end of the tube to your breast so the end is at your nipple. Be sure to sterilize everything you re-use thoroughly.

Supplemental Nutrition System (SNS)

Made in Switzerland (by Medela), this supplementer has two tubes. One can be taped to each breast to make it easier to switch sides while feeding. The rate of flow of the supplement can be altered by choosing one of three colour-coded tubes of different sizes. The neck strap is adjustable and changing the height of the bottle also helps adjust the rate of flow of milk. This supplementer can be sterilised by boiling.

It's available from Eurosurgical Ltd (01483 456007), for £17.74, including postage and packing and VAT.

The SNS is known as the Lact-Aid in the US.

BREAST-MILK BANK GUIDELINES
AND NEWSLETTER

Breast-milk bank guidelines are available from the British Paediatric Association, 5 St Andrew's Place, Regent's Park, London NW1 4LB, price £4.

A newsletter, 'Milk Banking: News and Views', is available

from Gillian Weaver, Human Milk Bank, Queen Charlotte's and Chelsea Hospital, Goldhawk Road, London W6 oXG.

BREASTFEEDING INFORMATION
ON THE INTERNET

Anyone whose work involves helping women to breastfeed is welcome to seek or exchange information about breastfeeding and lactation via e-mail on the internet. If you'd like to do this, use e-mail to contact: **LISTSERV@libraryl.UMMED.edu** and write in the message box: **Subscribe LACTNET,your first name, your last name** (but use no punctuation.)

VIDEOTAPE ON BREASTFEEDING ADOPTED BABIES

This video is available from Irene Elia, 68 Highsett, Hills Road, Cambridge CB2 1NZ (01223 561781), for £15, including a leaflet and postage and packing.

BREASTFEEDING EDUCATION PACKS
FOR SCHOOLS

'Breastfeeding' is available from Resource Material for Schools. Prices and mail order details from The Nottingham Breastfeeding Group.

OPEN-SIDED COT

The Bed-Side-Bed is a pretty, three-sided 'cot-bed' which can be converted into a four-sided cot, or a bed without sides, and makes night feeds much easier. With the cot right by your bed and the open side next to you, you simply slip your baby across into your bed, and slip him back when you're ready.

The Bed-Side-Bed costs £249.95 (including delivery and conversion kit). Mail order details 0181 989 8683.

FERTILITY PREDICTION

Lady Fertility Tester – If you're relying on breastfeeding and the sympto-thermal method for contraception, this microscope-like gadget the size of a lipstick can help by revealing the fern-like pattern in your dried saliva present only during fertile days. Priced £44.95, mail order details from PO Box 1185, Colwyn Bay, Clwyd LL28 4ZB.

First Response Ovulation Prediction Kit – This can be a useful additional guide for breastfeeding women also using the sympto-thermal method of contraception. Available from pharmacies and costing £18.99 for five tests, it can be useful when periods have returned to predict when ovulation is likely to return. This is because, when used towards the middle of the cycle, it indicates whether you are likely to ovulate by measuring hormone levels in urine. If ovulation is on its way, you can use additional contraception during the fertile days five days before and the day after ovulation.

If your periods haven't yet returned, it's too expensive to use each day but can be useful as an additional guide if you've observed changes in bodily signs (e.g. vaginal mucus) which indicate that ovulation is near.

Fertility Awareness Kit – This costs £19.99 and contains an explanatory video, thermometer and charts. Details from the Family Planning Association (01865 749333).

ORGANIZATIONS IN THE UK

La Leche League of Great Britain (LLL GB) – BM 3424, London WC1N 3XX (0171 242 1278): see page 152.

La Leche League has many leaders and groups, and also provides a wide range of information, including books and many leaflets and details of baby slings (see page 153).

Also *For the blind or visually handicapped* many publications in Braille, on cassette-tape or reel-to-reel. Ask for LLLI's (the international organization) special publications list.

For a price list send a stamped self-addressed business-size envelope. For information in languages other than English, ask for the translation list (No. 508).

National Childbirth Trust (NCT) – Alexandra House, Oldham Terrace, London W3 6NH (0181 992 8637), see page 152.

The NCT's Breastfeeding Promotion Group has many counsellors and a wide range of information including books and leaflets. It also has a register (the NCT Experience Register) of women who have breastfed in special situations and who are willing to discuss these with other parents. And in the UK it runs a workshop funded by the Department of Health to help midwives and health visitors explode their attitudes to breastfeeding.

NCT Maternity Sales (0141 633 5552) offers a wide range of nursing bras, underwear, night-wear, and various baby-care products.

The Association of Breastfeeding Mothers – PO Box 441, St Albans, Herts AL4 0AS (01727 859 189)

SOME OF THE MANY OTHER ORGANIZATIONS

The Nursing Mothers' Association of Australia – PO Box 231, Nunawading 3131, Victoria

La Leche League International – 9616 Minneapolis Avenue, PO Box 1209, Franklin Park, IL 60131–8209, US

International Lactation Consultant – 200 N. Michigan Ave, Suite 300, Chicago, IL 60601-3821, USA

A WORD FOR HELPERS

Helpers include relatives, friends, neighbours, voluntary breast-feeding counsellors, midwives, doctors and, in the UK, health visitors.

WHAT MAKES HELPERS EFFECTIVE?

1. Practical skills learnt from the experiences of success-fully breastfeeding women, from good teachers and, poss-ibly but not necessarily, from their own experiences of breastfeeding.

2. Up-to-date and reliable information about the benefits and practicalities of successful breastfeeding. If as a pro-fessional or voluntary helper you aren't offered in-service training, ask for it or arrange it yourself. However much you know, you can deepen your knowledge and broaden your understanding at any time – if you give yourself the chance.

3. Empathy – recognizing (through words, body language

and other unspoken messages) what a woman feels about breastfeeding and being a mother. Check this out with her and use your understanding at any time – if you give yourself the chance.

4. **Enthusiasm about breastfeeding** – all the while accepting that a bottle-feeding woman needs help and support as she feeds and cares for her baby just like a breastfeeding woman.

5. **The acceptance that every mother-baby pair is unique** and that the needs, behaviour and experience of every woman and baby are special.

6. **Encouragement.** A few words of encouragement can give confidence that may last a lifetime. One of us (PS) vividly remembers sitting in King's College Hospital giving our first daughter one of her earliest feeds. A midwife (Staff Nurse Benjamin) came and stood for a while, smiling with approval, as she watched. She said, 'Mrs Stanway, you're a wonderful mother.' Her warmth, generosity and encouragement have stayed with me ever since. If a woman has a breastfeeding problem, then identifying what she is doing well – and telling her – may help her persevere and find a solution by generating inner feelings of warmth, self-esteem and the belief that she can succeed.

7. **An awareness of their feelings about breastfeeding,** so that difficult and unresolved issues don't unwittingly adversely colour their advice. If these were unchecked, a helper might act out his or her emotional state by encouraging bottle-feeding. 'Sticking a bottle between baby and mother' would destroy breastfeeding – the trigger which makes these painful emotions surface (see below). We've already looked at a mother's (see page 246) and a father's

(Chapter 14) feelings about breastfeeding; these can apply to any helper who is a parent.

8. Satisfaction of their needs for nourishment and love. Without this, it's difficult, if not impossible, to be a good breastfeeding helper, as unmet neediness is likely to get in the way. Watching breastfeeding is a situation almost above all others that can trigger an awareness of having had insufficient love or nourishment oneself. An individual can expect to love others only as much as she loves herself. If you realize you are very needy, ask someone you trust either to help or to recommend where you can get some help both in coming to terms with your feelings and getting your needs met.

ESPECIALLY FOR HEALTH PROFESSIONALS

Several things are particularly significant for health professionals. Let's see how you can make the time you spend with pregnant and breastfeeding women into a time of golden opportunity for them and for you.

1. Be positive and enthusiastic – Being enthusiastic is important – *not putting pressure on women to breastfeed, bullying them, or putting them off with an evangelistic attitude,* but being positive about its benefits. Many studies confirm that an enthusiastic health professional can encourage women not only to start but also to continue. A woman who wants to breastfeed will also be much more prepared to overcome any problems if she knows you are interested.

Don't forget that people absorb ideas visually and

pictures of breastfeeding mothers in your clinic or consulting room will help you get your message across.

2. Be encouraging (see page 455) – Polish up your encouragement skills and learn to give well-focused, specific encouragement, describing exactly what a woman can be pleased about. This is especially important for a woman who is starting to breastfeed or having problems. There will be something you can encourage in every situation – even simply a woman's readiness to seek help.

3. Don't imagine you'll make women feel guilty – Some health professionals are reluctant to talk about the benefits of breastfeeding for fear of making those who don't (or can't) breastfeed feel guilty or inferior. This fear is best recognized and then put to one side.

It's only fair to respect each woman's right to make an informed decision but she can do this only if she has information. If she then decides not to breastfeed, that's her choice as an adult able to weight the pros and cons as she sees them. Hopefully she'll weigh them carefully and have confidence in what she believes is right for her and her baby. Just as if she were buying a car, she'll then stand or fall by her decision. It is *her* responsibility to decide and it is within her gift to live with the consequences.

Most women who choose to bottle-feed do so because they actively *don't want to breastfeed*. A woman may feel pleasure and/or regret, or indeed any other emotions resulting from her choice. Whether she feels guilty or not depends on whether she has come to terms with her reasons for bottle-feeding or feels bad or ambivalent about it. Professionals don't have the power to *make* women feel guilty, nor should we predict that they'll experience guilt rather than some other emotion. Women aren't little girls who need a parent-figure to take responsibility for their emotions. The effort to protect women from some proposed guilt they might feel is misguided at best and arrogant at worst. And it's a way in which some professionals unwittingly seek to infantilize pregnant and newly delivered women at the very time they should be encouraging and supporting them. Your responsibility as a health professional is to give pregnant women accurate, up-to-date and unbiased information about the benefits of breastfeeding.

The argument about the guilt (or disappointment) of the woman who *can't* breastfeed is another matter. First, most of those who 'fail' to breastfeed might have succeeded with better support, encouragement, information and advice. Only a very few woman physcially can't breastfeed. Also, virtually every woman who wishes to breastfeed can give her baby some breast milk and you can reassure her that a little is better than none.

Some bottle-feeding women know they are putting their needs first. Their emotions and concerns about their choice are far better acknowledged and discussed than hidden and seeping out as guilt.

It's important to consider whether the guilt you imagine a woman might feel could have more to do with you than with them. Do *you* think they *should* feel guilty? In other words, do you think they are 'bad' or 'naughty' because they don't breastfeed? If so, this may suggest that your whole life is too full of 'shoulds' and 'oughts' (both for others and for yourself) and that you'd be happier if you relaxed a bit. It isn't appropriate for someone who works with pregnant women and new mothers to apportion blame. And is your fear that women will feel inadequate if they can't breastfeed really a projection of your own fear of being an inadequate helper (see below)?

Women who want to breastfeed but find they can't may need to express all sorts of feelings, including anger and sadness, about the loss of the experience of breast-feeding. Our task is to support them in their mourning and help them grow both in their mothering skills and as human beings, empowered and enriched by dealing with their feelings and learning from their experience of 'failure'. Many women who want to breastfeed *do* see bottle-feeding as a failure, and learning to deal with failure is an extremely important task in anyone's personal development.

4. Become more self-aware – An important part of being a better listener is becoming more aware of our own emotions. We're unlikely to be able to help women over feelings which we've suppressed ourselves. And once we're aware of our feelings, we can put them to one side so they don't interfere with our work.

If we know in our heart that our advice tends to sabotage breastfeeding, we need to examine our emotions carefully. Talking about, watching and helping with breastfeeding may trigger painful emotions (in our mind or body) which unwittingly distort our advice about breastfeeding. Such emotions may stem from difficult and unresolved situations in our childhood or our current life. They may also reflect feelings about our own mothers and the mothering we had, and about the love and emotional nourishment we have or, indeed, do not have, today.

As an exercise, look at your feelings about breast-feeding, because just recognizing and naming them can be a great help.

When you're working with a breastfeeding woman, ask yourself these soul-searching questions:

1 Do I know what I'm doing and am I a good enough helper?
2 Do I at some level dislike breastfeeding?
3 Will I lose face if I'm not seen to be authoritative?
4 Will this baby starve?
5 Will it be my fault if the baby starves?
6 Can I bear it if this woman feels guilty because of what I tell her?
7 Will this woman dislike me if I tell her what she needs to do to breastfeed successfully?
8 What will my colleagues think if this woman doesn't breastfeed?
9 Can I bear giving up control to this mother and her baby?
10 Am I being unkind if I don't suggest that this woman with breastfeeding problems bottle-feeds instead?
11 Can I cope with the implicit sexuality of breastfeeding?
12 Do I want to watch this demanding baby who never seems to stop feeding?
13 Why haven't I got a baby I can love and who will love me?
14 Does my advice echo my personal experiences of breastfeeding?
15 Am I comfortable seeing this baby cared for so lovingly when no one seems to care for me and I don't feel I received the love and nourishment I needed from my mother?

If any of these questions rings bells for you, ask yourself how it makes you feel. For example, questions 1, 2 and 3 make some people feel afraid; 7 makes some feel helpless;

11 makes some feel jealous and unloved; 7, 11, 12 and 14 make some feel angry; 12 and 14 make some feel a sense of desperate longing and neediness; and 11, 12 and 13 make some feel envious.

If these emotions aren't familiar, either they don't apply to you or they may be suppressed in your unconscious mind.

Suppressed emotions usually stem from unresolved experiences in our infancy and childhood. We aren't aware of them because we've erected defences to stop them hurting us. But anything – and particularly the deeply significant act of breastfeeding – that disturbs these defences can stir up our suppressed emotions and allow them out. Sometimes this causes problems or, better, challenges.

One relevant challenge might be knowing that you often give poor breastfeeding advice (see below) even though this isn't what you consciously want to do. (Others might include compulsive behaviour – such as overeating, promiscuous sex, dependence on alcohol and drugs, or overwork – or depression or anxiety.)

So ask yourself whether rather too many of the women you advise choose to bottle-feed, or give up breastfeeding before they wish. If this is the case, could your advice be based on a need to avoid the painful feelings resulting from your 'yes' answers to the questions above? Are your difficult feelings, recognised or unrecognised, making you give irrational breastfeeding advice? By *not* giving sound information, advice and encouragement about breastfeeding, could you really be attempting to meet your own emotional neediness?

In other words, are you unconsciously seeking to separate a breastfeeding mother and baby by putting a bottle between them so as to prevent your own painful feelings?

Or are you even, unwittingly and symbolically, seeking to punish your own mother for being 'bad', under the guise of punishing all the mothers you meet by sabotaging breastfeeding?

This may seem fanciful to some readers but one of us (AS) has worked in depth in this area with numerous health professionals. It is astonishing how many health professionals who choose baby and child care have old wounds from their own past that so obviously need healing. Or perhaps it is not!

If you are aware of any problems in this area, you are certainly not alone. And if you work on your problems, you can use the insights you gain to improve the quality of your life in many ways. Many health professionals need to spend more time caring for themselves, listening to their inner voice and finding ways of getting their emotional needs met if they are to care for others more effectively. Otherwise, their own neediness could interfere with them being effective breastfeeding helpers.

Rescuers and 'wounded healers' – When we are unaware of our own needs and feelings, it's all too easy to seek to 'rescue' people from their predicaments in life. This is instead of helping ourselves, as we see our own problems only in others. However, being aware of our emotional pain can make us into 'wounded healers' who are more effective as helpers and better able to promote breastfeeding and support and protect breastfeeding women and their babies.

A 'wounded healer' is someone who has been emotionally 'wounded' but has taken steps to recognize painful feelings and deal with them effectively. The result is that he or she learns and matures emotionally.

The need for helpers to be aware of their own

emotional woundedness (and all of us are wounded in some degree) is rarely more important than in the fields of midwifery, obstetrics, paediatrics, mother and child care and breastfeeding. This is because these areas are, by definition, so primal and, as we've seen, so resonant with our own past experiences. As health professionals in these areas, we owe it to mothers, fathers and babies to be among the most aware of all health professionals.

Becoming more self-aware by 'listening' to yourself better is a big step towards improving your empathic listening skills and being able to listen to other people – including the mothers you work with – more effectively. In other words:

5. Share your feelings – If you'd like to come to terms with painful emotions triggered by helping women breastfeed, simple brain power and a wish to change may not be enough. You may need to discuss your feelings with a good and trusted friend or colleague. If you have the opportunity of discussing feelings about breastfeeding in a small group at work, it may be a more effective use of your time if you can work with a trained facilitator. Staff who make an awareness of feelings (both their own and those of others) a part of their professional skills can be a powerful source of expertise. A few helpers find they benefit even more from one-to-one work with a counsellor.

6. Polish your empathic listening skills – It's particularly important for all health professionals – not just those dealing with pregnant and breastfeeding women – to keep their listening skills well polished. Good listening skills enable you to help a woman recognise and understand how she feels about breastfeeding. Talking to you about her emotions may clarify things considerably for her. If she has difficult or negative feelings, recognizing and discussing them may enable her to come to terms with them and perhaps decide to breastfeed even though she had planned not to.

7. Practise what you preach – It's all very well talking about breastfeeding, but it's another doing it! If *you* have a baby, remember that how you care for and feed him will have an important modelling role for everyone who knows you are a health professional. If *you* breastfeed, they'll realize you think it's really worthwhile. If you don't, or you do it only half-heartedly, they'll find it hard to believe that you think much of it.

Some health professionals are often hard on themselves – and on their babies. And some work so hard that they have to squeeze out time to be with their babies, breastfeed them and enjoy them.

— A study in the US (1985) reported that health care workers (doctors, nurses and technicians) returned to work earlier than other employed mothers. And doctors whose babies were cared for in hospital crêches were often late for their feeds.

8. Remember you need encouragement and support too – You are a valuable person and a skilled professional caring for mothers and babies at a vitally important time in their lives; if you can find ways of polishing your self-esteem and your pleasure – in yourself, the way you live your life and the way you do your job – you'll help more effectively.

You might like to discuss the importance of well-focused encouragement with a group of colleagues and agree to find ways of encouraging each other. This might help balance the lack of time for each other experienced by so many health professionals.

9. Affirm yourself – Make time to recognize the good work you're doing and give yourself a pat on the back. It's surprising what a difference this can make.

10. Look after yourself – Take extra special care to look after yourself as you learn to recognize and adjust to your feelings about helping breastfeeding mothers.

Treat yourself as a valuable person who deserves an enjoyably healthy diet, regular exercise, time spent outside each day, and ample opportunity for rest, relaxation, entertainment and laughter. You well deserve it.

Index